AF634817

BEDLAM *at* BOTANY BAY

JAMES DUNK is a historian and writer living and working in Sydney, on Gadigal country. A research fellow at the University of Sydney and a conjoint fellow at the University of Newcastle, James is a frequent contributor to the *Australian Book Review*.

BEDLAM *at* BOTANY BAY

JAMES DUNK

NEWSOUTH

A NewSouth book

Published by
NewSouth Publishing
University of New South Wales Press Ltd
University of New South Wales
Sydney NSW 2052
AUSTRALIA
newsouthpublishing.com

© James Dunk 2019
First published 2019

10 9 8 7 6 5 4 3 2 1

This book is copyright. Apart from any fair dealing for the purpose of private study, research, criticism or review, as permitted under the Copyright Act, no part of this book may be reproduced by any process without written permission. Inquiries should be addressed to the publisher.

NATIONAL LIBRARY OF AUSTRALIA
A catalogue record for this book is available from the National Library of Australia

ISBN 9781742236179 (paperback)
9781742244556 (ebook)
9781742249025 (ePDF)

Design Josephine Pajor-Markus
Cover design Luke Causby, Blue Cork
Printer Griffin Press

All reasonable efforts were taken to obtain permission to use copyright material reproduced in this book, but in some cases copyright could not be traced. The author welcomes information in this regard.

This book is printed on paper using fibre supplied from plantation or sustainably managed forests.

UNSW
SYDNEY

CONTENTS

ACKNOWLEDGMENTS

When I began at the University of Sydney I enrolled in everything from chemistry, calculus and French to literature, government, and political economy. History came upon me almost by stealth, captivating me with its interest in people not as research subjects or examples of abstractions, but as they actually live and breathe. Richard White drew me into higher research, with his mixture of irony and sympathy, and he continues to be an encouraging and astute reader. As a graduate student I benefited enormously from Sydney's superb intellectual environment, and particularly from the guidance and friendship of Nick Eckstein, Sebastián Gil-Riaño, Chris Hilliard, Peter Hobbins, Miranda Johnson, Andres Rodriguez, Ricardo Roque, Penny Russell, and Ben Silverstein. Mark McKenna and Iain McCalman ran a striking seminar which left many of us passionate about the place of historical imagination in our writing. Alan Atkinson and Stephen Garton gave valuable early advice. Alison Bashford helped to establish my project and instilled a sense of the rigour and precision which history demands.

The extraordinary historian John Hirst had a powerful impact on many of us. In the seminars he hosted he insisted on the value of working word by word and line by line, trimming fat and sometimes carving down to the bone. An elder statesman of the historical community and a leading scholar on colonial

Australia, to me and other young historians he was a remarkably generous patron.

This book, like all historical work in this country, is underwritten by its fine cultural institutions, including the Mitchell Library, State Library of New South Wales, New South Wales State Archives, Libraries Tasmania, and the National Library of Australia, which hosts a vast collection of digitised newspapers that is the envy of historians everywhere. The cafes of the Inner West made their own investments in this book by overlooking my table for hours and sometimes days on end, and I recall them with fond thanks: Shenkin, Ralph's, Tripod, In the Annex, Ella, Toby's Estate.

A workshop in wintry Dunedin proved formative for my historical thinking: Volker Hess, Kathryn Hunter, Rebecca Lenihan, Jane McCabe, James Moran and I explored the ways that schools, armies, hospitals and asylums left paper trails which are now guarded in archives that withhold as well as disclose. The brilliant Sally Swartz stimulated us all to think more deeply, and Barbara Brookes, who brought us all together, remains a great friend and mentor.

Many exceptional historians have contributed their energies to help usher this book into the world. Hans Pols read through large swathes of text and helped me to think more adventurously about madness and empire. Christine Winter committed many evenings to reading through the entire manuscript, in an earlier form, and helped to clarify and extend its arguments. Hamish Maxwell-Stewart offered a critical reading and his firm support. Others, including many already named, read chapters at different stages and helped to sharpen and strengthen them: Jeannine Baker, Cath Bishop, Helen Bones, Emma Gleadhill, Chris Holdridge, Shane Greentree, Tom Griffiths, Claire Higgins, Katja Heath, Meredith Lake, Greg Murrie, and Alan Rome. In recent years, the members of our early-career writing group have been perceptive and heartening readers: Michaela Cameron, James Findlay, Rohan Hewitt, James Keating, Isobelle Barrett Meyering, Briony Neilson, Danielle Thyer, and Mick Warren. Billy Griffiths, Matthew Kennedy, Hugh Chilton and Cathy Perkins have also been wonderful companions in writing and researching.

Kirsten McKenzie has been an excellent guide through these years of reading and writing about Sydney, the sea, and colonial enterprise. Her hard-headed advice has been invaluable. Her brilliant story-telling about unlikely historical protagonists, and skill in drawing them into profound arguments about empire, were sources of inspiration for this book. Catharine Coleborne has been a wise and supportive mentor in recent years. Her work on colonial asylums and their place in forming southern societies is matchless, and she is a model of grace in an academic environment that can be harried and unkind. Much of the work here was made possible by Warwick Anderson, who is not only a luminous, world-leading historian but an exceptionally generous and considered mentor. His writing, which is elegant, unsparing, and audacious, continues to shape my approach to the discipline of history.

Phillipa McGuinness, at NewSouth, saw the potential in this book well before it took shape, and contributed a good deal to its form and style. Emma Hutchinson brought the book together with great dexterity and Tricia Dearborn helped to guide it through its final stages. Parts of Chapter 2 appeared in 'The Liability of Madness and the Commission of Lunacy in New South Wales, 1805–12,' *History Australia* 15, no. 1 (2018): 130–50, of Chapter 4 in 'Authority and the Treatment of the Insane at Castle Hill Asylum, 1811–25,' *Health and History* 19, no. 2 (2017): 17–40, and of Chapter 8 in 'Work, Paperwork and the Imaginary Tarban Creek Lunatic Asylum, 1846,' *Rethinking History* 22, no. 3 (2018): 326–355. I am grateful to the journal editors and reviewers for their suggestions.

More than many families my siblings and I stand against a storm – of our own making and the making of others. This book is a testament to our surviving this far, and I hope a gift to my mother, Joy, whose kindness has proven intractable. My brother Jonathan has been a close companion for three decades. His words are beautiful and startling, and his intelligence is incandescent. And to my own small family, which bears with me and shares everything with me, I owe more than I can say – to my wife Stephanie, my first reader, who has poured her intellectual, spiritual and practical support into me and into this book, and to my sons, Aubrey and Ira. Their warmth, humour, and curiosity teach me to trust in the future.

INTRODUCTION

'Pitt and Botany Bay!' the convicts cheered in Newgate Prison, at the news the British would create a penal colony in the half-mapped southern land. Or so quipped the London newspaper *Morning Herald*, piqued at the thought of its government carrying criminals halfway around the world.[1] Botany Bay divided people, even before the first ships set sail. It was a wild experiment, a colossal waste, a terror, a commonwealth of thieves – or was it a distant asylum, a place where the casualties of history could begin their lives again?[2] It was a place of contrariety.

Botany Bay has continued to divide those who have written about it. The notion that it was planned as a southern seat of empire appealed to the London-facing historians of the 20th century, reaching a climax in Alan Frost's progressive revelation of the historical fantasies of European Australia. He grew more trenchant – presenting the 'real story' of Botany Bay – after the art historian Robert Hughes conjured a southern gulag on the 'fatal shore'. John Hirst, an inveterate provocateur, looked hard and found 'freedom on the fatal shore'. From Canberra, Manning Clark had written in near-prophetic prose about the spiritual drama that unfolded in and around Sydney. Alan

Atkinson listened to the talk of those who came, and saw the transformative power of their writing, and the intellectual and spiritual work they did to make themselves at home. Grace Karskens unearthed the material traces of Aboriginal and European life and opened a marvellous new vision of *The Colony*, a place of natural splendour and rich humanity.[3]

The American Revolutionary War ended the slowing Atlantic market in convict labour, which made the prospects for those who fell foul of British justice in the late 18th century grim – chaotic prisons and nightmarish hulks, the near-fatal settlements in West Africa, or the gallows.[4] Botany Bay seemed like a southern arcadia in comparison. Convicts were to be carried across the seas, sentenced to remain for seven years, fourteen years, or for life. They worked for government, but, in those early years, they also built houses, fished in the harbour, tended gardens, and cooked their dinners. Striking opportunities opened to the new arrivals as those for the Aboriginal people who had lived in and cared for the land for longer than European imaginations could fathom rapidly shrank. The Eora people who lived around Sydney Cove were pushed aside by the Europeans as they 'settled', physically and then discursively. Trees were felled, crops and pastures were laid out, mud hardened into bricks. Convicts became free, soldiers and their wives set up small businesses, doctors and merchants built themselves townhouses and country seats.

If we slow down, however, and listen closely, we find that doubt, anxiety, grief, and despair intrude into these familiar stories. Some became irrational and could no longer govern themselves, or be governed by others. They erupted in mania, or lost themselves in memories and delusions. They cried in fury and tore at the walls of their cells, or stared slack-eyed into the distance. Some were consumed by the pressures weighing upon them, and killed themselves. Others simply wandered away. These were all signal problems in such a setting, where discipline, security and industry were fundamental to the business of a fragile government.

The colonists initially struggled to plant their northern seeds and raise crops. With an eye to the limited rations the ships had carried across the seas – food for a static population for two years – Governor Arthur Phillip sent the first fleet flagship, *Sirius*, to Cape Town for provisions. The ship sailed east across the Pacific, passing through the ice zone to skirt Cape Horn, and then cut across the Atlantic to the Cape. Shortly before the *Sirius* made the Cape, third lieutenant George Maxwell took the night watch through a desperate stretch of iceberg-strewn sea. A strong wind picked up but he made his men set more and more sail, wrote Jacob Nagle, a junior officer. The wind strained against the sails, forcing the *Sirius* to 'lay down' so far towards the sea that the captain was thrown from his hammock, and came spluttering on deck in his shirt sleeves. He had the crew take in the screaming sails, posthaste, and requested an explanation from Maxwell. He planned to 'tip all nines', Maxwell said, to see if the crew could raise the *Sirius* back out of the water. The captain saw that he was delirious, and sent him below.

It was not the first time. After leaving England, off the Portuguese coast between the Isle of Wight and Tenerife, Maxwell had become angry with the men on watch without reason, and had them thrashed. Hunter, when he heard, gave Maxwell 'a severe setting down' and Governor Phillip, who was also on board, warned that such behaviour would earn his severe displeasure. By the time the *Sirius* returned to Sydney from Cape Town, laden with supplies, Maxwell had 'got so raving' (in Nagle's blunt words) that the surgeons had no difficulty diagnosing him insane. He had been 'for a considerable time past in a melancholy and declining way', wrote judge advocate David Collins.[5] Maxwell was admitted to the settlement's hospital and placed in a cottage in the adjoining garden, at the foot of the sandstone crags on the western shore of Sydney Cove. While there, he received 70 guineas from England but 'in his fits', wrote Nagle, 'he went & buried it singly all over the garden'.[6]

People tend to try and isolate or contain madness when it emerges, but madness often breaks its barriers. Drought gripped the beleaguered settlement in March 1790, and Phillip sent the two ships at his disposal a thousand miles into the Pacific, to Norfolk Island. The harvest had been better on the island, and the ships carried a full third of the colony's people to its relative bounty.[7] Maxwell remained in Sydney, under treatment. Some weeks after the ships left he was found rowing a small boat across Sydney Harbour, perilously close to the sheer cliffs of Middle Head. He had been on the water for two days. As he was hauled ashore, men and women crowding around him, the *Supply* sailed through the Heads bearing the grim news that the *Sirius* had broken on the reefs guarding Norfolk. 'It was almost sufficient to have deranged the strongest intellect among us,' wrote Collins. 'A load of accumulated evils seemed bursting at once upon our heads.'[8] For a moment, the semblance of madness coalesced with the stark news of wreckage and the prospect of further isolation, and threatened the entire enterprise.

For Collins, and no doubt for others in the little colony perched at the edge of the vast Pacific, Maxwell's madness became a metaphor for the precariousness of their community. What is it to us now? Because he did not write or paint or draw through his illness we have little more than a glimpse of Maxwell's interior world, and we are left with questions. What was it like, confined below decks on the *Sirius* for weeks on end? What was he searching for as he rowed across the harbour so resolutely? What did he think and feel? What produced his madness, and what were its effects?

Madness is a beguiling and bewildering idea clothed in an expansive and unwieldy word. The word conjures up a wide range of symptoms, conditions and disorders which are experienced and interpreted in different ways. Madness came before medical treatises and legal doctrines, ran an ill-disciplined course through conversation, folklore and literature, and remains in use still, in the borderlands of societies where it undoes neat and artificial binaries like sanity–insanity. Whatever else it may be, it seems to me that acute madness, the kind we now medicate, is never less than a private suffering – something interior, perhaps incommunicable, which nevertheless clashes with the world around. As it does, it opens a new vein of history.

Eighteen months after Maxwell was hauled ashore, John Ascott also slipped into madness.[9] A private in Captain John Shea's company, he was servant to the captain, a man dubiously honoured as the first European to shoot a kangaroo.[10] After Shea died of tuberculosis, Ascott became servant to Major Ross, commandant of Norfolk Island, but he was promptly let go 'on account of his running after the women'. In Sydney, still in fear of starvation, Phillip reduced the rations of everyone in the colony, including himself, and by early 1790, they were running at 'a bare subsistence level'.[11] On Norfolk Island, the stores were dwindling; convicts were frequently caught trying to break in. Despairing of 'the supplies we have so long expected from Europe', wrote junior officer Ralph Clark, salt pork and beef rations were cut, and cut again. The following April the soldiers protested, perversely, by refusing their rations. Their officers responded by marching them to the store and forcing them to take their food. That evening Clark wrote that it had been 'one of the most critical days in my life.' Never was 'club law near taking place in any part of the world than it was in this', he said – never had he come so close to anarchy and the rule of violence.[12]

John Ascott had been the first to take his rations from the store, and 'the men had looked very cool on him since'. He was so fearful that he went round the barracks asking for a knife. None lent him one. Five months later, Ascott was 'quite mad' and his officers were 'obliged to confine him'. Clark felt for the private: 'I am sorry for him he does not like any body but me'. Notwithstanding the hunger, and anger, among the soldiery, Clark thought there was a specific cause for Ascott's suffering. 'It is all about a d... convict whore who has used him ill.'[13] (Clark, as Grace Karskens points out, 'called all convict women whores as a matter of course'.)[14] Whatever the cause, Ascott degenerated, and the next day a lean-to was made for him outside the guard station and he was placed there in a 'strait waistcoat'. These were standard issue, since the British Navy expected madness; sailors were some seven times more prone than the general population to it, probably on account of head injuries between decks, the shock of gunfire, and long-term inebriation.[15] Two days later Ascott was chained to a cannon in his lean-to, wrote Clark, 'quite gone', though he still had a measure of whimsy. 'Sent to speak to me,' Clark continued, 'and when I came he said my name was Mr. Clark and I was all in the dark.'[16] Ascott remained constrained in the dark until, after three weeks, he improved a little and was allowed 'to come out and walk under the colonnade of the guard in the day time – he ust to keep crying out that he was Phillip G. King governor of this island'.[17]

In the 21st century, the deep mental and emotional disruption of madness and its many mysteries are translated carefully into medical vocabularies of health and disease. Psychiatrists and psychologists work to constrain profound disorder within a series of categories, which are paired with psychopharmaceuticals, professional specialities and health insurance identifiers. Medicine has with difficulty established that mental illnesses operate, at least in some ways, like physical illnesses – outside moral logic – and much of the stigma has been stripped away. Others have worked to explain psychological damage not in the progress of disease but in the impediments created by trauma. There is a moral framework here, but guilt is located in social and political structures rather than in individuals.[18] Despite the many advances in ethics, neural science and psychiatric knowledge in the last two centuries, however, we have hardly mastered madness. The mind appears more complex the more we know about it, and our drugs and therapies are only partly effective, and cause unwanted effects. Madness remains a mystery to which artists, musicians and writers, as well as psychologists, psychoanalysts and epidemiologists, address themselves.

Madness generally entails a divergence between internal and external realities, which produces visible, audible friction. It registers in families and communities, in stories of eccentricity and silliness which are told and retold, in jokes and taunts, and in chains and straitjackets. It registers in sheds and locked cells which have housed not only those children and adults deemed insane but the fear, anxiety and shame which have often enough attended them. It is disruptive. Its unruliness makes it difficult for it to be contained, and demands always that work be done to define it. Like the fight against disease, or crime, or hunger, the confrontation with madness is a rich human drama which elicits compelling histories. But rather than doing battle with microbes, economics or ideas, it has been a struggle with persons and their demons – a struggle with ourselves.

This makes madness a powerful mechanism for writing history. Endlessly bewildering, interpretable in any number of ways, it always reveals subtler politics, formal and interpersonal.

Madness throws into doubt the fundamental qualities of personhood, but, since it also involves the possibility of physical harm to the self, to others, and to property, it demands that these doubts are resolved, and quickly. What philosophical principles, religious tenets, legal traditions or folk understandings are invoked in these resolutions? Studying madness shows the fault lines of societies. It is a subject which never loses its relevance because these fault lines still run around us like scars, the outward signs of an endemic disorder which reaches not only down into the belly of who we are but back into the paths we followed to get here.

TRACING THE DEVELOPMENT OF THE SCIENTIFIC STUDY OF the mind and of its disorders, many historians have been drawn into the lunatic asylums and psychiatric hospitals where that science took root. There, as in other hospitals, men and women became patients, and categories and labels took on substance. The charitable hospitals, which appeared irregularly in Europe from the medieval period on, quarantined madness and helped to define its parameters and to make it an issue with which states were obliged to grapple. Most famous was Bethlem Hospital in London, the name taken first from a fertility god but drawn into Christian tradition as the city of David and the birthplace of Jesus: the fount of peace. The asylum was nicknamed 'bedlam'. 'Bedlam' signifies uproar, chaos, pandemonium: words which refer as well to inner states as to the external effects of confusion, and to anything that seems to lack a compass or an even keel. Madness becomes a metaphor.

Madness also posed an intellectual and technological challenge. In the 18th century, the fabled 'age of reason', the old hospitals were joined by new institutions which, in their elaborate architecture, met the chaos of madness with a show of elaborate rationality. At the close of the century, entrepreneurs in England, France and Italy experimented with a range of therapeutic techniques which would come to be defined as 'moral therapy'. For the questionable obsessions with blood-letting, emetics and purgatives, 'heroic' interventions to re-establish equilibrium of body and mind, they substituted a prohibition on physical restraint, where possible, and provided a solid diet, comfortable furnishings, and early occupational therapies and entertainments. During the 19th century, medicine would come to dominate the knowledge and treatment of mental disease, but as it dawned doctors played only a supporting role. Many of the low-profile 'madhouses' and some of the larger institutions were managed by laypeople. Asylums have fascinated, even entranced historians for generations, but it has also become clear that the history of madness goes well beyond the asylum. There was madness before the asylum, madness outside its walls, and it remains with us long after the majority of asylums – now called psychiatric hospitals – were closed in the later decades of the 20th century. Recent histories have turned from the internal dynamics of these institutions to study the ways they have been used by families and embedded in communities, and the struggles of those communities to offer asylum after these closures.[19]

In New South Wales, madness bore only a tangential relationship with medicine and the 'lunatic asylum'. There was no asylum at all for the first two decades of colonisation, and the insane, whether convict or free, were housed in a gaol. The doctors attached to the military personnel stationed in New South Wales and those who formed the Colonial Medical Service rarely arrived with any training in mental symptoms and disorders. Moral therapy called for careful architecture, well-trained and well-disposed staff, and diverse entertainments, but the asylums that sprang up, late and under-resourced, were almost sickly themselves. The first, housed in a granary or a barn, was opened in 1811, run by a sapling botanist and by doctors under criminal sentence. It was very near devoid of medicine altogether, perennially on the brink of closure. When it was closed, after fifteen years, patients were transferred to the 'best, indeed the only means of accommodating' the insane, a parsonage in Liverpool fitted out as a courthouse. Its chief recommendation was that it was directly across the road from the hospital.[20] The staff of these institutions struggled against their patients' disorders, but also with their superiors' negligence, and with each other.

It would be half a century before the first purpose-built asylum appeared: Tarban Creek, built at great cost on a peninsula on Parramatta River at Gladesville, already known – uncannily – as Bedlam Point. Even here, as tendentious doctors and activist politicians were quick to point out, the insane were not entrusted to medical knowledge or sophisticated, scientific practice. Tarban Creek, and the madness of New South Wales, passed into the control of medical representatives in 1848, between the end of convict transportation and the achievement, in 1856, of the colonists' right to govern themselves through elected representatives. This was no coincidence. One means of pulling the colony into a convict-free future was to embrace medicine and its promises of cure.

Madness nevertheless stalked the colony, undeterred or perhaps encouraged by the lack of medical apparatus to accommodate it. Its movements were captured not, typically, by case files and patient registers but by other records produced by imperial representatives at the ragged edge of empire grappling with disruption. To establish sovereign order in Sydney, governors were equipped with a startling array of executive powers and supported by His Majesty's marines. At the right hand of the governor was the colonial secretary, a deceptively humble title for a role of enormous influence. The two worked together closely at Government House, on the slope rising from the eastern shore of Sydney Cove, passing letters, making recommendations, scribbling instructions, often from dawn until dusk, with few breaks. Together the governor and secretary administered all of the business of colonial government. In the management of madness, therefore, they coordinated the convict department, responsible for receiving, counting, clothing, feeding, and assigning convicts to private colonists and public projects; the amateur and unpaid magistrates, men of social standing entrusted with the rule of law and the discipline of convicts; the penal settlements which ringed the colony; the hospitals and medical service, by way of the principal surgeon; and the institutions which accommodated the vulnerable: widows, orphans and the elderly, the physically disabled, and the insane. The two sat, like spiders, spinning a web which stretched over the colony, and together produced a remarkable archive of government in a penal colony.

Madness also appeared in the satellite records of the convict department, as men and women were launched by British courts through the hulks and gaols, into ships and across the seas. On their arrival, the colonial secretary boarded each ship and organised the triage of convicts into government service and private assignment; later they might be drawn into gaols, gangs or penal settlements. Madness was largely overlooked until it became too disruptive, at which point masters, commandants and magistrates made decisions – summarily, perhaps, or in consultation with the governor and the colonial secretary, but with little reference to medical opinion. The colonial courts engaged with madness wherever it appeared to veer into dangerousness, or emerged from criminality, as elsewhere, and in civil proceedings, when families worried that it would ruin their estates. It was a pattern which appeared in other places, like the

Cape Colony, where government was similarly preoccupied with security and where social questions engaged with concerns about criminality.[21]

These records do not contain all the answers we might like to find. There was effectively no asylum until the final years of convict transportation. Certainly there were no psychiatrists. New South Wales offers an ideal setting for a study of madness 'outside the walls of the asylum'. It was a European society transplanted across the seas, from a culture which was rapidly developing an elaborate knowledge of madness in medicine, law, and literature. Many called it a 'peculiar' society: a delicate way of referring to the convicts that lay at the centre of its function. To preserve order among them, a strong executive government was installed, but no parliament of any kind. Courts were presided over by military officers, rather than answering to juries. It was an 'anomalous' society, in the words of the constitutional historian John Manning Ward.[22]

There are other absences. Women feature rarely in these records. Women remained a clear minority in the colonial population for decades, and were underrepresented in the selection of transportees, in colonial crimes, and in the more prominent business enterprises.[23] We know that there were female patients in the early asylums from the few surviving lists of patients and from passing references in government correspondence, but there is little to learn of the ways that gender shaped the description of symptoms or medical diagnoses. Where the madness of women appears outside the asylum, it does so predictably, as an intensification of male prerogative over their affairs, and we are otherwise left to wonder about the ways in which the particularly masculine bearing of colonial discourse and the gender imbalance, with all its pervasive implications, might have shaped the course of madness. Women do feature heavily in narratives of the madness of men, as carers for their siblings and spouses and as sufferers with them, trapped in claustrophobic households. Women were also accused of causing maladies, as in Ascott's case. There is still less evidence of Aboriginal people being drawn into European conceptions of madness, and they appear to have had little presence in the colonial asylums. There is much work to be done to properly situate the settler drama of madness in the broader history of colonisation.[24]

Similarly, the threadbare quality of the archival collections of the early asylums confound epidemiological questions about causation and correlation. Take, as an example, the brief exchange between William Bland, a naval doctor transported for duelling, who was surgeon at the Castle Hill asylum in 1814, and John Thomas Bigge, chief justice of Trinidad before he was appointed as commissioner of inquiry in New South Wales. There were between sixteen and twenty patients at the asylum while he was there, said Bland. Asked whether he could form any opinion as to the causes of lunacy – a tentative question – Bland said that two of the cases 'arose from the mere circumstance of transportation'. Bigge asked if their crimes had been serious. Both had been involved in the Irish rebellion, Bland said, and transported for their 'political opinions'. Others had become mad from religious fanaticism, intoxication, and a range of other causes, 'constitutional & otherwise'. Beyond such fleeting analyses, there was little effort to theorise the madness of the penal colony.

Many others who made decisions about madness had neither medical nor legal backgrounds. As they grappled with madness, however, they showed that they were familiar with its characteristics and contours. Their symptomologies and taxonomies were diverse, rich and inconsistent; they fixed upon symptoms, or behaviours, that fit their vernacular notions. Even in those rare instances in which symptoms were mapped carefully against prevailing medical or legal frameworks – in court, by lawyers or doctors, or in the columns of colonial newspapers – they often clashed with the common sense approaches of juries, judges and governors. These approaches tended to spring from the fear of violence associated with insanity, the need for economy, neighbourliness, or the maintenance of convict discipline.

Archives shape histories profoundly, and a closed door is an invitation to look elsewhere rather than a reason to stop looking. The records of madness at the beginning of European Australia are too slender for social history, which might show how madness cut across (but never forgot) class, age and gender, and too pragmatic to sustain psychiatric history. And yet the impossibility of writing this sort of history is also a kind of liberation, since it calls for a different sort of history. The literary scholar Laure Murat draws together a 'political history of madness' by mapping the intense tussle of revolutionary France with its insanity, building from the delusions and ravings of madmen and madwomen and the energies of their adversaries to the upheavals which rocked the great republic over a century. Asylum records, she concludes, 'are more conducive to literature than to math' – even those of the great Parisian asylums, and even in the midst of that other revolution of clerks, files and cabinets: the rise of modern bureaucracy.[25]

Late in 1836 Edward Hall wrote in his *Sydney Monitor* that half of the original (European) settlers on the Hunter had been dispossessed of their estates, 'and became vagrants, drunkards, lunatics, and suicides. The history of our Lunatic Asylum would tell some melancholy tales.'[26] So we might hope. But the lunatic asylum at Liverpool, the only institution which could have received those settlers, is survived by precious few patient records. Those that survive do not offer these tales – only glimpses of the suffering and breakdown of the mad, and of colonial efforts to impose coherence.

In this book I therefore avoid telling 'the' history of madness in colonial Australia. I avoid calculations and tables, given the dearth of records, and the difficulties of analysing data extracted from historical medical records, in which diagnoses rarely map neatly upon each other or upon our modern classifications of disease. Psychological diagnoses remain highly subjective, as the continuing travails of the *Diagnostic and Statistical Manual of Mental Disorders* project suggest.[27] I avoid carefully parsing the terminology in the sources, holding the descriptors lightly, just as those I write about did. They talked of eccentricity, incoherence and singularity, and registered more severe conditions either as permanent (stupidity, idiocy, amentia, feeble-mindedness), or temporary (derangement, mania, dementia, insanity, lunacy). In courtrooms they decided whether people were of sound or unsound mind, whether *compos mentis* or *non compos mentis*. In prisons and ships they said simply that men and women were raving, mad, or lunatic. Each of these words has a distinct history and suggests a particular symptomology, but this was not always reflected in their usage, which was often ill-informed, vague or careless. Sometimes they were used interchangeably. Instead, I render the stories of madness in the penal colony of New South Wales in the language of those who observed it, without inverted commas, which do little more than signal our discomfort.

These stories retain more details and eccentricities than other histories might, since they map the disruption of madness at every level. Those aspects which do not fit readily into sharp narratives are often the most revealing. My aim is to show the chaos madness produced in the colony and the chaos madness revealed in the colony. I examine the imperfect, uncertain qualities of legal and executive power; the importance of relationships and character traits or character flaws; the role of chance. This is a book which refuses to reduce madness into the attempts of others to rationalise it and render it knowable and manageable, to 'make the incoherent coherent'.[28] One means of achieving this is to show, where possible, the failure to recognise madness, and the failure to conquer it; to show people who lived with their illness, resisted treatment, escaped asylums. The chapters of this book are stories of madness and essays about its effects. Embedded as they are in the history of New South Wales, they show how, by disrupting families, communities and structures of colonial power, madness reveals them afresh, and shines new light on the peculiarities of the penal colony planted in Australia at the end of the 18th century.

HAVING PRESERVED THE NEW COLONY THROUGH ITS desperate first years, Arthur Phillip departed, leaving New South Wales in the care of the New South Wales Corps. Protected by governors drawn from its ranks, the officers established trade monopolies backed by coercive power. The naval governors who followed were unable to break apart these commercial interests, which were joined by a handful of private traders who expected a free rein in the colony. Government, which was occupied with the moral discipline of convicts and shoring up the sovereign authority of the crown, came into conflict with these interests, escalating into rebellion in 1808. Despite its weak initial response, the empire reasserted its sovereignty over the colony through the long and ambitious administration of Lachlan Macquarie, and the work of Ellis Bent, the first properly trained judge to hold office in the colony, who sailed out with him. It did so again through a commission of inquiry in 1819–21, which was tasked with a paradox: to assess measures for leading the colony into prosperity while it was remade as 'an object of real terror' across the empire.

This terror is one aspect of Australian history which brought madness to the fore, from the first. Many who were sent to the colonies had also first been sentenced to die, and the prospect of execution visibly aged those who waited for it, and worse. Some killed themselves under the strain, and others went mad. When they arrived, convicts were met with the 'bloody sight of corpses rotting from swinging gibbets on the harbour'.[29] In the 1820s, following Bigge's recommendations, the lash fell ever more heavily upon their backs. The acceptable number of strokes per flogging doubled to 100; a quarter of the male convicts were flogged each year. Pillories and treadmills were also introduced, so that mediaeval torture blended with modern torture. Most weeks a man or woman was hanged.[30] Around the settled areas, their semblance of British civilisation punctuated by pillories and scaffolds, were the chained labour gangs and penal settlements. The men, women and children sent to the colonies lived first under the threat of death, and then in its shadow. Even if they avoided the worst of convict discipline, they still lived in the fickle grip of masters, overseers, magistrates and governors, while the empire worked its policies out. The empire sought and achieved terror.

Free colonists found that they were not safe from the power the government wielded against convicts. This power was the cause of much tension in the early decades of the colonial presence, where there was very often a wide gap between the colonists' ambitions and the governors' assumptions. The laws shifted, in substance and as magistrates, judges, governors and London secretaries came and went. There was drama, and anxiety, and minds failed under the strain of life perched between a great unknown continent and the endless expanse of the Pacific Ocean. Madness emerged from the full range of human experience: there was grief, failure and collapse; there was even the madness which travels with success, laying waste to families, associations and businesses. These pressures were felt elsewhere, of course, but they were sharpened by the rawness of colonial society, the harshness of its politics, and the apparatus of state violence.

Little of the colony's madness was attributed at the time to the violence of colonisation. Nevertheless, we are painfully conscious of the ways that warfare and other forms of savagery typically etch their brutal stories in hidden places; what we cannot deal with in the present visits and revisits victims, but also perpetrators, partners, spouses and subsequent generations. We may wonder, through these stories about convict discipline, common grief, and business failure, how much of the derangement of New South Wales flowed from the violence of dispossession.

In 1828 a doctor and wealthy respected grazier who sat on the Legislative Council killed himself. After a difficult search, the man Governor Ralph Darling selected to replace him (since the council was not a proper parliament but an advisory committee appointed unilaterally) also tried to kill himself. 'Persons who have suffered from any temporary aberration of mind should not be sent to this colony,' wrote Darling, as his candidate recovered in hospital. 'If there is nothing in the climate which induces in colonists absolute derangement, there is undoubtedly something peculiar, which affects the spirits and produces extraordinary depression.'[31] A feature of the southern air or the waters of the Cumberland Plain, or perhaps, others wrote sourly, it was something in the style of government. Several years later another seat on the council became vacant when the far wealthier grazier John Macarthur developed delusions of persecution that turned him against his family. Even the council, peopled with the most educated and successful men in the colony, was haunted by mania and melancholy. Darling looked to the climate for answers, but there are other explanations for the madness of New South Wales. This book gathers together the scattered stories of madness at Botany Bay, and in doing so reveals how madness shaped the course of individual lives, families and communities, and spilled into courts, gaols and institutions for the insane, and into the broader structures of the colony, and the empire. It turns always back from madness itself to Botany Bay – that place of freedom and terror, of hope and grief, and contrariety.

1

THERE IS A WILDNESS

On 15 April 1803, a struggling young merchant named John Grant discovered that the woman he had been wooing, Anna Maria, had just married another man. At 4 o'clock that afternoon Grant loitered near St James's Palace in London outside the house of the lawyer who had thwarted his courtship. When the man appeared, Grant approached bearing two pistols, one pointing at the lawyer and one at himself, demanding an apology.[1] 'You damned villain,' he spat. 'You are the cause of destroying the happiness of my mind; take one of these pistols and you shall instantly shoot me, or I shall shoot you.'[2] Spencer George Townsend was in no mood for an apology or for a duel. He struck out at the pistols with his cane, turned on his heel, and fled. Grant shot him in the back, and as the lawyer lay propped on his side in the road, approached, swore, and shot him again. Townsend's butler rushed out at the sound of gunfire and apprehended the wild young suitor, who was arrested, and arraigned for breaking the peace.

The two pistols had been loaded with swan-shot, a fine, irregular stuff made for shooting birds by passing molten lead through a sieve. The damage had been so minor that Townsend had to consult a doctor to find out 'if anything had happened to him'. He had been shot in 'the ham', the meeting of the thigh and buttock, and suffered 'three superficial wounds' and 'three distinct marks'. And his jacket had caught fire.[3] Like the skin of the old lawyer's hams, the peace had been only very slightly broken.

Madness has blurred edges. Many people liked John Grant, but they also called him eccentric, wild, irrational, and simply mad. He lived on the verge of sanity, but having demonstrated the capacity for violence, he was caught up in British justice. This chapter follows Grant's difficult path to New South Wales and then Norfolk Island as a way of exploring the experience of convict transportation. It is an alien idea to modern western societies, which are now bent on incarcerating, or enclosing, those who are identified as criminals. What can we learn about its purpose and methods by listening to the words of one who was led by it off the precipice, into madness?

TWENTY-SEVEN-YEAR-OLD JOHN GRANT WAS WELL-educated and well-mannered, but when his father died his genteel family was left with little means. Grant apprenticed as a clock-maker with his uncle, and then traded as a chapman, a dealer in smallgoods. Together with his mother and sister, he moved into rooms in a house in Sloane Street, London. Next door lived Anna Maria Ward, daughter of the 2nd Viscount Dudley and Ward. Although she had been born while her mother was married to another man, Anna Maria was recognised by her father, and received a significant inheritance after his death.[4] The two became acquainted, and Grant sought a formal introduction to her through the family's lawyer, Spencer Townsend. Townsend said he was 'a foolish fellow' and told him to 'go about his business'. Unperturbed, Grant approached Townsend again, and again, and wrote some twenty letters, some appearing to threaten violence to the lawyer and to Anna Maria and her mother.[5] Townsend had Grant hauled before the Bow Street Police Court, where he was released on a bond of good behaviour.

Grant was declared bankrupt in 1802 after a crucial cargo was lost at sea.[6] He slept with the family maid, Betsy, who bore him a son, but continued to court Anna Maria. It is hard to know quite what passed between the two young neighbours. Grant was clearly besotted with Anna Maria, but her feelings are unknown. By his account, she suggested he should enrol in the army, and take out his frustrations on Napoleon and his men. He did indeed apply to the Horse Guards for an officer's commission in March 1803, but the bulk of commissions were allocated by purchase or patronage and the few remaining were earned in battle.[7] Owing to the 'number of candidates already on His Royal Highness' list', came the response, it was 'really not in his power to provide for you in the army'.[8] HRH was not in the business of tending the broken hearts of violent suitors.

Miss Ward became engaged to Major Horace St Paul, later MP for Bridport, Dorset, a man who obviously moved in the appropriate circles. After he had compromised his bond conditions, Townsend had Grant charged again, and in April 1803, proclaiming his innocence, he elected to spend twenty days in prison rather than admit his guilt.[9] Grant then learned that Townsend had told Anna Maria he 'wanted men and not women': a grave insult at the time, even if, as it seems, he wanted both.[10] Grant considered himself 'bred up as an independent English gentleman' with a sense of honour unparalleled even in the army or navy. He loaded two pistols with swan-shot and went to demand satisfaction.[11]

Anna Maria Ward and St Paul were married on 14 May 1803. Eleven days later, John Grant stood trial at the Old Bailey for breaking the peace. His lawyer, a man called Cockayne, dissuaded him from reading the twenty-page statement he had prepared – perhaps because it dwelt upon his injured honour.[12] A contemporary duelling guide held it 'assuredly just and reasonable to demand satisfaction when a personal affront has been received' but Grant had fired at an unarmed man, twice, and whatever sympathy remained for wounded honour in English courts, Grant was ineligible.[13] He had compromised the strict rituals both of duelling and of courting.

The violence had come about, argued Cockayne, because Grant's obvious passion had slipped into madness. No less than six witnesses were brought forward to testify to this 'hopeless passion for the possession of a female with whom he was deeply enamoured'. Some said the whole affair had been imaginary, that Grant had never even spoken with Anna Maria. One witness said he was 'extremely irrational, and deranged' on the subject of finances, and at the mention of Anna Maria became 'a complete maniac', raving and crying like a child; at such times he could have shot his own brother. Another told, quite wonderfully, how he had left Grant in a room with a caged leopard and returned to find him 'toying and playing with the beast, in a way that none but a madman would'.[14] London's Bethlem Asylum had closed its public viewing galleries a half century earlier, but lunacy trials continued to be immensely popular spectator events.[15]

Insanity has always occupied an awkward place in criminal law, since it complicates the relationship between action and responsibility. In medieval England, criminals who were deemed insane were found guilty, but not punished.[16] In 1736, Matthew Hale argued that while those over the age of fourteen could 'discern good and evil', 'absolute madness' compromised this capacity, transforming adults into 'brutes'. It could be partial, or intermittent, and acquittal of a crime required evidence of impairment at the time of committal.[17] The timing of Grant's trial was especially unfortunate. Three years earlier, in 1800, the veteran soldier James Hadfield had been acquitted of attempted regicide on the grounds of insanity after Lord Erskine introduced the concept of delusion into English law in a dazzling courtroom performance. Delusion meant that careful, calculated plans could be made without a proper grasp of moral consequences.[18] Many judges were outraged, and their interpretations of the law of insanity were especially stringent in the aftermath of the trial. These interpretations held great sway in these years, when doctors were rarely found in courtrooms.[19]

Grant had also shot too early to be able to call upon the jurisprudence of monomania, a category which allowed courts more flexibility. Coined in Paris in 1810, monomania combined the disordered faculties of melancholia and the 'exultance' or wild energy of mania. Its sufferers typically fixated upon one or more subjects or persons.[20] Because its symptoms were partial and intermittent, it presented an attractive criminal defence and quickly became a 'medico-legal nightmare' when it was introduced in British courts. A series of doctors might offer directly contradictory conclusions about the same behaviours in a defendant, all with great solemnity and each denying the validity of the other theories.[21] Juries and judges, meanwhile, made use of the expanding vocabulary of temporary, partial, and emotional insanities to secure acquittals for actions which were technically criminal but morally defensible – not unlike the generous response of earlier courts to proper duelling.[22]

John Grant fell between concepts and codes which might have helped him. Thinking, perhaps, of Hadfield, the judge demolished his insanity defence. Insanity was not 'an idle and absurd moodiness of mind', he said, 'arising from long-cherished resentment and hopeless passion, blazing out into desperation', nor 'that species of paroxysm, created by anger and revenge'. Derangement had to be proved 'in all common occurrences of life' and the matter boiled down to this: when Grant fired at Townsend in the alley, did he have the 'sanity and intellect to correct his bad intentions', or did he shoot him 'merely to gratify his revenge against a person whom he thought opposed his wild and hopeless passion'.[23] The judge's position was clear, the jury obliged with a guilty verdict, and John Grant was sentenced to death.

WAITING FOR DEATH CAN HAVE PROFOUND EFFECTS. The colonial reformer Edward Gibbon Wakefield planned his ambitious program of systematic colonisation during a three-year stint in Newgate. He had abducted a fifteen-year-old girl in a wild scheme of his own, hoping to obtain the patronage of her wealthy manufacturer father for a seat in parliament.[24] In Newgate, Wakefield saw men awaiting death for a month or more. 'Brown hair turned gray, and gray white. The smooth face of a man of twenty-five becomes often marked with decided wrinkles on the forehead, and about the eyes and mouth.'[25] Some were driven to kill themselves; others waited nervously on final petitions.[26]

As an execution approached, those under sentence of death were gathered around a coffin which lay on a table in Newgate chapel. They listened to 'a suitable sermon' and the Church of England liturgy proclaimed the mercy and justice of God.[27] The liturgy held out the promise of deliverance, but a beneficent monarch could intervene before the condemned met their maker. Like other desperate relatives, Grant's sister Matilda petitioned the royal princesses for clemency, and Grant also sent a petition to the king, attaching the signatures of thirty-eight London businessmen. Neither mentioned madness; both spoke of a young man's honour and the lack of real injury.[28]

Twelve hours before John Grant was to be executed, he learned that the petitions had been accepted and that his sentence had been commuted to transportation to New South Wales.[29] Grant was sent to await his transportation, crowded with twenty others in a small cell on an old French frigate moored on the Thames. He grew weak and emaciated. After refusing food for several days, he collapsed, and was sent to a 'hospital hulk'. Conditions for those awaiting transportation were abysmal. Even after a half century of regular transportation to the Australian colonies, a commissioner found that convicts waited weeks or months, 'much longer than they ought to', exposed to 'much bad association and many bad practices'. In the gaol at Aylesbury, Buckinghamshire, Ward found eleven prisoners awaiting transportation, thirteen awaiting trial, and three acquitted on the grounds of insanity, all rooming together. There were marbles, ball games and, apparently, a book of pornography; it was all 'highly improper'.[30] Ten years later, the hulks were still 'most disgraceful and discreditable'. Many of the prisoners received from other gaols were insane, especially from Millbank, the national penitentiary trialling the separate system and reportedly driving men mad. These inmates remained in the wretched hulks for long stretches, and there was little effort to move them to asylums.[31]

JOHN GRANT WAS CHARGED UNDER THE BLACK ACT OF 1723, the most severe in English criminal law history. It prescribed the death penalty for more than fifty crimes, and the great criminal historian Leon Radzinowicz describes it as an 'ideological index' to the criminal law, laying bare its class prejudice.[32] The frequency of English executions doubled during the 18th century, and increased again in the first three decades of the 19th. Foreigners were shocked at what they saw, and Whig reformers came to agree. Conservatives replied that these executions kept crime under control, that the 'lesson of the gallows' was a powerful one.[33] But the number of death sentences commuted to transportation rose still higher. Some 27 000 of the 35 000 sentenced to death between 1770 and 1830 had their sentences commuted, which allowed, writes historian Vic Gatrell, the law to acquire 'an appearance of mercy and justice while retaining its terrible threat'.[34] The contradiction also spilled into the administration of justice, where there was no clear logic determining which sentences were commuted and, of those, who was actually sent. The monarch, exercising the prerogative of mercy, had a different agenda to that of the courts and gaols. The courts were divided in various ways, and juries regularly, for instance, undervalued stolen goods to spare defendants the death penalty.[35] The penal colonies had different agendas again, since they were building societies rather than policing boundaries.

New South Wales was many things to many people. To Grant, who had watched his death approaching, and to others, the colony presented the chance to build a life. In a moment of special naiveté somewhere between San Salvador and Port Jackson, Grant wrote to his mother and sister: 'Upon the whole, when I seriously reflect, my emigration was the best step I could take, disappointed as I have been in favorite objects in England.' It was merely the 'manner of it' that bothered him, and the thought of leaving his creditors in the lurch.[36] He was rewriting his history, and in this he was aided by the suppleness of transportation, for that contrary, fluid logic spread from the courts to the hulks and gaols and ports, to the decks and cabins of the transport ships and even, in the early years, to the shores of Sydney Cove and the rivers and forests and plains beyond. It allowed John Grant to emigrate as a gentleman.

He certainly travelled as a gentleman, taking aboard his ship, the *Coromandel*, a black satin waistcoat and breeches – 'very beautiful' – expensive shirts, and a white hat, as well as chocolate from his mother, a small knife, a 'beautiful spun watch pocket' and a silver cream jug from his 'dear never-to-be-forgotten friend', Mrs Mallett.[37] He took his violin, too, and possibly a harpsichord, which would inspire a musical two centuries later, with Grant's poetry and prose set amidst music from his scoresheets, the sounds of the Australian bush, and the didgeridoo.[38] These perks, which showed the Grants hardly destitute, were likely facilitated by their connection with Mr Lane, one of the owners of the *Coromandel*, and by another friend who travelled aboard, a Mr Fielding.[39] Once aboard, Grant quickly befriended the officers, who were likely second or third genteel sons, and no doubt appreciated the respite he offered from the clamour of sailors and convicts.[40]

Grant envied the 22-year-old captain, John Robinson, the endless freedom of the sea. He invited Grant to share his cabin, where we might imagine him writing his sprawling letters home late into candlelit evenings. It was no small gesture; space on convict transports was highly contested. It meant comfort on a trying voyage, but also served as a status marker.[41] The wealthy convict George Crossley was able to accommodate his family in the cabin he paid for on his way out to the colony, as well as enjoying a measure of freedom, including to buy goods during the voyage. Henry Browne Hayes, who features later, paid three or four hundred guineas for 'respectable treatment and decent accommodation' in an already crowded ship.[42] Robinson's sympathies ran so deep, claimed Grant, that he offered him the chance to escape while they lay anchored at San Salvador.[43] Grant declined on account of his honour, but also, perhaps, because he had great expectations for New South Wales. The sea and the responsibilities of leadership – which Grant thought should never have been extended to one whose 'passion for toping' was known – proved too much for Robinson, who drank himself to death soon after the ship left Brazil, leaving a grieving fiancée at home, and his friend John Grant shocked that one 'in the prime of life' should perish 'in a state of madness': it elicited 'many serious reflexions'.[44]

The arrangements on the *Coromandel* remind us that convict transportation involved a wide range of experience. In an earlier tradition, it was indeed a form of exile which might be chosen in preference to death. It was part of what historian Alan Atkinson calls a 'conversation between king and subject', but the practice shifted across the 18th century, partly due to those who had accepted transportation breaking faith and returning. Transportation became instead a routinised banishment – not a conversation, but a lecture.[45] Shipping operators carried convicts to North America in exchange for a share in the value of their labour, which they sold on to established colonists, so that the lives of criminals were also shaped by the global labour market.[46] When Botany Bay was settled on after the American Revolutionary War of 1775–83, the system changed markedly. Because there was no existing European society able to absorb convicts, there was no market for convict labour. The government had not only to transport them across the seas but also feed and clothe them in the colony. As the society developed, and convicts were assigned to colonists, it was arranged primarily by government, not the market, and regulated by magistrates.[47] New South Wales was something of an experiment. In many ways a work of British imagination, its form and purpose, beyond transportation, were open.

NEW SOUTH WALES WAS A CLASS-CONSCIOUS SOCIETY. Lachlan Macquarie, who governed 1810–21, was eager to extend a second chance to those who had 'once moved in the ranks of gentlemen'.[48] Grant's journal and letters reveal the experience of a rare transportee, but also much about transportation more broadly, since he took a keen interest in transportation and in constitutional law. After complaining of the '199 abominable villains' the government had provided as companions on the *Coromandel*, he came to fight vigorously for those who had been ill-treated by the system.[49]

The respite Grant had found aboard the *Coromandel* continued in the colony. Those colonists of a higher social class tended to feel their isolation, while those who aspired to improve their class valued the company of the genteel highly. Educated convicts possessed rare clerical skills and overlooking or overturning a criminal sentence could be a small price to pay for the use of their services. In time, however, class would play out differently; colonists became more particular about their company, reformers insisted that penal discipline should be egalitarian. In the 1820s Governor Darling went so far as to send 'special', educated convicts to remote locations where they would feel more like convicts.[50]

In 1804, however, John Grant could apply his remarkable imagination in the space allowed him as a 'special' convict. In San Salvador his friend Mr Fielding had purchase a hogshead (60 gallons) of 'excessive fiery' spirits for him at 3 shillings and sixpence a gallon, as well as some sugar and coffee. He had heard that rum was 'so scarce and the sale so restricted as to almost amount to prohibition' – that it was 'prized more than gold'.[51] In his account of the colony published in 1798, judge advocate David Collins had claimed that the 'passion for liquor operated like a mania'.[52] Grant looked for a large profit margin, and planned to use the proceeds to buy sheep and cattle for a farm, or to partner with the 'opulent merchant' Robert Campbell and 'open a connection with India if possible'.[53]

The first governor of New South Wales, Arthur Phillip, had been forced to compromise on rum, and allow it to function as an informal currency. The interim governors who administered the colony in the three years after his departure did little to address this situation, but John Hunter, who governed from 1795 to 1800, sought to regulate the flow. His successor, Philip King, made the first serious headway in this and other areas of colonial disorder. One arm of his strategy was to undercut the rampant market by supplying spirits at a fixed rate.[54] The upshot of these rum politics was that King confiscated Grant's spirits on arrival, and gave him 8 shillings a gallon, little more than £20 in total instead of the £100 he had hoped for.[55]

Grant bridled at this interference, 'under pretence of attending to the health of the lower class', and dwelt upon it as he struggled to establish himself.[56] The realities of New South Wales were beginning to undo his narrative of emigration. Without capital, Grant had little chance of partnering with Campbell, and looked reluctantly for a salaried position in government or business. It should have been simple enough, since he was educated and bore letters of introduction from former governor John Hunter to some of the most prominent men in the colony: judge advocate Richard Atkins, James Williamson, former commissary, Major George Johnston, a senior officer of the New South Wales Corps, and William Cox, its paymaster.[57] Atkins, 'a little gentleman about 50, and most agreeable indeed', became Grant's first patron.[58] He talked of government positions and good connections, but his patronage may have harmed rather than helped; he was not well regarded in Sydney. In 1799 he had sued the popular surgeon John Harris for defamation; Harris had called him a swindler. Though Atkins won, it was a pyrrhic victory, and Harris pointed out that he could hardly do more damage to Atkins's reputation that Atkins himself. It was well-known that Atkins was an alcoholic, whose wife, as Grant learned, was 'forced to lead him to bed vomiting'.[60]

Cox, the paymaster, was fighting off bankruptcy, and was ordered back to England to account for his use of army funds, but one letter was more fruitful: James Williamson, a Scottish farmer, offered Grant a tumbledown cottage on his property at Parramatta, and some adjoining farming land.[61] The Williamsons welcomed him into their family, and the intimacy that developed between them helped preserve Grant's image of himself as an émigré. Their neighbour, Captain William Kent, also sympathised with Grant, and later petitioned the governor for his freedom.[62]

Grant called the farm 'an asylum', partly because the Williamsons were kind, but the farm also sheltered him from the convict system. This model had been tried the decade prior by a small group of political prisoners who were transported to the penal colony for their radical ideas about constitutional reform. These 'Scottish Martyrs' held that they were free men so long as they incurred no debt, and therefore purchased cabins for the passage out, which also afforded them 'the characters of gentlemen'.[63] Maurice Margarot, transported in 1794 for his seditious promotion of revolutionary principles, was joined in the cabin he purchased by his wife, which vexed the ship's officers.[64] In New South Wales, Margarot demanded his pardon, and though it was refused, he and the other Martyrs assumed that they were free in the colony so long as they incurred no debt from the government.[65] Governor Hunter found that 'they could not be compelled to work' and the government, suspecting that the law was on their side, opted to leave them to their own devices.[66]

Grant lived frugally at the farm, subsisting on bread and water and the kindness of Mrs Williamson. He had an 'aversion to cooking' but was also following the Martyrs' playbook. 'While I solicit no food from the Government,' Grant wrote, 'I am my own master in a certain degree, but, the moment I require provisions, I become harnessed and at their disposal as a slave.'[67] Rations were a crucial mechanism of control and discipline; the government had minimal control over those who by industry, capital or connections could stay 'off the stores'. The farm work was humbling, but not shameful, and it offered Grant the freedom to follow Atkins's advice, and embrace this 'temporary retirement to compose my mind'.[68]

AT ATKINS'S HOUSE, GRANT CHANCED UPON CHARLES Bishop, a master navigator and now trading partner of the explorer George Bass. The two were immediately drawn to each other. 'He is a person, who all his life hitherto, has been attached to the sea,' wrote Grant. Thirty-five years old, intimate with the governor and the social set, he was 'a gentleman of great respectability'. 'He possesses that openness of disposition you have censured sometimes in me, in a much greater degree,' he wrote to his mother and sister; his mind is as 'open and artless as my own'. Bishop invited Grant to live with him at his farm 'for the sake of mutual society'. It was possibly more than companionship. Grant had shared Robinson's cabin, and in Sydney he lived with two bachelors. Several years into their friendship, Bishop, reading the newspaper, said to Grant that he thought the execution of a naval officer 'for buggery' was cruel. 'Ah, if you go on as you have done this will be your fate,' Grant replied, enigmatically, and wrote in his journal: 'Bishop pretends to laugh this off but I hope it makes some impression'.[69]

Bishop was a 'pioneer of pacific commerce', writes historian Michael Roe. He worked the oceans between India and the Cape Colony, and Chile and China, exploiting the new markets emerging at the edges of the East India Company's monopoly.[70] He ventured into the sealing industry, making use of unskilled ex-convicts to beat, skin and boil down seals along the southern shores. In 1799, the year after Bass circumnavigated the continent with Matthew Flinders, he and Bishop entered a commercial partnership. They ran sealing expeditions at first, but the slaughter took its toll on the seals and the controls Governor King introduced in 1803 to conserve the population turned their attention north. They sailed to Tahiti to capitalise on the flourishing pork trade.[71]

Bishop, however, began to show signs of madness, and Bass left him out of his ambitious plans for 'a clandestine trade' with Peru.[72] 'Bishops ill health has thrown all cares & concerns upon my head both for ship & cargo and for some time they must remain those,' he wrote to his wife in November 1802.[73] He was rather less delicate to his father-in-law: 'Bishop has been totally useless to me and the concern for many months past, indeed ever since I left him at Otaheite in February … I shall leave him here to recover. It is more than probable he will be in the grave before I return.'[74] Although Bishop's health began to improve, Bass decided he was still unfit for 'strong undertakings', and so he remained in Sydney when Bass sailed their ship, the *Venus*, into the Pacific.[75]

It was in this state of limbo that Bishop received Grant into his home. He had been anxious for a companion for some months, after a violent attack by a gang of bushrangers, who had broken into his home, stolen his substantial arsenal and set the house on fire. 'If I had had a 2nd person to have stood by me,' Bishop wrote, to prevent them 'rushing at the back door, they would have been easily dispersed'.[76]

Bishop's cottage at Prospect Hill was set amidst verdant forest drawing on rich volcanic soils.[77] 'A beautiful farm,' wrote Grant, 'a fine farm … through the wood 5 miles from Parramatta.' He wrote happily of his first days 'in such a sweet house of his here (for I am now with him!)', sometimes going out 'shooting parrots etc. (with which the woods abound) in company with my friend Bishop', using the fibre of the paper-bark tree for wadding. Grant's poetry is interleaved throughout his journals and letters. Bishop was also literary: 'a man of noble mind', wrote Grant, 'tho' fond of women, an excellent navigator and a poet in his way – i.e. on sea-subjects'.[78]

As well as helping to secure the farm, Grant seems to have to filled the place Bass left in his partner's affections. The captain 'has a higher opinion of my strong mind (which he says is like Bass's) than of any other man,' wrote Grant. 'He advises me to accept no offers from Judge Atkins, but to wait patiently, to live with him, to keep him company, to amuse myself as I please.' Anything less than a position with Robert Campbell, Bishop assured Grant, would 'only lower me in the opinion of the respectable part of the colony'. Bishop's voice breaks into the diary: '"and why Grant!" (he will say) "will you be anxious about leaving me?"' He would make room for all of them if Bass returned. 'Adjoining my farm is another of 40 acres,' he said. 'You shall settle near me. Think no more of England, make this your adopted country, as I certainly shall do.' Grant was deeply moved. 'Bishop affects me much by his behaviour,' he wrote, 'which is so truly affectionate and delicate, for he knows I am poor but assures me I shall never become friendless while he remains in New South Wales'.[79]

Grant imagined that his life with Bishop would be therapeutic. 'He is subject to low spirits,' he wrote home, 'and myself also, so our mutual comfort seems to demand an increase of friendship.' But neither man was wholly at peace. Grant was anxious about the Napoleonic wars raging in Europe, which the French were winning. His mother was French, and French expatriates living in England were intensely unpopular. If the French won, that would be another problem.[80] Nor had he forgotten his 'disappointment'; he asked his sister to write immediately to him if 'Mrs St Paul' was widowed, by Napoleon or otherwise, for, he wrote, 'I am firmly persuaded her first affections were mine'.[81] Bishop was waiting for his partner, and news of their enterprise. Collecting some mail from him some months after Bass left, Matthew Flinders found him 'wholly dispirited'.[82] Bass's wife was waiting, too, a world away in England.[83] As the cottage filled with the music of Grant's violin and the poetry they wove together, it was also alive with the shadows of darker things. They were flirting with madness in paradise.

The *Venus* disappeared into the Pacific, together with George Bass and the enterprise, to become a maritime puzzle for adventurers and historians.[84] It was not uncommon for ships to wreck, and ruin businesses; the sea was a capricious silent partner in thousands of tenuous ventures. Bishop, however, who had already demonstrated symptoms of insanity, buckled under the strain. 'His grief about Dr Bass has tended to bring on madness,' wrote Grant.[85] Governor King had Bishop placed in a section of Parramatta Gaol reserved for the insane. Grant visited his friend often, and applied to lease and work his farm during his illness. He asked for help from King, expecting that his instructions from London to encourage agriculture would direct that a good farm should not go to waste. King was unenthusiastic, and requested a certificate of Grant's fitness from Bishop's trustees, then James Williamson and the chaplain Samuel Marsden, of Grant's fitness. They obliged, and Grant was allowed to work the farm, but without assistance.

He might have found a way to farm and live quietly and calmly, but, as Bishop wrestled with his mania in the gaol, Grant was drawn into the intense world of another set of politically active convicts, the United Irishmen. A liberal political group, the Irishmen were inspired by the revolutions in France and North America, and came into conflict with the law. Some were transported. Grant became close to Sir Henry Browne Hayes, who was not transported for his politics but actively supported his countrymen in the colony. A flamboyant and extravagant aristocrat who also dabbled in poetry, Hayes had been sentenced to death for kidnapping and forcing into marriage Mary Pike, a Quaker heiress; a false priest directed the rites in a dimly lit castle library. The sentence was commuted, and Hayes paid his way to New South Wales, where his life was notable, suggests his biographer Norman Lynravn, 'largely for his war against authority' – and for Vaucluse House. Its Italianate stone, and the grass he had shipped over from Ireland to protect from snakes, embodied his contempt for the convict role pressed upon him and for the very ground on which he stood.[86] Grant was intoxicated by Hayes, and joined him in this war against authority. Despite his limited means, he had a plough fashioned and hired oxen to work the ground with it, because to have men till the soil with hoes, under the threat of the lash, was to make slaves of them.[87] He had never been even-keeled, but his criticisms of the governor and the entire practice of transportation grew increasingly strident and reckless.[88] Others either transported for their politics or subject to discipline in the colony for them tended to rein in their activism where necessary, and survived the colony intact. Grant was not so lucky.

DESPITE GRANT'S DISAPPOINTMENT IN THE MATTER OF his rum, he still hoped for a job in Robert Campbell's thriving business at its dockside warehouses. Campbell's sister was married to commissary John Palmer, and was on close terms with Mrs Williamson, but nothing came of that approach; efforts through Richard Atkins and William Cox also failed, perhaps because both had poor reputations. Grant learned that Campbell needed someone 'to stand in his shoes' while he travelled to England, and thought Campbell refused to consider him for the position because he was still, legally, a convict (there may have been other reasons, like his former bankruptcy, or present eccentricities).[89] Fired by this rejection, and by the knowledge that King had pardoned some of the other *Coromandel* convicts, Grant intensified his efforts to obtain a pardon.[90] In October 1804, as Bishop's sanity failed, Grant wrote Governor King a letter, and asked his friend George Evans, the surveyor-general, to deliver it while he breakfasted with King. In it he asked the governor for a 'colonial emancipation' (a conditional pardon) and requested advice on how best to make a life in the colony, 'being equally unsettled in my mind, and in my views'. King visited Bishop that morning, but Grant was elsewhere. That afternoon he went to the governor's garden, where King was holding court.

Grant wrote home later: 'I waited upon him, surrounded by several Gentlemen in his Garden and said my name was "Grant".'

> King civilly touched his hat. 'Yes, Sir! I received a letter from you today.'
>
> 'I request a reply Sir.' But I was so hurt and agitated I spoke low and he did not at first understand what I said. I repeated 'I request a reply Sir.'

> Governor King then answered, 'I always like to take time to consider my replies, Mr Grant.' I very slowly retired.[91]

King's response was remarkable for its mildness, especially since he was known for his angry responses to any challenge.[92] It makes Grant's response, in a letter written that evening at midnight, the more startling. 'Why hesitate Governor King to do an act of Justice?', it began, and cited the case of Captain Bellasis, an officer of the East India Company army who had been transported for a duel in defence of his sister-in-law's honour.[93] The captain had arrived with a petition from 'the principal inhabitants of Bombay' and had been pardoned on arrival (in fact, as King replied, it was three months before Bellasis was pardoned). Grant was 'irreparably injur'd', suffering 'the vengeance of the law as a criminal who has yet done no harm!' King was the 'assassin of his peace of mind', and would not the gentlemen standing around him in the garden demand satisfaction at such grievances? 'I wish I could look on you in any other character than as my jailor and oppressor,' he warned the governor of New South Wales, 'but, if that is not to be the case, look sharp out, or I shall decamp and my arm may yet reach as far as home again – John Grant.'[94]

We can imagine the flame of Grant's candle dancing to the fury of his scratching and blotting, black ink splashing across the page. He had barely escaped the consequences of misreading the honour code at home, but here he was, rewriting transportation as a string of rights and wrongs, of threats and wounds. The letter survives because he copied it into his journal, to best 'express my feelings on maturely weighing Governor King's evasive answer'. There is a self-consciousness to his midnight writing, and even as he signed off it was clear he understood his transgression. 'If you imagine this epistle strange,' he wrote, 'I can only remark 'tis my native independence of mind which does not forsake me, tho' your prisoner, Sir!' But of course, as Evans made clear when he visited Grant several days later, 'King is governor, and will not be dictated to by any one'.[95]

Grant saw a colony divided. There was 'a very respectable body of *honest banished men*' in the colony, he wrote to his new friend Henry Browne Hayes, who were there for 'disputes in private life', 'political principles', poaching and perjury.[96] It was cruel of the government to place them on the same footing as the rest of the convicts. Like Hayes, Grant refused to accept the terms of transportation. 'It is only a proper respect I owe myself,' he wrote home, 'to keep *aloof* from servitude of every kind as long as I am considered a prisoner here'. He saw in both the civil government and the military apparatus 'a disposition to humble those who come here.'[97] He and his associates refused to be humbled.

Grant developed a critique of New South Wales similar to that of the Scottish Martyrs. Transportation amounted to banishment; any further punishment was an illegal act of oppression. He called to his aid the star of English jurisprudence, Lord Auckland, who argued that the crown renounced its claims on a criminal in the course of transportation, and William Blackstone, who had emphasised the inalienable quality of the birthrights of British subjects.[98] These fundamental uncertainties were expressed in hesitant and shifting policies on transportation and the discipline of convicts in the colony. Conditional or colonial pardons – effectively the release of a convict from formal custody and from any claim over their labour – were awarded by the early governors inconsistently, and sometimes arbitrarily.

Philip King awarded Grant a conditional pardon on 1 February 1805, some months after being interrupted in his garden.[99] The influence of Grant's friends, especially William Kent, and his letters of introduction were working in spite of his own efforts. But he had already come to despise the very thought of a 'colonial emancipation' – an 'atrocious bug-bear'. From what was he to be emancipated? 'Men arrived at their destination when banished are under the influence of the Grand Magna Charta of England', he wrote energetically, but it was 'violated' by the colonial authorities. The government behind this 'horrid system' was sinking into 'deep contempt in the opinion of all Englishmen'. Blood had already been shed – he meant the Vinegar Hill uprising of 1804, in which two or three hundred Irish convicts had marched on Parramatta and in which both Hayes and Margarot had been involved – and more would flow.[100] When Grant wrote to the governor about Bishop's farm three months later, he transgressed further boundaries. He would not present the 'ridiculous certificates' King had requested on account of King's 'contemptuous behaviour' at their last meeting. 'I wish never to see your face again,' he wrote. 'By what right do *you, make slaves of Britons* in this distant quarter of the globe?' He cited Lord Auckland, William Blackstone, the Magna Carta, and the skeletons of Irish rebels he had seen hanging in gibbets – and his rum.[101] To Hayes he was even more forthright: the massacre of the Irish convicts showed that King derived his real power not from the sovereign or the constitution, but from the New South Wales Corps.[102]

Grant had gone too far. On Saturday 18 May, a bench of magistrates assembled in the judge advocate's garden and demanded an explanation for these 'seditious and highly inflammatory' letters. He was so violently unrepentant that he was sent away for 'indecorous' conduct. On the bench, Atkins, George Johnston and Grant's friend William Kent expressed their disappointment that a man with such talents had applied them so poorly. When he was hauled back for sentencing, they denounced Grant's conduct as 'manifestly of a tendency the most absurd but not least dangerous in civil society'. Vinegar Hill had demonstrated the seriousness of the threat; Grant was sentenced to five years' hard labour, which he would spend on Norfolk Island, a thousand miles from the mainland.[103]

Ever the independent gentleman, Grant called upon Atkins the following day to remonstrate with him. He recorded Atkins's words in his journal: 'Mr Grant, you are acting so much against your own interests that I can guess the cause only in supposing you MAD – for, although your sentiments may be most righteous, why do you espouse in this way the cause of the prisoners? We have never treated you as a prisoner!'[104] Grant then wrote to Kent, bridling at the notion that his advocacy for convicts could only issue from 'insanity'. He had spent six months with them on the *Coromandel* and twelve more in the colony, he wrote, and he could hardly 'view the violation of the English constitution in their persons here! without lamenting their fate'. The free grew disillusioned, 'French principles gain ground', and the colony lived under the shadow of revolt. And Atkins, he hoped Kent would convey to him, was a drunkard and a traitor. 'A day of retribution will arrive.'[105]

This is the 'utter foolhardiness' which for Norman S. Lynravn reveals Grant's 'imbalanced mind.'[106] The civil authorities, respectable society, and even the governor had been willing to treat Grant as a gentleman, not as a convict, but fired by his grievances he had fallen in with the radical colonial resistance. 'The sickness and a second exile keep/Restrained a genius fluttering to soar', he wrote on 4 June 1805 as he was borne to Norfolk Island, in a militant ode marking the King's birthday. He was transforming himself into a martyr.[107]

THE REMOTENESS OF NORFOLK ISLAND NO DOUBT MADE it an attractive solution for a man who would not stay quiet. King had established a penal settlement at Coal River, Newcastle, for those who had participated in the Vinegar Hill uprising and others who proved especially refractory.[108] Though Sir Henry and Maurice Margarot were suspected of inciting the Vinegar Hill rebellion, they were sent not to Newcastle but to Norfolk, shortly after Grant. They were moved again three months later to Van Diemen's Land. King was wary of Margarot's 'secret mischief', and Hayes had nearly succeeded in setting up a masonic lodge and 'would very soon have made every soldier and other person Freemasons'.[109] He and several magistrates agreed to send Margarot, Hayes and the convict poet Michael Robinson, all 'suspicious' and likely 'dangerous' characters, to different penal settlements for the 'peace and tranquillity' of the colony. King included lines from a letter he had received from Grant and this agreement with the magistrates in his report to the Colonial Office. The magistrates and 'the colony at large' were eager, he said, to be rid of these 'incendiaries' who had been 'promoting discord and fermenting litigations' for years.[110]

Norfolk Island was not yet the place of penal horror it would become. Colonised at the same time as the mainland, it began as an unusual, egalitarian community which made decisions at communal meetings. By the early 1800s there was still little corporal punishment on the island, and Grant was assigned to John Foley to help him raise coffee trees and tutor his sons.[111] Foley's farm was one of the best on the island and it, like the Williamsons', became a 'refuge'.[112] Still, the commandants of Norfolk Island tended towards indifference to the law, and the convicts and free people placed under their authority easily became victims of the 'amateur' or 'frontier' law of the outposts and penal settlements. 'No British subjects,' argues legal historian Bruce Kercher, 'were further away from legal protection than the convicts of this remote island.'[113]

Grant continued his struggle against arbitrary power,

advocating for those who fell foul of John Piper, who was then commandant of the island. He narrowly avoided punishment for criticising the chaplain and the previous commandant, Joseph Foveaux, but when Grant confronted Piper in public, accusing him of continuing Foveaux's 'system of terror', the commandant ordered him flogged. The punishment was downgraded to imprisonment; Piper seems to have been reluctant to flog his gentleman prisoner. He had earlier treated the United Irishman Joseph Holt with respect, and earned Holt's in return. Foveaux had been known to employ force wherever possible.[114] To protest the chains he had been locked in, Grant gave up shaving. 'There are those who call me insane as a consequence,' he wrote.[115]

When Thomas Prosser, another United Irishman, was sent away from Norfolk Island for an affair with a married woman, it was announced that his effects would be auctioned off. Grant was so incensed at the injustice of this 'iniquitous and forced sale' that he attended the auction, even though he had been banned from the town centre. Piper saw him coming, and yelled to the gaoler, 'Put him in prison! Put him in prison!' Grant was suave: 'I, continuing on my leisurely way, saying not a word, accompanied by the gaoler enter prison for the second time!' His account could be lifted from *Don Quixote* except it lacks Cervantes' irony:

> I had not been in the prison yard an hour when a bell announces that the sale of Prosser's effects is to begin, before his embarkation. I am immediately filled with hot indignation, which lends wings to my feet (like another Mercury!) I leap to the top of the walls which surround me and, getting down on the other side, walk softly towards the place of sale, which had commenced. I shout at the top of my voice 'This sale is not lawful, and all those who buy goods here have no legitimate

> right to the property at all!' Everyone turns towards me, and I repeat this blunt statement and I've since been told that many men thought I was 'mad' both on that account and because of my beard, which I have never touched since the day I wore irons the 7th September last. I was soon seized by half-a-dozen constables and taken back to my gloomy cell for three hours!![116]

Grant was ordered to return to Foley's farm and not to leave it, or see Sir Henry or Maurice Margarot. Doing so would earn him a third exile to Phillip Island, 6 kilometres offshore. Grant nevertheless dined with his friends the night before they left for Van Diemen's Land, on 13 October 1805, and presented them with the 'Bond of Union' he had drawn up. Hayes and Margarot read its preamble: 'Whereas a system of government predominates in New South Wales and its dependencies, having slavery for its basis, tyranny for its action and consequently much oppression to His Majesty's subjects there'. Grant meant to solicit signatures from the colonists, who would then be obliged to prosecute the colonial governors and judges (with their corruption, 'pusillanimity', and 'habitual intoxication') when they returned to the United Kingdom.[117] Grant was so moved by his friends that he vowed to keep his beard in memory of them, and abstain from eating meat 'while tyranny 'midst Britons reigns'.[118] He kept his vow until July 1809.

Grant otherwise did as he was told, until, six months later, he helped John Morris write a formal complaint to Piper about his treatment. Morris had spent three months constrained by 'irons, chains and log' before opting to go to Phillip Island to be rid of them. While there he had gone three weeks without receiving provisions and water. Piper rewarded Grant with six days in gaol, during which he 'fainted dead away' before a doctor intervened.

'Thus you see, my Matilda,' he wrote home, 'your brother struggles for the unfortunate and for the establishment in these countries of the Whig principles of England.'[120]

Grant was irrepressible. Less than a fortnight later, he wrote to the island's schoolteacher, Mrs Mitchell, for details of a recent attack on her character. He was preparing a dossier of tyrannies which he would present to William Bligh, who he learned had been appointed governor. Piper learned of the letter, and his fury did away with whatever reservations he had left. 'The above letter,' Grant wrote tersely, 'occasioned Mr Grant to be publickly lashed in August 1806, besides, he has been repeatedly put in jail, his beard torn off his face by force.'[121] He was then rowed across the water to Phillip Island. Abrupt journal entries show that Grant meditated in the mornings and ate maize, refusing the 'pig meal' which would have compromised his vow. The island broke him in time. The historian W. S. Hill-Reid writes that after four months on the island Grant was found weak and almost prostrate by the man bringing provisions, having not eaten for ten days.[122] He was returned to Norfolk Island and to the 'sweet asylum' of the Foleys' farm.

GRANT HAD, HOWEVER, CONTRIVED TO COMMUNICATE his case to the incoming governor. In December 1807 Bligh instructed Piper to send a large contingent of those living on the island to a settlement north of Hobart on the Derwent, which would be called New Norfolk. 'There is an unfortunate person with you whose name is Grant,' he added. 'If he wishes to be here in preference to proceeding to the Derwent and there is the least chance of his mind being quieted by this indulgence let him come.'[123] Here was a governor, notorious for his sunburnished hardness, directing a penal commandant to consult the preferences of a convict serving labour for sedition – with care to his mental health. Bligh may have been particularly sympathetic on account of his daughter, Anne Campbell, then twenty-four, who suffered from epilepsy and was 'mentally afflicted'. She would later be legally declared 'a lunatic'.[124]

Grant wanted to see Bligh but opted for New Norfolk.[125] Bligh, having governed only eighteen months, was deposed on 26 January 1808, and imprisoned. Grant waited six months in Van Diemen's Land before returning to Sydney. Bligh, having deployed all his art to be allowed on board his old command the *Porpoise*, reneged on his promise to sail directly for England and ordered the captain, Grant's friend William Kent, to fire upon Sydney. (Kent refused, and was later court-martialled for insubordination.)[126] At length, Bligh travelled south to Van Diemen's Land seeking support from Lieutenant-Governor David Collins, arriving in March 1809, just after Grant's departure.[127] It was a wretched comedy of errors.

In Sydney, Grant approached George Johnston, who had once offered him assistance, then tried him for sedition, and had now deposed the governor. Grant asked for permission to return home. Johnston simply said 'No, I can't do that', and turned away.[128] He was beginning to apprehend the implications of the 'dreadful calamity' he had helped create, and would soon be ordered home to stand trial.[129] Grant recounted another meeting with Johnston in his journal. He told Johnston how a captain had approached him with the news that Anna Maria St Paul was a widow, that he had papers for Grant's pardon, and Grant was significantly in his debt. None of it was true. It was enough, Grant confided, to make a man shoot himself.[130] Johnston tried to extricate himself from the conversation, but Grant wanted to talk about 'the past and present and some ideas also about the future position in these countries'. 'Well Mr Grant – another time,' Johnston replied. 'But Sir I must have your permission first,' Grant said, 'that you will feel not offended at anything I may say.' 'Well – I will not,' Johnston said. 'And I now left him,' wrote Grant in his journal, 'perhaps he thinking me insane! for he looked droll.'[131]

Grant's journal is remarkable. Eloquent, warm and perceptive, it reveals the depth of his suffering in the colony. Alongside his private writing, with its window into the fitfulness of his thinking, the reactions of others are recorded – whispers, jokes and warnings. 'What Grant is that – what – Mad Grant?', Elizabeth Paterson (the wife of the ranking officer of the Corps) is quoted as saying.[132] When he canvassed support for his Bond of Union, the wealthy former convict Simeon Lord, who had employed and supported Grant, told him ''tis a mad scheme, and you will be taken up'.[133] Even his closest friends talked casually of his insanity. 'I must rebuke Hayes, who calls me regularly mad!' wrote Grant in January 1809.[134] Grant called this talk of his insanity a 'calumny' which had spread from Norfolk Island to Sydney, and through the ranks of the society he had once hoped to join. Another reading is that these were the words others used to describe a man they could not place – neither quite convict nor quite free, neither quite respectable nor quite a blackguard, and neither quite sane nor quite mad.

When Grant returned to Sydney he found Charles Bishop still confined in Parramatta Gaol as a lunatic. He begged Hayes to let Bishop stay on a sofa in his enormous house, but he refused. 'Everybody is reluctant for poor Bishop to remain among them in this country,' wrote Grant.[135] Thomas Jamison, who had replaced Marsden and Macarthur as Bishop's 'committee', decided that alternative lodgings would be too difficult and too expensive to obtain, and Grant began to think that Bishop should return to England to his friends and fiancée. He considered seeking a full pardon so that he could accompany Bishop, but Lord advised against it. 'You must first get your pardon,' he advised, 'and then you will apply about Bishop. If you blend your concerns with his and trouble them about him, they will throw you up.' Grant saw this was true, and 'retired up the stairs in tears'.

Samuel Marsden, chaplain, grazier and magistrate, must have taken to John Grant. On leave in London in 1809, he arranged a meeting between John's mother and Lachlan Macquarie, before Macquarie left to restore order to the rebellious colony. Macquarie was impressed by her, and arrived in Sydney well-disposed to her son. There he received a testimonial of Grant's good character, signed by John Piper (who had chained and exiled him), Elizabeth Paterson (who said he was mad), his friend James Lewin, Samuel Marsden, and other worthy characters. It was nevertheless six months before Macquarie met Grant, and another six before he awarded him a full pardon.[136] As he prepared to leave New South Wales, Grant wrote a final letter home, and added the postscript 'Christianity extinguishes anger! but the calumny of my insanity still predominates here.'[137]

WELL INTO THE HISTORY OF NEW SOUTH WALES, THERE was still room for profound disagreement on the nature of convict transportation – if not legally, writes Alan Atkinson, then in 'what might be called the moral economy of empire'.[138] A 'special convict', cushioned by the sensibilities of those around him, Grant was able to view his criminal transportation as an 'emigration'. He might have made a new life, but the adversity that clouded his trial in London followed him across the sea, so that he arrived amidst a flurry of political prisoners and violent unrest. In such a charged context, his strident, escalating and eccentric, if substantially accurate, critiques of the penal colony were treated severely, and penal discipline turned his eccentricity into something more pronounced.

But there was also room for compassion in the course of transportation, and even in secondary punishment. In Bligh's final week in the colonies before returning to England to testify against George Johnston, he asked the former governor for a certificate of his sanity, and received this statement:

> This is to certify that Mr John Grant is from all I can learn recovered from some mental derangement, and that during my knowledge of him has conducted himself in a mild and inoffensive manner and bears a moral good character. Given under my hand this 6th May 1810 – Governor Bligh[139]

Grant thought this certificate would 'tend most cruelly to countenance calumny', and returned it to Bligh with some suggested revisions. Bligh obliged him again:

> This is to certify that Mr Jn Grant is from all I can learn recovered from some mental uneasiness (arising from a double cause 1st a disappointment of marriage in London and exile for checking the man occasioning it. 2nd the forcing men to labour in New South Wales without pay for offences committed in England, notwithstanding and besides their banishment!)— and that during my knowledge of him he has conducted himself in a mild and inoffensive manner and bears a moral good character. Given under my hand this day of May 1810.[140]

What would he do with his certificate of sanity? Would he show it to his mother and sister, to prospective employers? Would he mount it and hang it on a wall? Perhaps it was intended as the *pièce de résistance* in the dossier he was preparing for the King on the subject of colonial constitutional abuse. The two certificates together form a remarkable document, which certifies that convict transportation and the penal colony of New South Wales drove men very nearly to madness. It may well be that Bligh, as he sailed home two days later, agreed in full.

When John Grant arrived in London in 1812, he carried a letter from Samuel Marsden to his own family asking them to help him, and a picture of one of Marsden's racehorses. Like those he bore when he first came to New South Wales, with his expansive hopes for the future, it included a character reference.[141] Grant had been 'transported to this country some years ago in consequence of firing at a gentleman,' it read, 'whom he had challenged and who had refused to fight him. The difference originated about a young woman to whom he was attached. His case was always considered a hard one in this colony. His conduct has been very good strictly moral and sober. There is a wildness about him probably occasioned by his troubles.'[142]

2

THE LIABILITIES OF THE SEA

John Grant thought of Charles Bishop, his friend and housemate, as 'a poet in his way – i.e. on sea-subjects'.[1] Bishop, a navigator and merchant, had been formed by the sea, and knew it intimately. Perhaps when his business partner, George Bass, sailed without him for South America, it aggravated his mental symptoms; perhaps when Bass disappeared in the vast Pacific, it felt like a personal betrayal. This is speculation, but sometimes speculation is called for. What form and shape did the ocean give to the town taking root in Eora country at Sydney Cove? What did it give, and what did it withhold? The people of Sydney heard the water at night as they waited for sleep, lapping against the oystered shore, and they heard it when they woke in the morning.

One Saturday in autumn 1794, just as the last of the salt pork was handed out and the doors of the store shut up, a ship was sighted at South Head. A signal was passed from the flagstaff there along the shoreline to the settlement. There was a great deal of interest. A ship was expected from India, and the people of Sydney 'looked daily' for the return of another from Nootka Sound, crosswise over the ocean. And 'we hoped for a ship from

England', wrote David Collins. Captain George Johnston took a boat to meet the ship in the harbour. He saw that it was flying English colours, but 'such a sea ran within the Heads; and the wind blew with so much violence' that it was forced out of the harbour with a split topsail. The hungry colonists had to wait another day before they learned that the first ship came from London with Irish pork and beef, the chaplain Samuel Marsden, and word of Arthur Phillip and the two Aboriginal men who had accompanied him, Bennelong and Yemmerrawanne.[2]

Newly arrived themselves, they continued to look out over the immenseness of the Pacific, for food, for news, for supplies. They took in convicts and soldiers in large numbers from ships that sailed into harbour and, if news travelled ahead, they waited eagerly for judges, colonists, chaplains and secretaries, and welcomed them with martial salutes. But the sea took as well as gave; the wreck of the *Sirius* off Norfolk Island in the midst of the 'hungry years' must have seemed a cruel work of the ocean among a people already feeling wretched in isolation. The sea was the wall of whatever sort of gaol New South Wales was meant to be, but it was a wall that could be scaled by those who knew its ways, like James Martin and Mary Bryant, who snuck out of the Harbour in the colony's fishing boat in 1791, with Mary's two infant children in tow, and made it as far as Kupang, at the edge of the Indonesian archipelago.[3]

Although this was a place where convicts were sent, a penal colony, it was also a fledgling society perched at the edge of the sea. It was intended that convicts not return, as they did from a prison or pillory. They were to build a new life *in situ.* The governor, in turn, was far more than a warden. He was the commander of an outpost which, though it had some of the trappings of a military establishment, contained a far more complex and varied population, and the problems that went with it. Around the convict ships and huts and barracks, there grew a peculiar, fluid society peopled in time by soldiers and officers as well as convicts – and their children. All were borne by ships that sailed through the Heads.

MANY OF THE OFFICERS OF THE NEW SOUTH WALES CORPS became the first voluntary colonists in Australia. Most of their military commissions had been purchased in England as investments in the colonial enterprise at Botany Bay.[4] They looked for profit, and found it in their coercive authority over the small society. After the first governor, Arthur Phillip, quit the colony late in 1792, a succession of interim governors plucked from the upper ranks of the Corps allowed its officers to establish a monopoly over colonial trade, purchasing all goods arriving in harbour wholesale and then selling them at exorbitant retail prices. Assisted by their enterprising paymasters, the officers saw impressive returns.

Robert Campbell (with whom John Grant dearly wanted to partner) broke apart this monopoly at the turn of the century. In 1795 he joined his elder brother in Calcutta, working for a small Indian Agency House, one of a number which were suffered by the East India Company to trade under licence into markets its directors considered too small for profit. The following year, the Campbells' firm sent a cargo of goods, including rice, sugar, salt meat, textiles, tobacco and indigo, together with some livestock and upwards of 105 casks of rum, two casks of brandy, and four 'pipes' of Madeira, to the penal colony of New South Wales. Their ship, the *Sydney Cove,* wrecked in Bass Strait in 1797. Sixteen men set off for its namesake, in a longboat and then on foot after the longboat also wrecked, off Gippsland, Victoria.[5] It was a tenacious outfit. Campbell himself travelled to Sydney in 1798 and bought land at Dawes Point. In 1800 he arrived again, this time to stay, in the *Hunter*, named after John Hunter, who had left behind his shirt sleeves to become governor. It was a winning strategy, and Campbell received permission to live at Dawes Point from Hunter, though never formal permission to trade out of Sydney. Campbell & Co. did so all the same, and flourished. By 1804 it reported goods worth £50 000 in its warehouses and wharves on the Harbour. This private trade broke the monopoly of the Corps, and Campbell developed a reputation for fairness, affordability and generous credit arrangements. He was lauded by all sections of colonial society, especially small settlers, who thanked him in stark terms in 1804: 'But for you, we had still been a prey to the mercenary unsparing hand of avarice and extortion'.[6]

The gradual opening of the colony to trade brought with it new problems and uncertainties. Visitors came selling goods and seeking advantage; officers built up businesses, typically through their wives, who tended to be convicts, or former convicts. This was a society with few precedents, comprised of second sons, felons spared the final penalty of the law, soldiers, and officers with their masculinist notions of good conduct. It was no military outpost, though it had the formal structures of one, but neither was it a small colonial outpost as in North America, allowed to grow organically. 'Botany Bay' was a site of mass immigration, but immigration of a certain kind, and its population skewed heavily male as well as criminal. Here were few of the conventional social structures: immediate and extended family, church, and charitable institutions were often pale shades of what they had been at home. Even that idea of home took on new qualities.[7] Within this novel, unsettled society there quickly developed a fundamental challenge to what the colony was, and what it was for, which ended in a coup, and the deposal of the governor in

January 1808. The 'rum rebellion', as it has been styled, is often viewed as a clash of incandescent personalities, which it certainly was, but it was more than egotism. It was the culmination of the clashing visions of the colony: an open gaol, receiving and disciplining the convicts of Britain; or a society where those who were born free, arrived free, and became free expected to enjoy liberty and property without despotic interference. Wealthy officers and settlers talked of tyranny and liberty as they arrested Bligh, formed a rebel government, and resumed their plunder, allotting land and privileges to each other.

We will circle back to the rebellion in Chapter 7, but it forms the backdrop here, as the governor and courts grappled with madness in order to bring it into the forming law of the land. The law of lunacy deals in the very rights at stake in the rebellion. What are the limits of individual agency? When could liberty and proper authority rightfully be revoked? What were the consequences, individual and communal, when someone was found incapable of governing himself or herself, and what if that person were an outsider? These questions coursed through the years of rebellion precisely because they were at the heart of what the Europeans were doing in Australia, as the representatives of the empire sought to establish sovereign order amidst settlers pursuing their own diverse projects. This chapter shows how they dealt with three mad men of the sea, and how they worked to set the colony on a surer legal and political footing.

WHEN CHARLES BISHOP DEVELOPED FULL-BLOWN MANIA in Sydney, John Grant found it difficult to care for him at Prospect Hill, and Bishop's old comrade, Governor King, decided that he needed to be removed to an institution. By the late 18th century, the lunatic asylum was part of the institutional landscape of European society, but colonies developed irregularly, in fits and starts, and European New South Wales was still in its infancy. When Bishop was removed, therefore, it was not to an asylum but to a section of Parramatta Gaol. In a prison which had no walls, where convicts were spread out through the plains and bushland, a free ill man was placed in one of the few secure buildings in the colony.

Although Bishop was 'admitted' in December 1804, it was fully ten months before twelve jurors were summoned 'to make enquiry upon view of examination of Charles Bishop and to say on their oaths whether the said Bishop is a lunatick'.[8] The procedure which finally took place was a crude rendering of the commission of lunacy practised in England and Scotland since the 12th century – a court procedure used by the monarch to implement the royal prerogative in the care of insane subjects. By the 19th century, the procedure was fairly standard. A petitioner, usually a family member, presenting affidavits and some semblance of medical advice, requested that the Lord Chancellor have a person examined for lunacy or idiocy. In the resulting inquisition, lawyers acted as commissioners, presenting evidence to a jury. Typically, witnesses who knew the subjects well were called and gave detailed testimony about their lives. Opposing lawyers might present the opposite case – for sanity – or the subject could defend themselves. A core component of the trial was the examination of the alleged lunatic. The jury finally decided upon his or her sanity, specifying if and when the subject had become *non compos mentis*, in which case they and their property were entrusted to a committee, normally some friend or relation who was willing to take on the burden. While one contemporary treatise argued that it was egregious to have a lunatic's heir at law serving as his or her committee ('because it is in his interest', a contemporary treatise put it bluntly, 'that the lunatic should die'), an heir was also the most interested in the success of the estate. A next of kin but not heir was ideally placed to manage the estate, but the confusion resulted in poor practice in the early 19th century.[9] Commissions were rarely held on married women because their estates were already controlled by their husbands. This would later place psychiatrists in the awkward position of speaking medically to the concerns of both patient and family – concerns which could be at odds.[10] The common law on the qualifications and powers of such committees was complex, but they were placed in control of the estate and could on the authority of the commission annul sales and contracts made while the subject was *non compos mentis.*[11] The Scottish commission of lunacy was similar, though with a slightly different lineage and vocabulary.[12]

The jury found Bishop 'incapable of governing himself, his chattels, lands, and tenements', and he and his estate were entrusted to a committee, in the form of the commission. The principal chaplain, Samuel Marsden, and the ex-officer and grazier John Macarthur were appointed as trustees, instructed to draw on Bishop's estate for his 'maintenance and support' and to preserve the estate. They were to pay Bishop's debts, receive what was owing to him, and keep careful accounts. Some historians have seen the empanelling of a jury, particularly, as a move towards civil liberty in a convict colony, but this seems optimistic. There were ten months of illegal confinement prior to it and the main interest seems to have been financial; little changed for Bishop himself.[13] The legal process likely helped with the question of John Grant's tenancy of the property at Prospect Hill, and the lingering problem of the uncertain fate of the *Venus.* The formal commission was pointedly public, since the person declared a lunatic became incapable of commercial contracts and transactions and this was important information. The *Sydney*

Gazette reported the result, and directly below the announcement was a notice from Marsden and Macarthur, requesting all who had furnished Bishop with 'necessaries for his immediate maintenance since his first committal as a lunatick' (in December) to present their bills. It may even have been these bills that precipitated the trial.[14]

Bishop's committee comprised prominent colonists because he had no family in Sydney, but there were persons interested in his estate. Although Bass was missing, Thomas Jamison was present. As well as agent to the partnership between Bass and Bishop, Jamison was principal surgeon, magistrate, and 'deeply embroiled in trade'.[15] He assumed sole responsibility for Bishop's person and property. Jamison was the officer who had complained about Henry Browne Hayes's privileges on the voyage to Sydney.[16] The following August, he printed an advertisement requesting 'any person having apartments in which Mr. Charles Bishop may be accommodated with lodging and board' to contact him.[17] Nothing came of it; Hayes did not want Bishop at Vaucluse, and in January 1809 Bishop was still in Parramatta Gaol. Jamison decided it would be impossible to find anything for Bishop, and his estate was in any case dwindling. 'Everybody is reluctant for poor Bishop to remain among them in this country,' wrote Grant.[18] The presumed loss of the *Venus* meant that Bishop became a liability for the government. Several months later the Royal Navy wrote to Sydney seeking to recover £84 12s 'from a Mr. Charles Bishop'. The acting governor replied: 'I regret to inform you that this unfortunate man is now insane, a pauper and confined in the gaol without, I learn, any funds to support him but the prison allowance.'[19] Jamison sailed home the next month, and it is unclear who, if anyone, sanctioned Bishop's repatriation four months later, or wound his estate up. The lack of ceremony and precision of the case lingers in the image of the governor visiting his 'particular friend' Bishop in a gaol got up as a lunatic asylum. 'I must do Governor King the justice to say,' Grant wrote, 'he behaves very tenderly towards him.'[20]

WHILE CHARLES BISHOP RAVED, THE COLONY WAS ENgulfed in a rebellion which thrashed out the key issues raised by his case: private property and personal liberty. Officers and colonists felt that William Bligh had undermined the sanctity of private property, and that his bad language and despotic mannerisms were indicators of a deeper despotism incompatible with the English constitution. Having gathered significant capital, the Corps officers had become deeply embedded in colonial commerce. Despite the common usage, historians rarely refer to the conflict as the 'rum rebellion' because rum, for all its symbolic power, was no longer central to the colonial economy when the crisis broke. Rum was not the impetus for the deposal. The rebels' resistance was not primarily to Bligh-as-tyrant but to the threat he posed to their profits with his strict militarist interpretation of his authority and the nature of the colony.[21] Alan Atkinson dubs the coup the colony's 'little revolution', since, to strengthen their case and widen their base the rebels clothed their economic interests in the language of property rights and common law, adding some more explosive natural law arguments for representative government drawn from John Locke and Thomas Paine.[22]

London took a rather more conservative view of the events in Sydney. The rebellion was repudiated, George Johnston was recalled to face court-martial, and John Macarthur spent eight years in exile after returning to England to bear witness, afraid that he would be arrested if he returned to his family and farms in the colony. A new regiment was commissioned to replace the New South Wales Corps and Lachlan Macquarie was appointed to address the constitutional, legal and political disorder which had precipitated rebellion and was then exacerbated by the rebel government. He was not simply to restore order, but to build a moral infrastructure which, reading the Colonial Office correspondence closely, was seen to have been lacking from the start. 'The great objects of attention,' Secretary of State Viscount Castlereagh advised Macquarie, were 'to improve the morals of the colonists, to encourage marriage, to provide for education, to prohibit the use of spirituous liquors.'[23] He would be aided, at least initially, by Ellis Bent, the new judge advocate with whom he had travelled to Sydney. Bent was 'a barrister of some eminence', according to the Colonial Office; certainly he was more experienced than his predecessors, having trained in Cambridge and practised on the Northern Circuit in England.[24]

When he arrived in Sydney in December 1809, Macquarie restored Bligh to power for twenty-four hours so that government could pass in an orderly pageant from one to the other. When the new year broke, Macquarie, guided by Bent, set about redressing the legal and financial wrongs of the preceding years.[25] All land grants made out by the rebel administration (and they had been made with abandon) were cancelled. All legal decisions were nullified. 'All trials and investigations' after the arrest of Bligh, Macquarie was explicit, had been heard 'before an incompetent jurisdiction' and were 'of none effect whatsoever in law or equity'.[26] But it was not only the rebels who had worked in the legal borderlands. It seems that Bent first addressed the precarious state of the governor's legislative powers, a problem pointed out in an 1803 pamphlet by the jurist Jeremy Bentham, though he suppressed it himself in fear of its volatile implications.[27] By the 1810s, this constitutional critique was gaining credence, and judicial officers were growing more cautious.[28] Macquarie was the first governor to submit proposed regulations to his judge advocate, and he issued 'proclamations' instead of the dubious executive orders of his predecessors.[29] Vigorous changes were also made to the Colonial Medical Service, which, like the rest of the colony, was in a state of disorganisation and disquiet.

Governor King had treated the disposal of the person and property of the mad – that is, personal liberty and personal property – rather offhandedly in Bishop's case. By 1810, such a casual approach had become untenable. The security of person and especially property had been foremost amongst the tensions that precipitated the rebellion. The partnership between Macquarie and Bent would eventually result in legal precision in cases of lunacy, but the first case of lunacy under Macquarie showed that this would not be a simple transition.

IN MAY 1810, THE WHALER *FREDERICK* LEFT ENGLAND WITH 'a handsome investment' belonging to the London merchant William Wilson. On 25 July the *Frederick* sailed out of Rio de Janeiro after a brief stop, as the *Hindostan*, *Porpoise* and *Dromedary* were entering the harbour with William Bligh and his supporters, en route to England and vindication. When the *Frederick* arrived in Sydney in late October, its captain, Alexander Bodie, was ill. Wilson's agent in Sydney, Richard Jenkins, wrote to the governor requesting a medical examination.[30] Bodie was 'in a state of mental derangement', wrote Jenkins, 'which disqualified him for the duties of a master of a ship and required personal care and attention to be paid to him to restore him to the use of his mental faculties'. Macquarie, however, was making his first tour of the outlying districts of the colony. The responsibility therefore fell upon the next ranking officer, Maurice O'Connell, commander of the 73rd Regiment replacing the disgraced Corps.[31] O'Connell promptly issued a Garrison and General Order instructing a medical board to meet the following day at Jenkins's house in Pitt Street, where Bodie was living. The goal of the examination was put simply, perhaps with military bluntness rather than civil delicacy: to ascertain 'whether it would be advisable to permit Mr Bodie to proceed to sea in his present state'. At stake were the *Frederick*, its crew, and its cargo.[32]

The board was led by D'Arcy Wentworth, who became principal surgeon when Thomas Jamison returned to London to testify against the deposed governor. He was joined by the regimental surgeons of the 73rd, since the rest of the colonial medical staff were absent. They found the captain 'labouring under serious mental derangement, which renders him totally incapable of performing the duties of his station'. The governor and his wife paused their tour in Parramatta, 'both a little indisposed after our late fatigues', to rest their servants and horses. While there, Macquarie learned of the examination and the doctors' conclusion, and scrambled to ensure the rule of law over the lunacy which the sea brought into Sydney. 'I deem it highly necessary and expedient,' he declared, 'under this representation of the unhappy circumstances of Mr. Alexander Bodie's indisposition to appoint a committee or trustees to take charge of the person and property of the said Alexander Bodie for and during the continuance of his said mental indisposition.'[33] Here, too, the language implied a temporary condition.

A still more formal declaration followed. Macquarie invoked the 'powers and authorities vested in me by His Majesty as Governor and Commander in Chief of this territory and as His Majesty's representative herein'. Until 1825, the governors of New South Wales, like other remote governors, were empowered by royal commissions which included provisions to deal with the person and property of 'ideots and lunaticks' locally, for reasons of expediency.[34] Macquarie appointed a committee to do what might be 'most conducive to the restoration of the said Alexander Bodie to the right exercise of his mental faculties and to the protecting all and singular the property belonging to the said Alexander Bodie for his own use and benefit and for the interest of all persons concerned therein'. There were persons very much interested in the property belonging to Bodie, and two of them were appointed as 'curators and committee' with Samuel Marsden: William Bodie, his brother and the third mate of the *Frederick*, and Robert Jenkins, the local agent responsible for that 'handsome investment'.

The *Frederick* sailed south to catch the whaling season, which ran from December to April in the coastal waters off Tasmania.[35] In Sydney, Bodie quickly recovered, and after four months at Parramatta Gaol wrote to Macquarie requesting his discharge. After three further letters, Macquarie replied, requesting Bodie be home the following day at noon for a medical examination. If he passed he would be freed from restraint and reunited with 'all your books, papers and property'.[36] The governor instructed D'Arcy Wentworth and William Redfern to examine Bodie and recommend whether he was 'perfectly competent to the management of his own affairs, and whether it would be expedient to release him from all those restraints which his mental derangement have rendered necessary for some time past'.[37] The doctors found Bodie sane, and Jenkins and Marsden were instructed to return to him all 'property of whatever nature belonging to him which may have fallen into your hands', together with 'a regular statement of the receipts and expenditures which have taken place on his account'. The account was to be settled in eleven days, and a copy of the statement, with signatures from the trustees and Bodie, forwarded to Macquarie.[38] (There was no mention of William Bodie.)

By the time Alexander Bodie recovered his senses in Sydney,

however, his investor in London, William Wilson, was bankrupt, on account of a protracted legal tussle with Robert Campbell, whose business had foundered when he was compelled to return home to testify for Bligh.[39] Bodie requested relief from the government, and was permitted, in September 1811, to land and sell 300 gallons of 'Rio spirits' to finance repairs to his ship. It was a concession, offered on account of 'the weighty expences you have been at with your ship *Frederick* since your arrival here, the disappointment you have sustained by her late unsuccessful voyage, and the embarrassment you must be under with respect to drawing bills on England' following Wilson's bankruptcy.[40]

It appears that William Bodie and Richard Jenkins had some knowledge of a pre-existing condition. Their approach to the government, the conclusion of the surgeons, and Macquarie's formal declaration all anticipated recovery. This was by no means standard. Perhaps Alexander, who worked and lived with Bodie in the belly of the sea, knew his brother's irregularities and allowed them until they crossed some threshold of incoherence or aggression. A manic captain was a fearsome thing at sea. Certainly Bodie's behaviour after leaving Sydney, convalescent, was erratic and cruel. The *Frederick* sailed in October 1811 with letters of marque, permitting it to engage French ships if it came across them.[41] With them travelled several Māori who had been living with Samuel Marsden and been taught his faith. Reaching the coast of New Zealand, Bodie agreed to take the Māori home after a season whaling, but after six months the *Frederick* sailed straight to Norfolk Island, where the Māori were left, some 1500 kilometres from their homes, in a settlement which would soon be abandoned. Bodie retained the services of single young Māori man, who is recorded weeping for his countrymen. On the return voyage, in Sri Lanka, Bodie landed eleven sailors to be tried for sedition, and precipitating a fresh mutiny. His was a ship of disorder, and it seems likely enough that before and after his committal as a lunatic in Sydney, his mind was precarious. He was killed when the *Frederick* was captured by a French privateer the following year.[42]

ESTABLISHING LEGAL AND SOCIAL ORDER IN THE PENAL colony of New South Wales – a remote outpost drawn into the mercantile and exploratory networks of the Pacific – was a challenge. The rebellion made this challenge urgent. Madness, presenting in the men of the sea who sailed in and out of the Heads and also circled around the more remote parts of the colony, was a dramatic test of the integrity of this order. It invoked the very concerns that fuelled the rebellion: what protections to person and property were applicable in a penal colony – or rather, which rights should be dispensed with? Madness brought into relief the fragile balance between a strong, military-style government, the discipline of convicts, and the private projects which took root nearby.

In January 1812, the brig *Active* anchored at Port Dalrymple, at the mouth of the Tamar River on the north coast of Van Diemen's Land, the southernmost outpost of the colony, which separated in 1825 and was renamed Tasmania in 1856. Jonathan Burke McHugo went ashore and began to sell his cargo of Calcutta goods with reckless abandon. The commandant, George Alexander Gordon, took 'three cases of wine', Captain Kenny 'a considerable quantity of goods', and three others bought further goods worth £667.[43] McHugo made it known that he was a military general travelling incognito, and a royal to boot, tasked by the home government with surveying the colonies. Major Gordon relieved his command to the visitor and, according to oral sources drawn on by the historian James Calder in the 1920s, anarchy very nearly engulfed the town – Gordon and several settlers were nearly hanged.[44] Junior officers broke the chain of command and sent Burke McHugo to Sydney under guard, bound in his cot to prevent injury to others.[45] When the *Active* arrived in Sydney, the naval officer boarded the ship to find Burke McHugo deranged, a patient–prisoner on his own ship. The governor 'deems it expedient', wrote colonial secretary J. T. Campbell, 'that a medical consultation or survey should be held on this unfortunate gentleman'. The doctors were to proceed aboard the following day and 'take the usual professional means of reporting on Mr. McHugo's case' and recommend what was 'best calculated for his recovery'.[46]

Jonathan Burke McHugo represented a clear financial liability for his own investors. He represented also a significant liability for whoever took responsibility for him, since he, like Bodie, was liable to regain his senses and demand an account, and after a firesale like the one in Port Dalrymple the accounting would have been complex. But, just two years after Macquarie arrived to restore order and with the coup still raw in colonial memories, this arrival in the south presented a more serious threat because, in his madness, Burke McHugo had managed to wreak havoc on the imperial infrastructure at its vulnerable periphery.

Macquarie's account of the affair to London suggests a chaos he could scarcely credit. The commandant had 'suffered himself to be so far imposed on by the wild and extravagant nonsense of Mr. McHugo as to imagine him to be one of the royal family incog.,' – the words as if he could barely set them down – 'and possessed of authority at pleasure to supersede all governors commanders, etca., etca., wherever he pleased to visit'.[47] Gordon had 'actually surrendered his command to Mr. McHugo, who was likely to have made a very alarming use of the power so yielded to him', if it had not been for the junior officers.

Macquarie's instructions for an examination of Burke McHugo are striking for their composure.

Although no-one was indelicate enough to mention it, it seems likely that Gordon himself was mad. Calder, who confesses to embellishing certain details, put it down to sunstroke.[48] It could have been anything. After Port Dalrymple, Gordon had further trouble. In September 1812, after being relieved of his command in Van Diemen's Land, he was posted to Sri Lanka. He was forced to resign four years later, however, after he was discovered drunk on duty.[49] The 73rd Regiment had served in India and fought in a series of critical battles before being appointed to New South Wales. There is a wide range of possible sources of delusion or psychosis in such colonial and military settings.[50] Gordon was rather gentler on himself five years later, when he defended his actions from Old Slaughter's Coffee House in St Martin's Lane, London (the haunt of William Hogarth, Henry Fielding, and Samuel Johnson). Gordon had simply received Burke McHugo 'with the usual attention due to a stranger and a gentleman, his manners being prepossessing and appearing to be well-informed and intelligent'.[51] Prepossessing indeed.

The governor's commission rendered 'ideots and lunaticks' a legal liability, to be cared for in the colony in which their symptoms manifested. Madness created other liabilities, too: Charles Bishop had become, eventually, a financial liability, after his wealth vanished in the Pacific – a pauper drawing from the gaol fund for his board and treatment. Alexander Bodie had represented a private liability to his investors, but also demonstrated the liability of recovery to government. The prospect of his recovery had been flagged from the outset, which might have encouraged Macquarie to take care with his effects. The proximity of agents who represented the investors and partnerships which stood to lose most from this madness reminded governments to pay due attention to 'interested parties' in their ventures and estates. These layered liabilities rose incrementally to the fore as the governors of New South Wales dealt with the string of madmen sailing into the Harbour.

Efficiency was one feature of a government so centralised. Burke McHugo sailed into Sydney Harbour, bound to his cot, on Wednesday 29 January. On Thursday 30 January, Macquarie called for a medical board to test his sanity, and on Saturday 1 February, Wentworth and Redfern found that Burke McHugo clearly laboured 'under a severe mental derangement rendering him totally incapable of attending to any business'. They recommended 'his being brought on shore in order that such measures may be adopted as may be deemed conducive to his recovery'.[52] Burke McHugo was to be received from the sea, formally to invalidate him from further ruining his business venture.

The governor, however, had no immediate authority to bring Burke McHugo ashore. The colonial secretary's instructions gesture to the legal procedures, which would take some time to arrange. In the interim, a 'professional' medical report would provide legitimacy for treatment. Macquarie wrote to judge advocate Ellis Bent for advice on how to proceed. This time, everything would be strictly legal. On Sunday 2 February, Bent replied, 'I have inclosed to you the form of the commission necessary to be issued in the case of the poor lunatic on board the *Active*.' He would have petitions and affidavits ready for the committee members to sign the following day, which would then need to be lodged in the secretary's office, and 'the commission above mentioned will be declared to them & by them to me: I will then immediately take the necessary steps for summoning a respectable jury to assemble at the court on Tuesday morning & conclude the business'. Aware that they were breaking new judicial ground, Bent described the process meticulously, but colonial government was intimate, and his precision mingled with humbler concerns. 'I am very lame this morning,' he wrote, 'and my foot is so painful that I fear I have gout.'[53]

The following day, Bent interviewed members of Burke McHugo's crew and prepared the commission of lunacy. English commissions typically proceeded on petition by a family member, but could also follow from information offered by some member of the public. Bent wrote to Macquarie that he had thought best to proceed by information, since Burke McHugo was alone in the colony.[54] The master of the *Active* provided the information: Burke McHugo was deprived of his reason and unable to manage himself or his affairs.[55] He and the first mate stated under oath that they had been 'well acquainted' with the subject for five months and had been confident to sail with him from Calcutta, but that from the second week of January, their frequent observations of his 'behaviour, words and actions' led them to conclude he was 'a person deprived of his reason and understanding in a very great degree'. The master said that Burke McHugo 'acted with great violence, and talks incessantly of being put upon his lid [sic] and wanting papers for his defence'. He was 'in no way capable of governing himself or his estate'.[56] 'I have every thing now ready,' wrote Bent, 'and wait only until the commission, which must be under the territorial seal, is delivered to me. The jury will be assembled tomorrow at ten o'clock here, and the whole proceedings will occupy but a very short time.' The aim, at least in Bent's view, was not to test Burke McHugo but to demonstrate and declare his madness publicly.

With documents prepared by Bent, Macquarie formally commissioned the judge and two colonists, Alexander Riley and Gregory Blaxland, to enquire 'whether Jonathan Burke McHugo late of Calcutta merchant owner and supra cargo [sic] on board a certain Brig called the *Active* of Calcutta, aforesaid now at anchor at Sydney Cove in this territory, is a lunatic, or enjoys lucid intervals so that he is not sufficient for the government of himself, his tenements goods and chattels'. If indeed he was a lunatic, they were to ascertain 'from what time, after what manner and how', and whether he had disposed of anything while in that condition, 'and if so … to what person or persons, where, when after what manner and how'.[57] The interest was overwhelmingly in property – even the symptoms of illness were tied to goods and chattels. Illness was phrased in the language of self-government and the government of estates; once established, the questions focused on the specific liability to the estate.

The jurors, a combination of merchants and esquires not otherwise specified, met at the courthouse on Tuesday 4 January at 10 o'clock. Aside from misspelling their subject's name, the document was precise and comprehensive. Burke McHugo was 'of an unsound mind and doth not enjoy lucid intervals so that he is not capable of the government of himself' or his effects, and had not been for at least three weeks, though 'how or by what means the said Johnathan Burke McHugo so became lunatic the jurors aforesaid know not, unless by the visitation of God'. Burke McHugo had no relations in the colony, they found, and no lands, but held 'a certain interest in a certain brig called the *Active*' and in its goods, wares, tackle, apparel, furniture, sails, boats, guns, and ammunition.[58]

On Wednesday 5 February, the colonial secretary issued a Government Public Notice reporting the inquisition, naming the judges and the authority under which they conducted the commission – the Great Seal of the Territory – and the presence of the jurors. 'The said Jonathan Burke McHugo is of an unsound mind,' he wrote, correcting the spelling, 'and not capable of the government of himself, his tenements, goods, and chattels'; a 'special grant' was announced to appoint Campbell, the merchant Richard Jones, who was connected with Calcutta through the Riley brothers, and Captain Thomas Cripps of the *Ruby*, currently anchored in Sydney Cove, to 'the care and custody of the person of the said lunatic', and the management of his estate. Anyone connected with the estate was to declare it.[59]

It was a procedural triumph. 'My dear Sir,' wrote Bent to Macquarie as the documents dried, 'I have much pleasure in returning to you in the form usually practised in England, the Commission of Lunacy lately issued by you', with the custody documents for Burke McHugo's person and estate. The original inquisition with the actual signatures and seal, Bent noted, had to be filed in his office, but the members of the committee ought to have a copy of the commission and inquisition from Macquarie's secretary. 'In England', Bent pointed out, committee members 'generally find security for the due execution of their duty but this is a matter of discretion with yourself'. The business of lunacy was couched within the other functions of colonial governance. 'Mr Woodhouse informs me he has taken up the precept for the appointment of Major Geils,' Bent went on, and added on the reverse, 'Riley has left me only this scrap of paper to write upon which I trust you will have the goodness to excuse. E. B.'[60]

MACQUARIE AND BENT WERE RIGHT TO BE CAUTIOUS. FIVE years later, in March 1817, Jonathan Burke McHugo entered the Police Court in Bow Street, London, and made a deposition. He spoke of a merchant venture gone awry; a Calcutta brig which he owned, heavy laden with goods, taken from him in New South Wales. He sought £8350 in losses from the Colonial Office, including '*four thousand pounds* at the least' after his investors were paid out.[61] He pointed out his '*undoubted* and *yet undecided* constitutional rights', as heir to the throne, and complained of the 'infernal doses administered to me at South Wales' and the appalling food at the asylum at Calcutta.[62] Given his eccentricities, it is remarkable that he obtained an audience with the secretary of state for the colonies, Earl Bathurst, and still more that the secretary took him seriously.

Earl Bathurst's response gives a glimpse of the substantial liability which colonial governors themselves posed for metropolitan governments. While 'subject to occasional fits of derangement', Burke McHugo did appear to have been in New South Wales as he said, Bathurst wrote to Macquarie, with a vessel and cargo, and was now in England without a penny. 'I am sure you will not consider his infirmity as entitling him, if his claim is well founded,' he added drily, 'to less consideration than he would otherwise have received.' Macquarie was to report 'fully both as to the causes which led to the seizure of the *Active*, the legal proceedings under which the vessel was condemned, and as to the manner in which the produce of the vessel and cargo was disposed of'.[63] Burke McHugo wanted his property, and Bathurst wanted order. Macquarie, having learned from the cases of the others who had sailed mad into Sydney Harbour, and wary of the extreme delicacy of questions of liberty and property in the post-rebellion colony, had taken every precaution – the medical board, the committee of trustees, the accounts.[64] The curators had remitted £7015 17s 2d and Burke McHugo himself to Alexander & Co. in Calcutta. Receipts were attached.[65] The procedural enthusiasm of Macquarie and Bent in dealing with lunacy – part of their wider efforts to establish order – protected the colonial government from Burke McHugo's recriminations, and the imperial government from colonial scandal.

GEORGE MAXWELL HAD WASHED, ALMOST, IN FROM THE sea, having been struck down by it off the Cape of Good Hope. He was found rowing back and forth across the Harbour, as if he were trying to return to it. Charles Bishop, Alexander Bodie and Jonathan Burke McHugo were all men of the sea, too, so that the geography of the oceans and the vagaries of maritime trade become part of the story of their madness. The sea made them, and broke them with its wind and waves and in cabins crowded with club law and the threat of commercial failure. The sea also shaped the response to the madness of these men. The efforts of first mates, constables, lieutenants and lawyers to declare and contain their madness remind us that the people they administered were all dependent upon the sea. They looked out over it in hope and dread. And through the Vice Admiralty Court, the governors of New South Wales were entrusted not only with the people of Sydney and the lands which ran off their faltering maps but with imposing order over the sea.[66]

Lunacy helps to reveal the anxieties of such a place, which gathered around criminality, as the first chapter suggested and the next will explore further, but also around mobility and fixedness. The commission of lunacy, used in England chiefly to mediate disputes in inheritance law, was introduced here to limit the liability presented by the madness of captains and merchants – a mobile, fleeting and, in certain senses, dangerous class. Settler colonial society was defined by the curation of mobility, as the historian Catharine Coleborne argues in her study of social institutions in Australia and New Zealand. These institutions represented the heaviest application of the power to contain and categorise undesirable elements – 'fugitives, restless wanderers, men without women, remittance men, alcoholics, the desperately lonely and dislocated'. These were men deemed to have failed, financially or morally, and to have rejected the colonial 'imperative to settle'.[67]

Coleborne draws on the work of historian of science and medicine Warwick Anderson to suggest that we learn much about 'the operations of colonialism through its perceived weakness'.[68]

In 1812, New South Wales was far from a settler colony. Much of its population consisted of forced emigrants and temporary sojourners. The 'imperative to settle' was present, but came from above, with a heavy hand, rather than from within a colonial society seeking stability, and projecting its anxieties onto 'homeless wanderers'. Here the relationship between settlement and mobility was more fluid. Emancipated convicts, free settlers and military officers were all residents of uncertain fixity, as were their children. This meant that mobility did not threaten settler identity so much as colonial governance. Escapees and deserters were a regular vexation, joining with sealing and whaling crews that plied the southern seas and making their way to New Zealand or the Americas. The British were wary of foreign vessels and unsanctioned traders partly because of their brazen complicity in such schemes.

In September 1812, Thomas Cripps, captain of the *Ruby* and one of the trustees in Burke McHugo's property, 'in a most daring and piratical manner effected his escape' from the colony aboard the *Cyclops*, bound for Calcutta. He was 'in direct violation of the port regulations' and he left several investors in the lurch. The colonial secretary called for the 'utmost vigilance' to prevent such occurrences; the naval officer would now board each departing ship and remain until the Heads were cleared.[69] The ocean, on the other side, was more an open corridor than a barrier.[70]

Madness threatened profits from trade ventures, and when governors took custody of the insane as their commissions directed, they accepted the cost of food, board and medical treatment, which could blow out.[71] The real liability, however, was to the rule of law and to imperial authority, which Macquarie was tasked with establishing. The law, and its relation to settlers, soldiers, convicts and merchants, was the 'perceived weakness' in post-rebellion New South Wales. It is this anxiety which breaks through in Macquarie's account of the events in Port Dalrymple. But it posed a far more serious threat to colonial order. The commandant of Port Dalrymple had 'actually surrendered his command' to a madman who claimed to be vested with all authority of parliament and the crown. A medical board was assembled, a commission of lunacy executed, and the subject was placed in the hands of a committee, all within a week of his sailing through the Heads.

Drawing a comparison might help us to see this narrative in a different light. Kirsten McKenzie's *Imperial Underworld* focuses not on the networks which stretched around the world, mostly through the careering of elites and professionals, but on a single agent who slipped quietly across the oceans, very nearly besting the imperial bureaucracy.[72] In an inversion of the standard approach of the new imperial history, McKenzie peels away the intrigue around the subversive 'imperial career' of Alexander Loe Kaye, or William Edwards, a lawyer, escapee and volatile libertarian. He and others like him were 'astute enough to link their personal ambitions and vendettas to highly charged contemporary debates about imperial liberty and despotism'.[73] The mad men of the sea in this chapter showed no such ambition or astuteness, but, as McKenzie demonstrates, this approach can show not only the way marginal figures drove the business of empire, but the way they reveal colonial developments in new ways.[74]

Following this line, early efforts to deploy law to deal with colonial madness show the resonance of Sydney's local disorder, expressed most vividly in the 1808–09 rebellion. Legal historians

Lauren Benton and Lisa Ford argue that the rebellion brought 'despotism talk' into the imperial spotlight, where it would remain, as the 'rage for order' cut across the empire through the 19th century, delivering, after a complex labour, the system of international law.[75] William Bligh's despotism was supposed to reside in his disregard for private property and independent justice, in his indifference to the rule of law in the colony. Benton and Ford argue that the treatment of the rebels in the wake of the rebellion was lenient not because the charges were trivial, but because their rebellion tapped into fundamental constitutional issues. The empire was being remodelled, including a significant expansion of crown power, and this made the despotism of vice-regal officials, like colonial governors, increasingly sensitive. The commission of lunacy was introduced into New South Wales in the immediate aftermath of this clash over the administration of law in the colonies, and dealt specifically with those touchstones of the rebellion – liberty and property. These imperial concerns loomed in the background of the local, even idiosyncratic, developments around Charles Bishop, Alexander Bodie and Jonathan Burke McHugo. The commission of lunacy here was burdened with local disorder; it was a portent of the coming 'rage for order'.

3

MADNESS AND MALINGERING

Daniel Gordon, also known as Janel or Jack, a middle-aged West Indian man, was liberated from slavery in Charleston, South Carolina in 1779. Six years later he was found guilty of stealing clothes to the value of 7 shillings in Winchester, Hampshire, and carried away from England in the first fleet of convicts bound for Botany Bay.[1] Barely a month after he arrived, Gordon was sentenced to death for stealing eighteen bottles of wine with John Williams, 'Black Jack'.[2] Williams was pardoned because he was 'an ignorant black youth'. Gordon, however, was taken to the gallows and read the last rites by the harried chaplain Richard Johnson before, at the last minute, being reprieved.[3] He and two others were sentenced to exile on South East Cape, in Van Diemen's Land: the southern island of the southern land, at the very limits of European imagination. It was a fantastical sentence which the government lacked the means or will to execute. Instead, the government instead installed Gordon and his companions on Pinchgut Island in Sydney Harbour, now Fort Denison.[4] This 'little sterile island, or rather rock', wrote First Fleet surgeon John White, was to serve 'until a place of banishment could be found'.[5] Reserved for 'particularly refractory convicts', it was the first in a long line of prisons, islands and remote penal settlements which the British used to create terror and order among the convicts of Botany Bay.[6]

Governor Phillip celebrated the King's Birthday, 4 June 1788, with an extraordinary act of liberality. He pardoned all crimes committed in the colony, including those of 'the four unhappy wretches labouring under sentence of banishment' on Pinchgut, as the perceptive and eloquent lieutenant Watkin Tench noted. Gordon and the others were 'freed from their fetters, to rejoin their former society'. The sovereign munificence washed over the colony, erasing their sins from afar. The celebration had a special significance for the young settlement struggling to establish itself. 'Hours of festivity, which under happier skies pass away unregarded, and are soon consigned to oblivion' were here more prized, and, no doubt, with crops failing and the rule of law precarious, held onto longer.[7] Later that month, Gordon was reported as 'penitent', and even prevented the rape of a convict woman in September.[8]

A year later, however, Gordon stole some shoes, shirts, pork, worsted caps and nine pints of pease from a group of convict huts at Major Ross's farm, on present-day Milson's Point. But when he stood before the court to plead, he appeared to be delirious. Surgeon John White examined him and thought his pulse, warm temperature and cold sweat indicated delirium, or possibly intoxication. The court adjourned, but the next morning White found the same 'appearance and delirium and wildness'; Gordon's pulse was irregular and his tongue was unusually white, contracting in a manner White could not remember reading about. He concluded that Gordon had 'more the appearance of idiotism than madness'. Then a sergeant called Clinch, who had guarded Gordon before the trial, testified that he thought him perfectly sane. It was only after Gordon was called up to plead, according to acting provost-marshal Henry Brewer, that he began to mutter incoherently, and appeared not to understand instructions. When the court adjourned, Gordon was watched closely and acted uniformly like 'a person delirious'. Despite these doubts as to the genuineness of the affliction, the court found that Gordon was 'not in a state of mind to be put on his trial' and he was put in the little hospital in the Rocks.[9] 'It was generally supposed,' Collins wrote in his journal, that the prospect of punishment 'occasioned the derangement of intellect'. Collins learned that many of the prisoners gave Gordon 'credit for the ability with which he had acted his part, and perhaps he deserved their applause', but the court's 'humanity would not suffer them to proceed against a wretch who either had not, or affected not to have, a sufficient sense of his situation'.[10]

In a case of apparent feigning it was initially deemed better to err on the side of mercy, even in Botany Bay. Although Arthur Phillip thought highly of David Collins, and his successor, John Hunter, called him 'a most valuable and excellent officer', he had no training in law.[11] This is part of a broader pattern. Although convicts enjoyed the status of free persons in court – suing, being sued, and giving evidence – the configuration of the courts acknowledged the distinctive nature of the colonial setting.[12] Officers sat in judgement with the judge advocate, as in a military outpost, since trial by jury would entail convicts deciding the fate of other convicts. But these officers, typically untrained, were also called upon to innovate as they applied English law to 'the circumstances and situation of the settlement' (Tench quoted from the constitution of the criminal court).[13] In law as in other fields, the military and civil officers of the colony frequently worked from first principles. This mixture of inexperience and consciousness of the novelties of the colonial situation meant that something like madness was dealt with differently than it was in established societies – and not necessarily more sternly.

In Sydney, therefore, in 1789, Daniel Gordon was not subject to formal sentencing, but simply sent to hospital. The historian Cassandra Pybus, convinced of Gordon's disingenuousness, suggests that the transfer of convicts and soldiers to Norfolk Island in early 1790 during the grip of famine 'gave Phillip an excuse to deport serial offenders like Daniel Gordon, who had miraculously recovered his senses'.[14] It is possible that this kind of casual exile was deployed in the grey space between criminality and insanity. Norfolk Island certainly served this function in the wake of Vinegar Hill. Gordon's original sentence expired on Norfolk Island but he remained for some time as a free man – a tailor, writes Pybus, 'patching the ragged uniforms of marines that were literally falling off their backs'. He later moved to the Hawkesbury, where he died in 1818, aged 80.

Where modern legal and medical expertise failed, decisions about madness could be made summarily, or discretionarily, according to a form of common sense reasoning. Psychological research shows that juries tend to approach the law in this way, and that in insanity trials, especially, jurors make decisions using their own notions of culpability, rather than the precise models offered them by legal precedent.[15] Military officers acting as judges may be assumed to have taken a similar approach. Common sense reasoning could also more readily incorporate the possibility that convicts, who had a clear object of avoiding punishment, might be feigning illness. The vagueness in the measures taken to curb and contain madness, both here in the borderlands of law and sovereignty, and in other settings where the law held a tighter grasp, may well have been deliberate. Under such a regime, punishment could be mixed with care in responding to the presentation of madness. Lacking prisons large enough to contain the unruly convict population, authorities looked to the Australian geography, and the expanse of the Pacific, to impose order and contain turbulence; they relied on the bush itself, and its fearful countenance to those unfamiliar with it, to deter convicts from escape.[16] Departure from English precedent issued no doubt partly from ignorance, but also from the peculiarities of New South Wales, as those in authority responded to the disorder of early colonial projects, the unruly convict community, and the new possibilities presented by the scale and shape of land and sea.[17]

WHEN CRIMINAL SENTENCES WERE PASSED AND MEN AND women entered into the custody of the British government, the government accepted a duty of care over them, which in the 19th century became a robust mixture of surveillance and intervention. This is apparent from the string of parliamentary inquiries which guided reform in British prisons across the 19th century.[18] The transportation of convicts across the seas anticipated these reforms, however, at the turn of the century. 'Botany Bay' was a bold departure from standard practice, a grand experiment: a large-scale, ambitious public venture in criminal justice, not to send criminals away but to carry them across the sea in an elaborate and expensive global redistribution of labour.[19] The project's principal architect, Viscount Sydney, hoped that the labour might be more than productive, as Alan Atkinson writes so compellingly – that it might instil morality and industry, but also offer entry into a society which might reward those virtues materially.[20] Foundational to these London dreams was the elimination of those who were presently living in the great southern land, with their own cultures of labour and justice and their own moral economies.

If the British were indeed engaged in an ambitious colonial experiment, the research subjects would need to be in fair health for it to have a chance of success. Before convicts were embarked, hulk doctors were required only to ensure that they were bathed in warm water and soap and had a haircut. After several particularly fatal voyages, the position of surgeon–superintendent was created in 1814, incentivising medical care through bonuses for convicts delivered in good health.[21] The surgeon–superintendent's responsibilities began with the inspection of the prisoners selected to travel on their ship, conducted with the medical officer of the hulk or gaol. The inspection was not designed to select the strongest or best-equipped convicts, however, but to check that those who were sent were not infectious and had a good chance of surviving the voyage. Neither 'old age or bodily infirmity', doctors were explicitly instructed, disqualified prisoners from transportation.[22] The examination was 'very unsatisfactory', complained one doctor named George Fairfowl in 1830 – the convicts were 'anxious to get away, and the surgeon equally anxious to get rid of bad or troublesome cases', so that both parties with the relevant knowledge were 'interested to conceal any symptom of disease'. Many set sail who never should have, and even some that Fairfowl had rejected, 'a piece of ingenuity not found out until too late to be remedied'.[23] As late as 1851, after a particularly trying voyage, a surgeon complained that the medical officer at an Irish prison was 'much to blame' for allowing a patient to embark in 'a lucid interval'. She proceeded to 'attack the nurses, bite and otherwise molest them' and at night disturbed 'every person in the ship'.[24]

Prisoners might also be keen to stay where they were, like the ex-soldier James Deery, who was found deliberately irritating his leg ulcers and swallowing a large amount of tobacco to avoid being transported. He was sent, regardless, with the surgeon–superintendent struggling to save his abused leg during the voyage. Others tied cords around their limbs to induce swelling, or feigned epileptic fits.[25]

When the transport ships arrived in the colonies a similar inspection was performed by the colonial secretary, and the ill were sent to the hospital or asylum. Convicts were in general well nourished and tended to by the doctors engaged by government to treat them.[26] The expectation that government would see to the health of the convicts is clear in the practice of assignment. Colonists agreed to feed, clothe and accommodate convicts in exchange for the right to their labour, but medical care remained the remit of government. The chief agent of the Australian Agricultural Company, in charge of its famed million acres, complained in April 1830 that there was no government medical service within a reasonable distance, which meant that the company was deprived of a 'very material advantage' enjoyed by private masters.[27]

Convict diets were also better generally than those of the poor at home. Dried northern rations were supplemented by fresh meat and vegetables from the public garden at Parramatta, the governor's garden in Sydney, and from the gardens which convicts were encouraged to cultivate themselves. Other foods were sourced from knowledge shared by Aboriginal people.[28] At one point convicts refused to accept the maize allocated them, which demonstrates not only their sense of entitlement but a striking food security.[29] Discipline was harsh and work could be blistering, but for many convicts their criminal sentences afforded them entry into a better dietary and healthcare regime than they could have expected without it.

However, if the colonial doctors assumed that illness disqualified convicts from certain types of labour, particular locations, or corporal punishment, they quickly joined the convict authorities in their scepticism about the symptoms with which convicts presented. This suspicion developed to such an extent that a special room at the Sydney Hospital was reserved for convicts who reported sick, and they were confined there for the workday.[30] And no condition was so slippery and challenging as madness.

IN HIS PRIZEWINNING ESSAY ON *FEIGNED OR FACTITIOUS Diseases*, the Scottish physician and sanitarian Hector Gavin cited a dizzying range of people who were liable to feign insanity: those hoping to avoid military or naval service; those already in the army or navy and wanting out; those in prison, or facing it; those exaggerating injuries so as to increase the punishment of others or the compensation due to them; and, in former times, slaves. To these credible categories he added 'those who prefer idleness to industry', 'sycophants', fanatics, those indulging in 'animal magnetism' – mesmerism, or vitalism – or 'influenced by the principle of imitation' (an unconscious, mechanical copying of behaviours), the hysterical or otherwise too nervous, the ambitious or attention-seeking and, finally, those who 'assume the semblance of disease from some inexplicable causes: these are chiefly females'.[31] 'And other causes may be imagined,' wrote the baronet physician Henry Acland, in another prize-winning essay – including the prospect that feigning the effects of illness could be a symptom of genuine madness.[32]

We typically only become aware of illness as a mechanism of avoidance through the comments and policies of sceptical authorities. The very language of malingering, and feigning, simulation and shamming, cloaks an evaluation of character through the assessment of symptoms; medicine working as an adjudicator. These lists, of course, reveal as much about the limited empathy and the class and gender sensibilities which drive discussions of malingering as they do of the behaviours they seek to describe. What is clear is that situations of coercion give rise both to malingering and the spectre of it. Gavin cited the military as well as prisons; few men entered His Majesty's service by choice, as A. T. Thomson pointed out at the University of London lecture in 1837, and 'their anxiety to get off induces them to feign diseases'.[33] The American physician Thomas Blatchford wrote that mania was 'pretended by sailors and soldiers, who would rather be in an asylum' than endure the discipline and deprivations of the navy and army.[34]

New South Wales was more fundamentally a site of punishment and coercion than the army or navy. In such a place, it is not surprising that illness appeared to convicts not only or perhaps even primarily as an affliction, but as an opportunity. In 1820 Principal Superintendent of Convicts William Hutchinson reported that feigning illness was widespread, especially amongst recent arrivals. The missionary Lancelot Threlkeld found himself besieged by insubordinate convicts at his mission station on Lake Macquarie. Feigning sickness was one tactic in a more general resistance. They also pretended not to know how to use their tools, stole meat rations, and told Threlkeld plainly that they wanted to be sent back to Sydney.[35] Convicts feigned madness on Norfolk Island, where Henry Graham was surgeon in 1841–44. After a stabbing on the island by a convict known to be violent and troublesome, Graham had been 'very doubtful as to his state of mind particularly, as I know it is a practice among some prisoners to feign insanity for the purpose of evading punishment, or in the hopes of being sent to the Lunatic Asylum'.[36] This instance appeared genuine, after close observation, but others were not. Sudden violence registered especially, since many simulators were under the impression that 'real madness was characterised by violent conduct and vociferous language'.[37] 'It is not insanity that an impostor can or will imitate,' wrote Acland in 1844, a world away, 'but the popular idea of it'.[38]

For the convicts of New South Wales, illness might promise escape from specific places, duties or punishments, or, if cards were played well, escape from government custody altogether. Feigning madness in a prison or penal outpost could accomplish removal to an asylum. Not only was there minimal labour at the asylum, it was minimally guarded and, in the early period, dilapidated to the point of insecurity. The asylums at Castle Hill and Liverpool were on the edge of European settlement, but nowhere near as remote as the penal settlements which ranged across the south-eastern seaboard using geography as their security.

Like convicts, the soldiers stationed in New South Wales had restricted choices and freedoms. They conducted their duties under a disciplinary regime in some respects more draconian than that applied to the convicts, and they too faced the stringencies of colonial life. Six soldiers were hanged a year after the Europeans arrived for stealing from the public store – 'the flower of our battalion', wrote Lieutenant Watkin Tench grimly. Flogging, which is heavily associated with convict life, was also a standard punishment in the British army, and continued to be practised long after it fell out of favour in civil society.[39] Simulation was not, therefore, only to be found among serving convicts, even in a penal colony.

The courts, which were in the colonies as they were at home the gateways between penal and free society, also saw illness put to use. Mania was commonly feigned to 'escape the sentence of law', wrote Blatchford, 'or to mitigate the severity of punishment'.[40] The amateur legal environment in the colony allowed the largesse of untrained judges full expression, but also plenty of space for other outlooks. Patrick Shannan, or Shannon, was middle-aged, moderately wealthy and well-connected. It is unclear whether he arrived as a convict. By the early years of the 19th century he appears to have fallen on hard times. In 1804, while living at Chapel Row (at the corner of Castlereagh and King streets in Sydney), Shannan advertised the sale of 30 flood-free acres at the Hawkesbury – 'pleasantly situate' and 'truly desirable', with 6 acres clear, 3 felled, and a farmhouse and barn.[41] The following January he sought to sell a 'capital and commodious' weatherboard in the Rocks, with a large back-yard and garden. He appears to have been in a state of some private and public strife; in July 1805 he was tried by a bench of magistrates for assault and battery.[42] The year after, he advertised 15 acres of likely the same 30-acre property at the Hawkesbury: 'Lamb's Farm', also 'pleasantly situate'.[43]

On 1 July 1808, Shannan was indicted for a second 'violent and unprovoked assault'. He was released on a substantial bail, but the next day stole a pound of thread from Isaac Nichols's shop in Sydney.[44] Standing before the court, Shannan did not answer the charge against him. Witnesses testified that he 'had laboured under a mental derangement for some time previous to, and at the time of his committing the theft'. Anthony Kemp, a New South Wales Corps captain acting as judge advocate, was keenly aware of this possibility as he observed Shannan. 'It must obviously be attended with evil consequences to society were such a plea to be countenanced,' he pontificated; it would 'afford to other delinquents a prospect of offending with impunity'. There was little of David Collins's humanity here, or of Arthur Phillip's liberality, only fear of the disruptive power of insanity. Insanity did not present itself to Kemp as a misfortune or an illness, but as a tactic 'craftily resorted to as a subterfuge for eluding the stroke of justice'. If he had trained in law the captain might have known that the legally insane hardly eluded justice. The

Criminal Lunatics Act had been rushed through parliament following the acquittal of the attempted regicide James Hadfield in 1800, but it was a miserable refuge. He and others like him were detained 'at the pleasure of His Majesty'. Indefinitely.[45]

But this court was full of other people who participated in the proceedings far more than they might elsewhere; these people knew Shannan, and knew that the law here was fluid. The representatives of 'society' over which Kemp fretted testified both to Shannan's virtues when sane and to his present insanity. John Harris, a prominent and wealthy colonist of impeccable credentials, gave a character reference.[46] Several acquaintances suggested that Shannan's symptoms were produced by a downturn in his business interests. Kemp eventually agreed that Shannan was 'unhappily deranged', and at this juncture 'a solicitation' was presented noting that 'it might be considered dangerous to suffer the prisoner to go at large' and requesting his 'present confinement'. It was all rather civilised, and vague. 'The application was considered reasonable, and was acquiesced in by the Court.' Kemp gave instructions that 'every attention should be paid to the proper treatment of the unfortunate man'. There was, however, no obvious place to confine Shannan, since there was no asylum in the colony. He may have been admitted to Parramatta Gaol, where a handful of others wrestling with madness were confined, like Charles Bishop – or perhaps one of those who spoke for him took him in.

Shannan's trial was an approximation of English legal procedure, just as Gordon's had been. 'In a colony so peculiarly circumstanced,' Major Joseph Foveaux wrote several months later, it was 'impossible to regulate the dealings between man and man by the strict letter of the law or to judge of them by any other criterion than that of sound equity and common sense.'[47] It is not clear, however, if he was referring generally to the vagaries of a convict colony ruled by a military government, or to more particular circumstances. Since 26 January that year, New South Wales had been in the midst of a constitutional crisis after the governor had been deposed, and Foveaux had reluctantly taken over the administration of the colony.

Shannan, like so many others, slipped entirely out of the public record, for while its convict indents and musters were path-breaking and at points even breathtaking, New South Wales was a pre-bureaucratic state. These trials show a colonial legal system which was not systematic in its dealings with madness, concerned less with precedent than with practical solutions to immediate problems arising from its distinctive population and situation. Legal officers (by appointment, rather than by training) bridged the gap between their expertise and the problems confronting them by invoking common sense notions of symptom and disorder.

WHEN MARTHA SMITH, WHO HAD 'DECOYED' A TODDLER and was caught stripping his clothes, with 'two children's bonnets and a little jacket' on her person, was arraigned for trial at the Police Magistrate Court in 1834, she looked to be insane. She was remanded for further information, however, because the chief magistrate thought 'there was some method in it'.[48] Before anything was proven, *The Australian* reported the incident as one of 'feigned madness'. Suspicion had become standard. The phrase 'method in madness' has entered the vernacular, gathering an innocuous meaning – logic in apparent chaos, an apology for idiosyncrasy. It was born, however, as a suspicion of the common symptoms of madness. There was a method which could be deployed to simulate madness, and this method spread through penal New South Wales. A secret scheme between bushrangers to feign insanity was unearthed at the penal settlement in Newcastle. It shows that some convicts, at least, were familiar with how and where madness was dealt with in the colony, and the escape it might offer.

William Geary, an engineer or gunner, arrived from Limerick in 1814, aged twenty-five. Within three years he became a notorious bushranger and leader of a successful gang based in a cave near Gordon, 15 kilometres north-west of Sydney, which robbed houses and held up carts returning from the markets.[49] Geary was captured in early 1817 and sent to Newcastle penal settlement, although the details of his sentence did not accompany him. Geary 'had some appearance of being insane', wrote commandant James Wallis, requesting information. That August, Geary attacked two other convicts whose lives were saved only 'by the knife taking a different direction'. Wallis was working hard to bring order to the settlement and had struggled to manage a man 'so very treacherous' as Geary. He concluded that the bushranger was feigning.[50] The sparse human geography of the colony meant that penal commandants typically made decisions locally, and then informed central government, but in this case Wallis wrote to the colonial secretary, J. T. Campbell, for instruction. The convict 'should either be tried for his life or confined to a mad house in a straight waistcoat', he recommended, 'as he is to [sic] dangerous a character to be at large'.[51] It was the standard conflation of illness and criminality; the role of the straightjacket was clearly sub-therapeutic. Campbell gave orders for Wallis to be sent to Sydney, and Wallis obliged, reiterating that, 'whether a lunatic or not he is a dangerous man to be at large … he should either be tried for his life before the proper tribunal or be confined for life in a madhouse'.[52]

Campbell instructed the keeper of Sydney Gaol to collect Geary from his ship and 'keep him in safe custody until further orders' in November 1817. It is unclear what transpired next, but Geary was returned to Newcastle the following October.[53] The violently insane, or those whose violence took the semblance of insanity, were difficult to handle, but they also threatened a more insidious disruption, since, if they succeeded, other prisoners might follow their example. James Morisset, who had replaced Wallis as commandant at Newcastle and imposed a more severe regime of labour and discipline, wrote in alarm to Campbell in 1819. '*Gough* [another bushranger] and *Geary* two of the gaol gang agreed to commit a *murder*. Geary who was at one time insane was to perpetrate the act, Gough borrow'd a knife and gave to him, saying we shall both get up to *Sydney*, I shall be a *witness*, and will swear you are mad, and the worst they can do to you will be to send you to Castle Hill where you were before, and I shall remain in Sydney.' Taking the knife, Geary 'waited an opportunity' and stabbed another prisoner, but again 'the knife was turn'd from its direction by the hip bone, which saved the man's life, who is in the hospital doing well'.[54]

Morisset's account reads as if Gough sought to manipulate Geary, but the infamous bushranger was hardly a pushover. He was a leader, a man with clear agency and initiative, and his loyalty to his comrade bushrangers, even to the end, seems likely to have produced loyalty. Did one of the bushrangers break after the knife turned; or did another convict come forward who had overheard them whispering in the night? As with all malingering, it was only in failure that it could be identified as malingering. Though the plan was hardly watertight, it clearly shows how notions of madness could be manipulated, since the bushrangers assumed that because Geary had been admitted to Castle Hill previously, an act of irrational violence would make authorities think him insane again, especially if another prisoner bore witness. But the episode also reveals the limits of official credulousness.

Morisset inquired whether Geary's current sentence had expired. It had not; he was serving a life sentence.[55] Geary was not mad, the commandant decided, and sent him to Sydney for trial. It seems likely that he never had been mad, and that the previous asylum admission and the 1817 attack at Newcastle, were both efforts to evade punishment. The fact that neither attack was fatal – that both blades turned uncannily aside – may suggest both that Geary was sane and that he aimed, as other bushrangers did, to avoid civilian injury.[56] When he was finally captured and retried, he emphasised his aversion to violence. The judge took this as no more than a bid to avoid the death penalty.[57]

In his wildly popular journalistic novel *For the Term of His Natural Life*, Marcus Clarke recounts a scheme similar to the attack at Newcastle, in which three convicts drew lots. The longest straw was the 'lucky' one; the one who drew it would be killed by the one who drew the mid-length straw, and would receive the blessing of the gallows. 'The unlucky one was the witness. He had, of course, an excellent chance of being hung also, but his doom was not so certain, and he therefore looked upon himself as unfortunate.'[58] There could be a wide variety of method in murder. Some have seen such intense dramas as evidence of the wretchedness of the penal settlements, but historians have been sceptical that such 'suicide lotteries' ever took place.[59] Still, it is perfectly plausible that death appeared attractive to long-serving convicts serving hard labour in stark places. The justice system offered release without calling down the judgement of which Irish Catholics, particularly, shuddered to think. There is evidence for several cases of such 'state-assisted suicide' on Norfolk Island, minus the rigmarole of straw-drawing or the pathos of Clarke's narrative.[60]

Eighteenth-century gaols were derided by social commentators like Henry Fielding as 'schools of vice' and 'seminaries of idleness'.[61] The bushrangers' scheme suggests something like a schooling. Did they take the opportunity to practise their pretence, perhaps late at night? The image of the two contorting and convulsing, and offering each other whispered pointers, is both fantastical, but also plausible. Outlaws may well have pieced together strategies, identified weak points in legal procedure, and even shared their knowledge of life in lunatic asylums, noting compassionate or lazy doctors, or gaolers easily gotten to. This kind of exchange was understood, and feared, by army surgeons. 'It is not only the loss of one man that is to be guarded against,' wrote a reviewer of Henry Marshall's 1828 guide for young army doctors. The knowledge of attempted feigning spread through a regiment, and after it the threat of imitation. Shamming was as infectious as typhus, and worse; 'if it is known that the surgeon has been once deceived, the fear of detection is naturally diminished'.[62]

In New South Wales, networks formed among convicts, along routes of regular communication and commerce and in institutional hubs which brought either reoffenders or those with particular skills, like mechanics, together for a time. And there were the bushranger gangs which hovered at the edges of settled society, some commanding loyalty not only internally but among the communities of the 'interior', where those who had come free or been born in the colony mixed with those who had served out their sentences and with Indigenous populations. There was a certain sympathy for those who lived outside the law from those who had once felt its weight.[63] Other gangs simply inspired dread, but there was a dominant bushranging culture – antisocial, in certain respects, and incendiarily anti-authority – which might easily lend itself to something like schooling in feigned madness.[64]

Geary was irrepressible. Having escaped by some other scheme, he was recaptured in February 1821 with six gang members and some settlers who had harboured them. In July, however, a gaoler reported the escapes of two of the 'immense number' of prisoners at Sydney Gaol, including the 'notorious bushranger' Michael Ryan. The following evening, prisoners forced out the metal struts behind the chimney and broke through the bricks while others simultaneously attacked the walls securing 'the three notorious bushrangers Geary, Smith and Wiseman (commonly called the Flying Barber)'. On 7 July, Geary and another rushed on and 'fastened' a constable, escaping one last time. The provost-marshal recommended that a handbill offering a reward of £20 or £25 be drawn up. Perhaps this helped precipitate the capture of Geary and many of his gang two months later. At the trial, Geary 'was determined on criminating himself in every charge'. He and four others were hanged six days later.[65]

THE DETECTION OF FEIGNED MADNESS WAS A CONTEST between medical knowledge of 'genuine symptoms' and a more practical knowledge of imitable symptoms.[66] Doctors have long been well acquainted both with mental illness and the means of simulating it, as a range of treatises and guides demonstrate. 'The original must be known,' wrote Acland, 'before the copy can be criticized.' The more practical guides balanced increasingly precise descriptions of mental illness with strategies for outwitting those who were feigning them. There was a wide range of mental symptoms which could be copied, but violent symptoms were the most obvious signifiers. They could backfire, however, since the delicate boundary between violent insanity and mere violence could easily blur in the eyes of overseers. The subtler symptoms, and quieter categories of madness like melancholia, appear to have rarely been simulated. There were two classes of insanity in the popular imagination, wrote Acland: mania and dementia. Both were assumed to be easily recognised. 'Genuine insanity', however, was more complex, even though it did fall roughly into the two categories – excitement (or mania) and depression. The success of feigning depended 'not more on the skill of the simulator than on the incompetence of the judge', warned Acland, and offered a set of 'aphorisms' for doctors who aspired to competence.[67]

There was, in fact, a vast array of signs which the many 19th-century treatises on insanity urged practitioners to observe if they wanted to distinguish between real and simulated madness: the onset of symptoms, overacting, response to surveillance, repudiation of symptoms, abstinence from food, sleep, countenance, the ability to look at an examiner, memory deficiency, alienation of affection, absurdity, insensitivity, hesitation and premeditation in conversation, impropriety, and odour.[68] As for detection, the more elaborate techniques involved either specialist equipment or sophisticated training, neither of which was much in evidence in the colonies. Physicians were encouraged to entrap a suspected feigner by one of three methods: looking for imitation of symptoms they had suggested; the capacity to repeat behaviour; or written intelligibility. Or they could use strong drugs, to which the truly insane were understood as being resistant, or they could simply tell the patient that they would never be believed, seeking a reaction. More controversial were the threat of violence or violence itself. Hot irons, hot wires, flagellation, intoxication and dousing in cold water were all considered effective, but 'the most certain test', suggested Professor A. T. Thomson in his London lecture, was the 'whirling chair'. Suspected feigners were strapped in and violently spun. 'Few men can act a part after such discipline.'[69] The ethics were obviously complex.

Henry Acland thought that 'if the phenomena of insanity were fully understood, they *could* not be simulated.' With 'the light we even now possess,' he continued, 'it is nearly impossible for an impostor to escape.'[70] But most were less sanguine. The prospect of simulation added guile and cunning to an already difficult diagnostic, navigating the convoluted terrain of the mind. Working at the turn of the nineteenth century, the French physician Philippe Pinel thought that only sustained, intimate observation could reveal simulation, either in overacting or the absence of accepted symptoms like quick eye movements and insomnia.[71] Modern medicine looks for repeatable, randomisable tests, but some suggest that close scrutiny of patient and case history, as Pinel advocated, may be the only means of confirming mental illness. Other strategies have proven unscientific and even moralistic.[72]

LIKE THE COURTS, THE HOSPITALS AND ASYLUMS OF NEW South Wales were shaped by the peculiarities of a penal colony. This meant that doctors were called upon to be both less and more than medical professionals. Their expertise was often disregarded, as when Major West, surgeon at Parramatta Gaol, found that three men he had discharged as sane were returned to the asylum even though none had shown symptoms of insanity after their discharge.[73] Their only 'symptom' was violence – maiming cattle, robbing orchards and 'putting the neighbourhood in bodily fear'.[74] West discharged them again, 'being very proper objects for Government labour', but within six months, two were returned yet again to the asylum. One had previously tried to kill William Bennett, the superintendent, several times, and on his third admission, beat an old patient 'unmercifully'.[75] West told commissioner Bigge that he 'never knew an instance in which the surgeons at Castle Hill have decided upon the sanity or insanity of persons sent there'. Patients were sent by surgeons at the various institutions around the colony, or directly by magistrates. William Bland, surgeon at the Castle Hill asylum in 1814, said that patients came 'frequently without order', but otherwise generally by direction of the magistrates or by the principal surgeon, likely on instructions from the colonial secretary.[76] A succession of doctors were outraged by the failure of government to place the lunatic asylums in their hands and, generally respect their medical judgement.[77]

Doctors were also placed in the ethically perilous position of judging illness in a context where it was presumed feigned until proven genuine. A reviewer of Henry Marshall's *Hints to Young Medical Officers* wrote drily of the military surgeon's burden, 'to guard against the various, well-conceived, and long sustained stratagems, by which those who have had enough of a life of glory endeavour to escape from it'.[78] Convicts, in similar fashion, sought often to escape the glories of the penal colonies, and doctors were required to watch and guard them, and then, only if it was appropriate, to treat them.

Van Diemen's Land was a remote territory of New South Wales from 1803. It became a separate colony in 1825, received the bulk of convicts in the following decades and the entirety of transportees between 1840 and 1868.[79] It inherited the suspicions of its parent colony. Upon opening Port Arthur penal settlement in 1833, Lieutenant-Governor George Arthur set down instructions for the officers. The 'most difficult duty' of the surgeon, he warned, was 'to distinguish feigned from real illness'. A surgeon must 'not exempt any individual from labour or receive him into hospital, without taking down for subsequent report a minute detail of the symptoms of his case'. The report had to then specify 'the reasons which induced him to conceive the disease not to be feigned but real'.[80] In this way, working backwards from the assumption that all convicts were feigning the illnesses they presented with, Arthur neatly reversed the surgeon's vocational tendency.

Sometimes doctors simply opted out. 'In Newcastle Gaol there was a man named John Johnson,' Attorney-General John Plunkett reported in 1837, 'who had been for a length of time in custody on a charge of bushranging.' Likely a convict, Johnson had been treated for insanity at the gaol, but 'the medical gentleman would not certify whether or not he was possessed of his intellects'. Plunkett therefore had him discharged, on account of the long period he had already spent in custody.[81] Lacking the guidance of medicine, the representatives of colonial law might fall back on their particular politics and inclinations in decisions about convict and criminal madness.

Convict madness was dealt with primarily by convict authorities – masters, magistrates and governors – as long as convict transportation continued. Such brushes with the courts and law officers show the fluidity in the application of legal concepts, precedents and sentences. They also, however, show the strong and lingering influence of Botany Bay, of the idea of a penal colony, in the evaluation of insanity.

Late in 1845, in Van Diemen's Land, where the transportation of convicts continued, a convict and former inmate of the New Norfolk Lunatic Asylum named Thomas Judd stood before the Hobart Supreme Court accused of theft. A Dr Crook testified that Judd was 'a decided monomaniac' from heavy drinking, presenting in 'a strong tendency to pilfering'. Even during a lucid interval, the defence argued, those with such a 'confirmed aberration of intellect' might break into manic behaviour at the slightest disturbance. The solicitor-general, acting as prosecutor, and the judge were both appalled. If 'pilfering monomaniacs' were not accountable for their crimes in patently lucid intervals, 'all the "cranky" men in the colony might perpetrate all kinds of offences with impunity,' Justice Horne glowered, 'to the great injury and evil of the community'.[82] In its report of the trial, the *Observer* took a different view of the penal colony. Medical treatises demonstrated that lucid intervals could also be fluid, it pointed out, and 'in a community like ours,' wrote the editor, 'in which we have not only much crime, but … much that is the fruit of mental weakness or derangement', it was particularly crucial to consult the best medical literature.[83] The jury, however, sided with the judge and the solicitor-general, and Judd was sentenced to twelve months' hard labour.

Free colonists would eventually see the need for concepts like monomania and lucid intervals, and would work for greater legal protections against government authority, for the sane and insane alike. They would need to weed out the suspicion which had gathered around illness, and remember that madness was not primarily a refuge or a subterfuge, but an affliction.

4

THE 'LUNATIC ASYLUM' AT CASTLE HILL

A social institution like a lunatic asylum is more than a building – it is an idea, clothed in people and resources and walls and history, one which very nearly has a life of its own; conceived by an active mind or by a parish committee, perhaps in the flush of an intellectual revolution or in the long half-life of an old convention. It is not an organic growth, but the physical expression of the answer to a question. Central Railway Station, Royal Prince Alfred Hospital, the Benevolent Asylum – these words are shorthand for complex entities with distinctive histories in which all kinds of historical strands meet: intellectual, social, economic, political and biographical.

The 19th century was the age of the social institution in Europe. The Enlightenment continued its progressive transformation of the world, spreading outwards from the salons and scientific societies. Questions were asked, with the expectation that societies could be improved with the answers, and new institutions were built from developing theories in order to solve social problems: poverty, crime, sickness, disability and abandonment. The lunatic asylum moved people more deeply than its counterparts. Born in the mediaeval period from theological convictions about what humans were and how they should live, asylums proliferated in Western Europe at the beginning of the 19th century. By mid-century, the asylum was an imposing presence in metropolises and rural towns, in architecture and literature, and as a practical solution to the problem of madness. We remember the asylum as the boldest ambition of a surpassingly ambitious era, as the repository of the deepest fears and desires, and the guardhouse which societies placed between themselves and oblivion.

But was it? The building which was renovated in 1811 to house the mad of the penal colony of New South Wales had no formal name, no special architecture, and no particular therapy. It had no clear authority structure, and kept no obvious records. Soon after it was opened the government talked of closing it, and after a decade the one who had established it and heralded its humane qualities, Lachlan Macquarie, placed it in inverted commas as if he was not sure quite what it was.[1] This chapter searches for the lunatic asylum at Castle Hill. What was it, and what was it for?

HISTORIAN ALAN ATKINSON ARGUES THAT HUMANITARIANism was 'the force, both good and bad, which shaped authority among the first Europeans in Australia'. The criminals who formed the bulk of the colonists were just 'the kind of human raw material which seemed to cry out for the order which humanitarianism offered'.[2] They were ripe for experimental work. This was also the view of James Mackintosh, a jurist, politician and historian, whose career ranged across the British Empire. In 1807, he was recorder, or chief judge, of Bombay, but eager to escape India for New South Wales. He had 'heard, read, and thought' a great deal about the 'extraordinary colony' and the great challenges faced by its governors: 'While on the one side the experiment of a reforming penal colony is, perhaps, the grandest ever tried in morals, it is one which is perfectly safe; for the settlement never can be worse than it is now'. Mackintosh thought that if he could not get a seat in parliament he should like to be 'lawgiver of Botany Bay'. He would lay down a constitution, 'introduce law and morality', and 'rescue at least the children of the convicts from brutality and barbarism by education'. If an 'enlightened governor' was not appointed very soon, he prophesied, 'success will be impossible'.[3]

Such belief in the power of social reform was characteristic of the Scottish Enlightenment, that subset of the broader movement which emphasised common sense policymaking and saw civil society as something like perfectible. Its advocates believed in the power of institutions, particularly, as a 'practical support for improving the social structure'.[4] Between the walls of libraries, factories, gaols, courts, hospitals, cultural institutions and lunatic asylums, society could be transformed.[5] Mackintosh was a man of the Scottish Enlightenment, but one ill-equipped to offer practical support. 'No man doing so little,' wrote one contemporary, 'ever went through a long life, continually creating the belief that he would ultimately do so much.' Forming government in 1830, Charles Grey found that he could not appoint Mackintosh to a position of responsibility because for all his talents 'he was, practically, quite useless'.[6]

Lachlan Macquarie, a close acquaintance of Mackintosh, was more practical. Appointed to bring order to the penal colony after it erupted in rebellion in 1808, Macquarie was the last of the 'autocratic' governors invested with extraordinary powers. Nevertheless, during his extended administration, which covered the years 1810 to 1821, he developed a reputation as a humane and visionary governor. After he arrived in New South Wales, Macquarie demonstrated the Edinburgh influence, establishing charity schools and orphan institutions and even visiting classrooms to present medals to skilled readers and hard workers.[7] He also interested himself in the conditions of the incarcerated, opening a poorhouse and frequently visiting the gaols of the colony. He was president of the Benevolent Society and Bible Society.[8] He also set up the Native Institute and the Blind Institute.[9] With such material to work with, posterity has been kind to Macquarie, especially during the 20th century, when Macquarie began to be celebrated by some as the 'father of Australia'.[10] But Macquarie was no philosopher. A career soldier, he left Scotland at fourteen, and whatever he knew of the Scottish Enlightenment did not come from an Edinburgh education. Much of it likely came from James Mackintosh, since, by a twist of fate, Macquarie lived with him in Bombay. Macquarie was military secretary to Jonathan Duncan, governor of Bombay, and since Duncan was a bachelor, he invited Macquarie to take up quarters at the expansive Government House. Mackintosh, recorder of Bombay, joined them for a year.[11]

Macquarie did not please everyone. His notions about convict reformation offended many free colonists, but in London it was his propensity to spend British money on buildings in Sydney that caused the most trouble. Macquarie was 'extremely desirous', as he announced in 1810, to do whatever would 'in the least degree contribute to the ornament and regularity of the town of Sydney'.[12] This expensive building program, assisted by convict architect Francis Greenway and Macquarie's wife Elizabeth, helped precipitate a commission of enquiry, and the end of his tenure in the colony.[13]

The asylum at Castle Hill was not quite part of this program. A large barracks had been built at the government farm in 1803.

One hundred feet by twenty-four, and built on stones set in mud mortar, it was the first of its kind in the colony, and was intended as a sort of quarantine station to contain the convict sedition which the government feared was brewing, especially among the Irish arrivals. In fact, by concentrating so many convicts on the outskirts of the settlement, it probably exacerbated it, and the following year hundreds of convicts marched on Parramatta. 'We then learnt that Castle Hill was in flames,' wrote Elizabeth Macarthur; ladies like her were encouraged to evacuate to Sydney. The rebels were betrayed, however. Their leaders were killed in battle or executed afterward – there were other means of dealing with sedition.[14]

The structure of the economy was changing, and the government farm was shut down in 1810. In its last years the farm had housed fewer and fewer convicts, operating mostly as a depot from which convicts were assigned out. The barracks was referred to as a granary or barn, and in 1811 it was one of the few large buildings in the colony. Macquarie fixed upon it as the site of the new asylum. The colonial secretary, J. T. Campbell, ordered minimal renovations: a garden laid out behind the building for the patients' exercise; the old cooking house of the farm revived; a fence built from timber salvaged from one of the dilapidated wooden outbuildings. For Campbell, this was enough to make the building into 'an hospital'. As soon as work finished, the six 'lunatics' then 'confined at the jail in Parramatta' were to be transferred, 'attended by Cullen their present keeper and by the woman who now acts as cook to them'.[15]

'Commiserating the unhappy condition of persons labouring under the affliction of mental derangement,' the *Gazette* announced on 1 June, Macquarie had ordered 'an asylum to be prepared for their reception at Castle Hill'. The patients had already been transferred from Parramatta Gaol, and 'every provision that humanity could suggest has been made for their accommodation and comfort'.[16] History books refer to this hastily renovated barracks, granary or barn as 'Australia's First Psychiatric Hospital', the first ray of the 'Dawn of Australian Psychiatry'.[17] But by 1814, when the convict doctor William Bland arrived at the asylum, there was no medicine in stock, patients escaped frequently, notwithstanding the new fence, and obtaining even trifling supplies was a great challenge. The buildings were in complete disrepair, Bland recalled, and 'in all other respects the establishment was as bad as possible'.[18] He left in disgust. The asylum continued to be plagued by staffing issues and shortages of food, medicine and other supplies, including lime and brushes to whitewash the walls against vermin.[19] The bed bugs multiplied so much that, by 1824, most patients were sleeping naked. Those with 'a little sense of feeling, or decency, prefer lying in their day clothing, on the bare boards'.[20] The institution's clearest function was to draw lunatics from elsewhere, to empty other buildings of madness and its disruptions, but even this proved difficult, as patients frequently escaped. Benjamin Sparkes, who escaped in February 1822, was typical: recaptured within a month and placed in Parramatta Gaol until an asylum keeper came to collect groceries.[21]

The rhetoric of the *Gazette* matches poorly with the hasty renovations, the almost complete lack of therapy, and the absence of dedicated staff. The incongruence begs the question – what did Macquarie mean by a 'lunatic asylum'? He was, indeed, the last autocrat, and so had a good deal of discretion; it matters what he thought an asylum was. What did he hope for it? What purpose did he envision for it? These questions are part of a larger discussion about the residential social institution as it was deployed at home and in the colonies to shape and reshape society.

Perhaps the language offers a clue. At the turn of the

19th century, the word 'hospital' was unlikely to raise the images of precise and clean medicine it has now accrued. The word 'asylum', however, was a powerful one, imbued with hope and peace and associated with the prospect of refuge, like the celebrated new institution at York, The Retreat. The institutions which followed, shaped by the precepts of moral therapy, would choose the imagery of asylum over that of the hospital. Moral therapy eradicated many of the chains and other methods used to restrain the insane, and encouraged them to develop self-control and rejoin society. It seems significant, then, that Macquarie used the same language to describe New South Wales itself. He thought of the colony as a 'penitentiary or asylum on a grand scale', where the chains of 'children of misfortune' could be discarded as they worked towards restoration to society. Michael Robinson, that 'incendiary' convict poet, was appointed poet laureate by Macquarie (the only one ever appointed in Australia). He, too, wrote of the penal colony as 'an asylum for unhappy convicts'.[22]

But was the building at Castle Hill really a place of refuge? Macquarie's colonial experience may have tempered his ideals. He travelled widely before his appointment as governor, so that few of his adult years were spent in Britain or France, where moral therapy was emerging, and the Enlightenment proceeding apace. He was in Bombay when the Retreat opened its doors. Soon after patients were freed from their chains in Paris, at the Asylum de Bicêtre, he left India for Cairo with a colonial army. He moved through Sri Lanka, China, Egypt, Russia, South Africa and Saint Helena. But he served longest in India, and it was likely there, working and living with the governor and recorder of colonial Bombay, that he came to see an asylum not as an ambitious social institution, but as a building which received and secured the ungovernable from society.

The earliest Indian asylums applied European ideas about the mind and its afflictions in very limited ways. Little is known about them; they remain shrouded in ignominy. In Bombay, the insane were placed in a small institution on 'Butcher's Island' in the harbour, 4 miles offshore (now Jawahar Dweep). They were moved at the turn of the 19th century to the house of surgeon R. Fildes on the island of Kolaba. Twenty years later the building was in alarming disrepair, in 'such a wretched state' that renovation was not feasible. Poor ventilation had caused 'agonizing suffering' among the patients. The European insane were, accordingly, sent to England and the calmer Indian patients removed to a nearby general hospital.[23] Racial ideas heavily influenced the treatment of insanity in India, with administrators concerned that the image of white madmen might belie their rhetoric of racial superiority.[24] Indian psychiatrists later proceeded to reject many of the cultural assumptions that underwrote the discipline, as part of a broader scepticism of psychiatry's role in western imperialism.[25]

Staffing and funding are other ways to gauge the nature and significance of an institution; an important institution, a substantive answer to a problem, is placed in the hands of a person of some merit who is entrusted with responsibility and with the authority and resources appropriate to their task. It is a measure of the ambiguity surrounding the first asylum in New South Wales that historians have not been able to establish with clarity who first ran it.[26] Patrick Cullen and the unnamed female cook who arrived with the first patients from Parramatta Gaol ran the institution under the superintendence of the commandant of Parramatta, Robert Durie, who had also been tasked with its renovations. Durie was replaced by Captain Haddon Smith in 1812, who received 'occasional reports' to assist his oversight.[27] When Smith left the colony with his regiment in 1814, his office was abolished, and the asylum passed into the hands of the chief magistrate at Parramatta, Samuel Marsden, who was to give whatever directions he thought 'advisable for the care and comfort of the lunatics'.[28]

Marsden was a busy man. He was principal chaplain to the colony, a conscientious and successful farmer, and took his many magisterial duties seriously. He was also at this point turning his evangelistic energies towards New Zealand, frustrated by the lack of conversion among convicts and Indigenous Australians. He established a society in 1813 for the 'protection' and 'civilization' of the Māori, and left on his first of seven voyages there in November 1814.[29] It seems likely that Marsden, whose Protestant, middle-class work ethic was formidable, would have had little interest in an institution like Castle Hill, where industry and progress were difficult to gauge. Marsden saw receptivity to the Christian gospel as tied closely with industriousness in other spheres of life, and concentrated his energies accordingly.[30] This meant that he had little time for the asylum, and thus he arranged to have it removed from his responsibility.[31] The only overt measure he seems to have taken was to report a pre-existing arrangement to Macquarie: a third of the patients' meat ration was being exchanged with the store at Parramatta for tea, tobacco and oil. Macquarie ordered that the 'bad practice' cease immediately.[32] The superintendent later reported that small comforts like these did visibly help 'to allay and calm' patients suffering from mania and melancholia.[33]

By 1814 the patient population at Castle Hill had grown from six to sixteen, and in September Macquarie appointed a superintendent and surgeon, both resident on the asylum site.[34] George Suttor, a neighbour and friend of Marsden since 1802, was made superintendent. He was a struggling amateur botanist, who had sided with William Bligh against those who deposed him and accompanied him to London in 1810 to give evidence.[35] The post came with £50 salary, a weatherboard cottage on site, and some of the fields which had comprised the old government farm. William Bland, who we met in the Introduction, was appointed surgeon of the asylum. A naval surgeon and the son of a distinguished English obstetrician, he had thrown a glass of water at a much-despised purser *en route* to a post in India. The purser challenged him to a duel and was fatally wounded. Bland was court-martialled, but with a recommendation to mercy, and he and his second were transported for seven years. They both took up residence at the asylum, and farmed land previously worked by the overseer.[36] Bland's quick temper had not been curbed by British justice, as Suttor would soon discover.[37]

The two officers, superintendent and surgeon, were appointed with parallel authority, and the division of their responsibilities was indistinct. Suttor's instructions made some of his duties clear. He was to keep the patients clean and well-fed, with rations 'properly dressed and served out … at proper hours'. No one was to 'defraud' the patients of their food. Suttor was to set up a kitchen garden, providing the patients with amusement and exercise as well as fresh vegetables. He was responsible for ensuring that no 'unnecessary severity' was deployed and that the patients were 'at all times treated with mildness, kindness and humanity. The keepers and other attendants are to receive strict orders to this effect'.[38] These instructions suggest something of the rhythms and priorities of The Retreat, with its religious and Enlightenment precepts emphasising the humanity of the insane, and the gentle treatment which would guide them back to sanity. They also show that the system was not gentle in everything; kindness to the patients was to be achieved through severity toward the keepers – who were almost certainly convicts.

The instructions to both officers addressed the fragility of the situation. 'It is hoped,' Macquarie wrote to Suttor, 'that you will pay every proper attention to that gentleman' – William Bland – 'and to his instructions in regard to the treatment of the patients in your joint care.' It was this problem of joint care that would haunt the institution. The surgeon was given responsibility for 'the health of the unfortunate patients', and instructed to 'cultivate a good understanding' with Suttor, 'co-operating with [him] in the care, management and proper humane treatment' of the patients. It was 'of the utmost importance to the good management of the asylum that a good and friendly understanding should subsist'. Bland was sent a copy of Suttor's instructions to this end. Each was to make minimal monthly reports to the governor, the surgeon on the number and health of the patients, 'and whether any are likely to recover', and the superintendent, simply, on 'the number and state of the lunatics', noting any 'casualties, increase or decrease as may have occurred during the preceding month'.[39] The surviving reports offer two or three clipped sentences on the patients, and note any staffing changes.[40]

There had been a vacuum of authority at the outset, and now everything was pressing in on the little asylum. The governor who had shown little interest in the previous three years now laid down its intimate rhythms. Patients were to wash their hands and faces each morning and to 'shave and put on clean linen twice every week, namely on Sundays and Thursdays'.[41] And two officers had been appointed and told to cultivate a good relationship while circumstances guaranteed that they trod on each other's toes. It was hardly surprising that 'a state of ill-will soon developed', as W. D. Neil writes in her history of the asylum.[42] After five months, in February 1815, a small conflagration over religious worship offered a glimpse of the institutional tension. Bland, learning that Suttor was conducting a service with the patients, stormed in crying that he could 'read to the bare-wall for not a dam'd soul of them should stop' for the liturgy.[43] Both men wrote to Macquarie in protest. The reply was diplomatic; permission had in fact been given for the services, but perhaps there had been some failure to communicate this to the surgeon. Bland was no doubt irked at the request he would 'therefore have the goodness to promote this object' and encourage whatever patients 'as may be in a suitable state of mind for devotion' to attend.[44] Appalled by conditions at the asylum, and further vexed by the staffing arrangements, Bland managed to quit while still a convict under sentence, in August 1815. Macquarie gave permission for him to live anywhere in the colony he liked, and on receiving his pardon in October, he set up a private practice in Sydney, though maintaining an interest in mental health and recognised, in time, as a specialist.[45]

Bland was replaced by another serving convict, Henry Ravenscroft, a naval surgeon who had been transported in 1813 for petty larceny.[46] Ravenscroft worked at the asylum between August 1815 and March 1817, when he was caught embezzling patient bedding.[47] Another convict followed. Arriving in Sydney in early 1816 on the *Fanny*, Thomas Parmeter was part way through a seven-year sentence for bigamy. Parmeter was anxious to improve his circumstances, and petitioned Macquarie for a pardon immediately on arrival.[48] In May 1817, a month after he began at the asylum, he again requested a pardon on the grounds that the patients would give a free doctor greater respect.[49] New South Wales was an unusual society; while historians have disproved the standard 19th-century claims that asylums were staffed by the dregs of society, here asylum attendants were highly likely to be current or former convicts,[50] since the doctors in authority over them were. It has been suggested that it was this aversion to convicts that lay at the root of the conflict between Suttor and Bland, and then Suttor and Parmeter.[51] Certainly, given the qualms expressed elsewhere at patients being treated by persons of lower social standing, Castle Hill cannot have been attractive to families of the free insane. Macquarie was apparently unperturbed by the divisions in the staff and patient population, however, and Parmeter's pardon was not forthcoming.

The relationship between Suttor and Parmeter quickly became toxic. Just six months after starting at the asylum, Parmeter looked for the support of the medical department, and the principal surgeon, to establish his supremacy at Castle Hill. He was 'anxious to try the effect of medicine', he said, but was 'more and more prevented by the grossly ignorant and improper actions on the part of the Superintendent from effecting the purpose of so excellent an institution'. The patients, he wished someone would tell Suttor, 'ought to be entirely under my direction'. With a few more partitions and a coat of whitewash, the asylum could house double its current number in comfort (some were at this point 'sleeping in a hot kitchen'), who could in turn be properly classified as manic, melancholic, epileptic – or female. This would 'facilitate my attempts to recover or relieve their several maladies' and even render the asylum worthy of a visit by the governor and principal surgeon. 'And I should feel delighted admitting', added Parmeter smoothly, 'that I had that complete management of the asylum … being fully authorized by His Excellency the Governor to have the entire management of the patients, and to be obeyed by the keepers.' Suttor would need 'confining … to the very letter of his instructions – that is of delivering out their rations and keeping the patients clean &c'.[52] It was an innovative interpretation of Macquarie's instructions.

In the 1850s, the influential American superintendent Thomas Story Kirkbride wrote about the difficulty of sharing authority in a lunatic asylum. He derided the physician 'who voluntarily confined his attention to the mere medical direction of the patients'. Such a man, he continued, 'must have a very imperfect appreciation of his true position. He becomes, in reality, a very secondary kind of officer, and his functions will be pretty sure to be considered by many around him, as quite subordinate in importance.'[53] Parmeter, by contrast, appreciated the doctor's role perfectly.

Suttor had some altercation with Parmeter, possibly on learning of these industrial machinations. Parmeter complained to the principal surgeon, who in turn complained to the governor. 'I shall send for Mr Sutter,' Macquarie replied (misspelling his name), 'and reprimand him severely for his outrageous and insulting conduct to poor Parmeter; and shall warn him that he will be dismissed from his situation in case he ever insults Dr Parmeter again.'[54] The specifics of the dressing-down were not recorded, but its tenor is quite clear.

The asylum continued as the battleground of its two senior officers. In June 1818, some eight months later, while they were collecting firewood, a Portuguese man called Francisco kicked Griffiths, 'an idiot', in the shins. Griffiths struck Francisco three times in the back of the head with an axe, and 'the Portuguese maniac' was found lying on his face outside the asylum walls, surrounded by several patients. The keeper meant to attend them had been given some other task by Suttor. Parmeter requested urgent repairs to the asylum walls to help prevent anything of the kind happening again. 'I will make but one simple remark,' he added after his report, written that evening. He had objected more than once to the patients fetching firewood, 'particularly when the superintendent has two government men and a cart' that could be put to the purpose. 'Assuredly so long as patients can be put to labour, in defiance to my instructions to the contrary,' he finished, 'the desired influence of the surgeon, is but a secondary consideration, in the minds of the keepers of the patients.'[55] He gave another turn of the screw at the coroner's inquest which followed: '[I] conceive that Francisco might yet have been alive, had my repeated regulations (in conformity to His Excellency the Governor's instructions) been attended to.'[56] And he made yet more from Francisco's demise by writing the 'melancholy catastrophe' into verse: 'The Portuguese Maniac', a movement in his longer work, 'The Asylum'.[57]

The situation at the asylum grew tense. At the general muster of land and stock at the Red Cow Inn, Parramatta, in November 1818, Suttor told a friend that he would sacrifice all of his property to see Parmeter ruined. Parmeter, meanwhile, informed the governor that patient rations were being exchanged for tobacco. Macquarie was 'cross' about it, crosser than he had been in 1814. He enclosed with his reply 'an open letter of reprimand to Mr Suttor', which he hoped, rather blithely, would 'be the means of restoring peace and harmony between them'.[58] Instead, Suttor made formal charges against Parmeter, and the governor, no doubt annoyed, instructed Hannibal Macarthur, as magistrate at Parramatta, to investigate. At this point, Parmeter, who had already delegated many of his asylum duties to an untrained youth called Peter Cook, left the asylum altogether. Suttor 'might be damn'd and the place, too', Suttor recalled him saying. 'He did not care a damn for the thirty pounds a year', had only taken it as a favour to the principal surgeon, and had asked repeatedly for a new position.[59]

Macarthur conducted an inquiry in December 1818 and January 1819 at the Court House, Parramatta. Suttor told of how Parmeter had misappropriated soap, wine, tea and other asylum stores for his own use. Patients and the asylum laundry had been forced to do without soap for weeks at a stretch. Parmeter was visiting less and less frequently, so that even dying patients had to do without medical assistance or the comforts that only Parmeter was authorised to prescribe. His defence and countercharges were delivered in a written statement that has not been retained, but their thrust is clear enough from his witnesses. The image emerges, between questions and answers, of Suttor showing a rather too flexible notion of occupational therapy, with patients working at his own property to cultivate the garden, wash sheep and bring in the harvest. He seems to have invited patients to drink cider with him and his wife after work; perhaps his wife drank too much.

Much was made of Suttor's angry words at the muster. Not denying that he had said them, Suttor asked each witness in turn whether he had actually sacrificed anything to ruin Parmeter and whether he, Suttor, 'was a maliciously disposed fellow'. He had not and was not, each witness confirmed, except for his neighbour Thomas McDougall, who said simply: 'I am of opinion that Mr Suttor is.'[60] The response is curious, since when McDougall's mother had died that month, Suttor had been one of the few friends at the burial.[61] Suttor was also found to have dismissed a keeper for obeying Parmeter against his express orders and going to Sydney.[62]

It seems that Suttor, Parmeter, and even Bland sought modest advantage through mild exploitation of the asylum patients, though Suttor claimed that Parmeter had done it with abandon, refusing to discharge recovered patients in order to retain their labour as 'emoluments'.[63] The asylum salaries were hardly lucrative, but they were secure. (Parmeter entered private practice after he left the asylum, but suffered a serious riding accident and slid into penury, to wrote ruefully in time of his 'easy birth [sic]' at Castle Hill.)[64] Parmeter appears to have also been misallocating wine, sugar, and soap. His more serious failing, however, was his pursuit of authority at the expense of every therapeutic ideal. Bryan Newland, a patient who said he had been '*perfectly well*' for some time and 'long wished to be *discharged* from the *asylum*', complained that when he had refused to work for Parmeter at his house, '*the Dr shaved his head* thro' spite'. When Newland said he would have revenge when he left the asylum, Parmeter replied that 'he would take care' that he 'never should be discharged', and placed him in solitary confinement for a day and a half. David Tennant, another patient who appeared 'perfectly sensible and sober and perfectly in his senses' to the court, verified Newland's complaint and added his own. For eight of his twelve months at the asylum he had run errands for Parmeter to Sydney, the Hawkesbury, Portland Head, Cabramatta and elsewhere, driving cattle and collecting parcels. He had also ploughed 6 acres at Parmeter's house. He had never been paid, and when he once refused to work, the doctor had his head shaved.[65] Head-shaving was a common means of standardising and sterilising inmates in 19th-century institutions; pupils, prisoners and patients found themselves shorn en masse.[66] Wherever it was not standard, however, as at Castle Hill, shaving served as a punishment, demonstrating the control of authority even over the body of the inmate, producing shame. It was most powerful, and culturally revealing, when practised upon women.[67]

A keeper corroborated these accounts and offered a chilling fragment of conversation. 'If I say you are mad to day,' the surgeon was recorded telling Newland, 'you shall be mad, and if I say you shall be well tomorrow, you shall be well, and if I order you to walk upon your head, you shall walk upon it.' When Newland said he did not 'want to be kept in the asylum, as I am not mad', Parmeter replied that he would remain 'as long as he was surgeon'.[68] He had another patient whipped for stealing clothing, tin pots and plates.[69]

For Francis Willis, the famed specialist who treated George III, once a patient was initially 'impressed with the notion of fear', even the 'menacing look of a very expressive countenance' was enough. Therapeutic power emanated from the superintendent's 'eye'.[70] Parmeter was either less proficient, or his patients were less impressionable.

Although these measures appear to have been intended to demonstrate mastery, they may have actually undermined Parmeter's authority. Self-control was crucial to the semblance of authority in early psychological theory: a superintendent might need to express calmness and anger in turn, but he must remain always in control of his emotions. Johan Henrik Seidelin, who developed a 'mental cure technique' based upon fear in the 1810s, was dismissed from the Sankt Hans Hospital near Copenhagen when he lost control in a therapeutic beating, 'screaming continuously that [his patient] should shut up and stand still'.[71] The new moral therapy hinged upon training patients in self-government, which required an unerring 'presentation of self'.[72]

The conflict emerging in the court of inquiry clearly confused the keepers about the division of authority at the asylum.[73] Joseph Cooper, the convict keeper who was dismissed by Suttor and arrested after running an errand to Sydney for Parmeter, said plaintively, 'Having two masters, I did not know which to obey.'[74] Another 'even declared', Parmeter complained, 'that he has orders not to obey any instructions I may give him provided Mr. Suttor thinks proper to countermand them'.[75] Parmeter's volatility, and the impossible orders to obey or disobey one or other of the officers, meant that there was no clear authority within the asylum.

Parmeter's campaign for therapeutic reforms and for a singular medical authority over the asylum appear to have been a mask for his careerism. His rhetoric is belied by his actions, and the inquest found little evidence of any form of therapy at Castle Hill. Hannibal Macarthur concluded that both parties had neglected their duties, and Macquarie reasserted the authority of government, dismissing both men on 15 February 1819. He then appointed a new resident superintendent and a surgeon to visit the institution from a safe distance.[76]

Though Macarthur's report and Macquarie's actions suggest that these higher authorities were perplexed at the state of affairs at Castle Hill, it is hardly surprising in retrospect. In the former therapeutic ideal, the asylum was to be under the strict control of an authority figure who would terrorise the patient into submission. In the new ideal, the asylum was the site in which rational, calm interaction could be modelled, underwritten by the authority and charisma of the superintendent.[77] In both formulations, singular authority was fundamental to the institution, modelled and even exaggerated by the complete obedience of asylum staff.

At the zenith of moral therapy in the mid 19th-century, Thomas Kirkbride wrote emphatically about the importance of the superintendent's absolute control of all facets of the asylum.[78] He developed complex organisational structures to establish and protect this authority, which extended to the most minute details at the establishment.[79] 'The simple possession of adequate authority,' Kirkbride wrote, 'often prevents the necessity for its being exercised. It may be unseen and unfelt, and yet a knowledge of its existence, will often alone prevent wrangling and difficulties in the household, and secure regularity, good order, and an efficient discipline about the whole establishment.'[80]

By the same token, the absence of 'adequate authority', as manifest in major disputes and public reprimands but also in minor infractions and a steady stream of whispers and accusations, undermined therapeutic space. Conflicts between asylum staff were frequently catastrophic.[81] Every aspect of the asylum – the interactions between staff, and between staff and external officials, as much as the medicine and therapies – had a powerful effect on patients that was 'not readily appreciated by a careless observer'.[82] Even a careless observer, or an underkeeper like Joseph Cooper, could readily appreciate that dividing authority between two officers led to industrial conflict; it does not appear that anyone linked this division to the patients' chances of recovery – except for Parmeter, whose motives were suspect.

The tenor and extent of authority were natural concerns in institutions which sought to wrestle with human will, first violently, and then with a paternal authoritarianism. The petty conflicts between the inferior officers at Castle Hill may be partly accounted for by the difference in their conditions, as Best argues in his article on the asylum, or by the mercenary undercurrents in colonial society.[83] Suttor was a free settler, while all the doctors he served with were current convicts, no doubt anxious to assert their authority in the face of their 'condition', and all apparently eager to obtain pardons and quit the small-time asylum with its lay superintendent. Focusing on the therapeutic significance of authority, however, opens the view from these conflicts to reveal the broader forces shaping the treatment of madness in New South Wales.

Like Kirkbride's careless observers, perhaps, these colonial authorities did not 'see' the need for a careful configuration of authority within the asylum. Neither fear nor strong authority featured in the treatment of the colony's insane. It is possible that this assertive, military-style government left little room for authority at the peripheries. Certainly other forms of authority struggled to find purchase, including the authority of an independent judiciary, the moral authority of the press, and the agency of private citizens. The therapeutic deficiencies of early Australian asylums issued, finally, from the legal and political structures established for a penal colony and from the preoccupations of colonial government. These conditions impinged not only upon abstract political institutions but upon concrete social institutions and the men and women who inhabited them. Critically, they manifested in the theoretical and practical efforts of men like George Suttor, William Bland and Thomas Parmeter, as they each vied for the authority they felt was necessary to manage the patients at Castle Hill, and to attend to the mental illness of a penal colony.

When John Thomas Bigge conducted his commission of enquiry into New South Wales in 1819–20, he reported on the medical establishments as well as the numerous other facets of colonial society. Between October 1819 and December 1820, twenty patients had been added to the thirty-nine in the asylum. Of these, five had died, eight were discharged, and ten had escaped. Thirty-six remained.[84] The death rate was high; the rate of escape was very high. The figures suggest inadequate care and inadequate structural attention. It was not a satisfactory asylum, and Macquarie told the commissioner of his plan to close the asylum, first mooted five years earlier. Bigge said this should 'be effected with all convenient expedition', since the patients had little medical attention and the building was 'dilapidated' inside and out.[85] The plan they thought best – to remove prisoners from Parramatta Gaol to a new building 'with better accommodation and stronger walls' and to turn the old building into an asylum – was not without irony.[86] In one of the two main rooms of Parramatta Gaol, the floor, window shutters, and gratings all bore the scars of the 'wanton mischief of the prisoners'. The whole was 'old and very ill-built'. Part of the encircling wall had fallen down, and four prisoners had escaped through the grating of one of the privies. It was perfect.

BIGGE'S REPORTS WERE CRITICAL OF MACQUARIE, AND IN 1820 the Colonial Office accepted the resignation that Macquarie had been trying to submit for years. Returning to London in some disgrace, Macquarie worked hard to defend his reputation against his detractors. 'I found the colony barely emerging from infantile imbecility,' he wrote, 'and suffering from various privations and disabilities.'[87] He had worked to treat its ailments and to build up the society, through physical institutions as well as more subtle measures. For a man who took great pride in his work, however, he found little pleasure in the asylum. It was near the end of the list of 152 construction works he had completed in the colony which he sent to Earl Bathurst in 1822. After Sydney, and Parramatta, and the little settlements circling out from there, the last place listed before the distant outposts of Newcastle and Port Macquarie was the site of the old farm.

> At 'Castlehill'
>
> The old government barn, new roofed and repaired and converted into a '*lunatic asylum*,' being properly fitted up *as such* for the accommodation of 30 patients with a court for the lunatics to walk in, surrounded by a strong stockade …
>
> N.B. – 'Castle Hill' is distant seven miles from Parramatta.[88]

Even cast in its best possible light, it was hard to see the asylum as a proper institution for the treatment of the insane. Bigge, in his report, called it the 'receptacle of lunatics at Castle Hill', which is more accurate, although, with the frequency of death and escape, not entirely correct.[89]

Macquarie's departure, and the censure of the bulk of his public works by Bigge and the Colonial Office, made future spending difficult. This broader censure militated against many of Bigge's recommendations, so that no new gaol was built, and the patients remained at the 'lunatic asylum' at Castle Hill. Arriving in late 1821, the new governor, Thomas Brisbane, pursued more moderate policies in the colony, and more moderate public works, although, according to Edward Hall, writing in the *Monitor*, Brisbane quickly 'became deeply impressed with the necessity of building a lunatic asylum'.[90] None was built, however, and by early 1825, a delegation of local colonists found the lunatic asylum in a dire state. Far too small for its forty patients, there were still few subdivisions, making classification nigh impossible, and the building was in an 'extreme state of dilapidation', in a 'ruinous condition'. It was patently inadequate to comfort or even keep its patients.[91] In August a second deputation, including George Suttor and his son, reiterated 'the total inadequacy of the building to the purposes of the establishment'. It was too far from fresh water and from medical attention, lacked supplies and comforts, and housed thirty-five lunatics under the charge of one 'keeper' who was frequently called away to other duties. A copper boiler for the laundry was needed, and a cart for drawing firewood (more than a year after it was plaintively requested).[92]

The nature of the institution at Castle Hill was never made clear, and, with talk of abandoning it beginning soon after it opened, it had never been a place of fixity. It was nebulous and undefined, like the madness it was meant to secure. At the periphery of the colonial township, the building which had failed to contain convict sedition failed to contain madness. Even the refuge it might have offered was compromised by the frustration, and probable neurosis, of its officers, thrust into a situation that was hardly tenable by a governor who commiserated with the unhappiness of the insane but, between Enlightenment ideals and colonial realities, did not know what to do with them. When the governor who had created the asylum in 1811 enclosed it in inverted commas in 1822, it was a testament to the indistinct nature of the institution. It points also to the way that its substance finally eludes us in the writing of history. The asylum at Castle Hill was an absence, an empty shell into which individuals and authorities poured their expectations. We, too, have filled it imaginatively with what might have been its intellectual and material heritage, and used it for something other than care – to show how, lacking medicine, supplies, and the requisite authority for effective treatment, it suggests there was little real effort to treat madness in the colony. Always inadequate, always in the shadow of evacuation, its requests denied and its staff left to manage irrational patients but succumbing to their own internal flaws, the lunatic asylum at Castle Hill was little more than a vacant space where an answer might have stood.

5

THE POLITICS OF A PENAL COLONY

In 1787, King George III entrusted the figment of British imagination referred to as New South Wales to Arthur Phillip, a post-captain with a reputation for honesty, bravery, and self-sacrifice. He would lead the colonisation of the Australian continent as the head of a military-style government.[1] New South Wales was constituted as a crown colony and governed with the same limited rights and liberties as those which were ceded by conquest. This system was used, with modifications, wherever a colonial society was considered so immature or divided that representative government would be problematic.[2] It was hard for those in London to imagine a society where self-government would be more dangerous: the 'first fleet' consisted almost entirely of convicts and soldiers, groups drawn from similar social backgrounds. More convicts arrived each year, and those who served out their sentences generally lacked the means to return, and sometimes the inclination. It was considered that proper respect for law or government was unlikely in such a 'commonwealth of thieves', and metropolitan suspicions of Botany Bay remained strong for half a century and longer.[3]

Crown colonies had a strong executive government, a weak judiciary, and either a feeble legislature subordinate to London, or, like New South Wales, none at all. Autocratic governors operated under precise instructions from London; so precise that the crown colony configuration in Trinidad was castigated as 'colonial office government'.[4] And this was not far off the mark. Crown colonies lacked representative local government, and policy was made by a secretary (or minister) and a handful of parliamentary undersecretaries in London via a governor *in situ*, none of whom answered to those they governed. In New South Wales, established as a place of penal discipline, the governors were entrusted with particularly expansive powers, and, from Arthur Phillip through to Lachlan Macquarie, had more power than those who administered other colonies, and more power within New South Wales than any English monarch since the 16th century.[5]

Madness, when it manifested, challenged even such robust powers as these governors enjoyed. Disruptive, difficult and unpredictable, it divided people, including those ranged in positions of authority in the colony, from the governor and colonial secretary through to the institutional superintendents and subordinate staff and the magistrates who wielded much of the effective power. Working around these official authorities, with their commissions and instructions, were those who made the quieter decisions which history does not always notice: the mad themselves, whom we often cannot reach, and their families, who suffered with them. All of these actors, agents and decision-makers were held in the firm, shrewd grip of the Colonial Office, which cast formal and informal lines of power across the globe. New South Wales was a tiny colony at the edge of the Pacific, but its politics – high, middle, and low – were complex, and, in places, perverse. By demanding urgent, decisive action, madness brought these politics into view and often revealed the contradictions that inhabited them.

MICHAEL HOARE AND JAMES GILCHRIST 'FELONIOUSLY and burglariously' broke into the schoolhouse at Kissing Point, in what would become Ryde, in October 1815 and stole some clothing and other sundries; in time this event would resound throughout the empire. Although they pleaded guilty, each was sentenced to one year in solitary confinement at Parramatta Gaol, two years on a gaol gang, and then transportation for life to a penal settlement.[6] Samuel Marsden, who as chief magistrate at Parramatta had oversight of the gaol where they would begin their sentences, warned Macquarie that these 'very extraordinary & heavy punishments' would kill the prisoners. Worse, they had been published in the *Sydney Gazette* and were likely to 'attract the eye of some person in power & call for public notice & animadversion'.[7] Macquarie was not prepared to interfere with the ruling of the court. He had been tasked not only with restoring order in New South Wales after the rebellion, but with establishing a clarity which the rough configuration of colonial law and government had never enjoyed. To interfere in the sentences of the criminal court, he told Marsden, would be to 'interpose what would be justly termed an illegal and tyrannical exercise of the powers vested in me'.[8]

For all the power enjoyed by Lachlan Macquarie, his government was subject to the direct authority of London, and it was responsive, in turn, to the demands of colonists with influential connections, and to shifts in British politics. These played themselves out not only in direct exchanges in the colony, but in the many carefully written letters which crossed the oceans. Scholars associated with the 'new imperial history' work to map the networks into which these letters fed – humanitarian, scientific, military and administrative networks, which, as they show, stretched across the empire. The success of colonial projects typically depended on the reach of these networks, but so too did the business of governing the empire. There was the formal correspondence between officials in London and the colonies, but an older school of undersecretaries also encouraged their colonial counterparts to write to them unofficially.[9] This layered government correspondence competed with a continuous volley of unsolicited letters as people of every rank sought leverage from their connections – aristocrats, members of parliament, church leaders, prominent scientists and military officers.[10]

In early March 1816, dissatisfied with Macquarie's response, Marsden took a disgruntled colonist on a tour of Parramatta Gaol, where the first phase of those extraordinary punishments had begun two months prior. His guest was Nicholas Bayly, a second son in an illustrious family who had been favoured with a free commission in the New South Wales Corps in 1797. After a string of missteps in the colony involving alcohol and cruelty to his convict servants, he resigned his commission in 1803. He nevertheless lent strong support to his former comrades in the 'little revolution', and was rewarded with public office and a large land grant.[11] When Macquarie arrived to reassert imperial control of the wayward colony, winding back the rebels' cronyism and cancelling such land grants and appointments, Bayly's grant remained intact, perhaps due to his family connections.[12] He was not, however, a successful merchant or grazier like other rebels, and without a salary he was left with a large estate he could not afford to maintain. After six years of Macquarie's administration he therefore returned to the offensive, dispatching a scathing letter to Henry Bunbury, undersecretary of state, which reported on the suffering of prisoners at the gaol. 'Horrid to relate I saw a prisoner who had nearly lost the use of his limbs and faculties by confinement on bread and water', and in another cell, 'a prisoner perfectly mad, chained to the wall'. Bayly drew attention also to four 'dreadful sentences', including those of Hoare and Gilchrist, and pointed out that a bread-and-water diet had been proven to damage the faculties in less than six months.[13]

The year prior, a parliamentary committee had exposed a wealth of abuse in English asylums and madhouses, forcing the superintendent and apothecary of Bethlem Hospital to resign.[14] The Retreat in York had been established in 1792 by Yorkshire Quakers after similar abuse was uncovered against one of their brethren in the local asylum. Its methods and critiques were receiving new attention after Samuel Tuke, grandson of the founder, published an account of it in 1813.[15] Prison reform was also a growing parliamentary force, building on the work of advocates like John Howard, the prophet of the prisons and workhouses, and George Onesiphorus Paul, a pioneer of separate imprisonment and prison medicine.[16]

Bayly's letter drew upon this reformist energy, but to connect these abuses with Macquarie was to invoke also the spectre of colonial despotism. Despotism loomed over British domestic politics, argues legal historian Lauren Benton, because it cast doubt over the legitimacy of empire. The character of governors represented political capital – or political liability – for the home government, and charges like Bayly's were 'potent political weapons in conflicts over the structure of rule'.[17] This may be why Earl Bathurst, Bunbury's superior, became so interested in the suffering of prisoners in Parramatta Gaol. He sent anonymised extracts to Macquarie, warning, as he did, that they reflected 'to a great degree your character and conduct in the administration of the colony'.[18] Macquarie had already shown a tendency to over-brisk governance in various public clashes with the judicial officers of the colony, and the memory of William Bligh lingered.[19] He received the extracts in late August 1817, finding the accusations 'very insulting', as he told his wife.[20] He set about gathering evidence, and had affidavits prepared by the key actors: the judge, the constable, the magistrate, the asylum superintendent and Michael Hoare, who was not the 'perfectly mad' prisoner Bayly had written about, but quickly took centre stage.

Before legislation called for direct medical input, it was very often local magistrates who were responsible for judging and acting on madness, in the metropole and colonies alike. This is why, in January 1816, after only thirteen of his 365 days of solitary confinement, when Michael Hoare showed symptoms of violent insanity, the gaoler reported it to Samuel Marsden. As chief magistrate at Parramatta, Marsden had the oversight of both the gaol and the asylum at Castle Hill – and the power to move inmates between them. The local surgeon, Major West, spent little time at the gaol, burdened by other duties and chronic illness. He would not visit for days or even weeks, according to Marsden, and in consequence the gaol hospital was 'in a state of great filth & disorder'. Marsden examined Hoare several times with Henry Ravenscroft, surgeon at the asylum, who thought he should be admitted there and sent a keeper and cart. Marsden ordered the gaoler to 'let Hoare be sent', subject to the agreement of Major West.[21] Bringing an emaciated Hoare to the asylum on 29 January 1816, the keeper, quite remarkably, told superintendent George Suttor that Hoare had been very violent 'but was supposed to be an impostor'.[22] Supposed by whom? Suttor treated Hoare guardedly, with 'all the indulgence and care that the lunatics received', but came to agree: the man spoke rationally and behaved well, though he had a 'weak understanding and an irritable mind'. At one point he was handcuffed after threatening a keeper and became 'noisy', but promised he would be quiet if he were released. And he was. 'He exhibited no signs of insanity,' Suttor decided, 'and was an impostor.'[23]

Suttor reported back to Marsden, but one of the keepers told Hoare that his sham was up and that he would be sent back to gaol. He promptly escaped, on 2 April 1816, taking with him 'a considerable quantity of cloathing' belonging to another patient.[24] That he could do so, despite the staff's suspicions, indicates the poor security of the building. Within a fortnight he was caught being 'burglarious' again, and arrested at Gregory Blaxland's farm. Returned to solitary confinement, he brazenly reprised his earlier tactics and was rewarded with heavy irons, and chained to the wall. The gaoler called on Marsden again to say that those in and near the gaol were being 'greatly disturbed by his violent noise night and day, but particularly in the nights'. He had wrenched an iron bar loose from his window and used it to destroy most of his cell. 'If something were not done with Hoare,' he warned, 'he would pull down the end of the gaol.' After examining him, Marsden thought he was ill. 'I at this time believed the prisoner to be raving mad,' he later recorded, 'and that he ought to be returned to the lunatic asylum.' Instead, he ordered Hoare into the gaolers' lodge with proper food and 'a little extra attention' – whatever was 'best calculated for his support under such a situation'. It was a course of treatment offered to a patient, not one of discipline imposed on a prisoner, and Hoare indeed 'became more rational'. Marsden, clearly following events closely, then ordered Hoare into the main gaol with freedom to exercise in the yard, and 'under this treatment he recovered from his real or apparent insanity'.[25] Many doctors would have prescribed the same: food and exercise, trust and a respectful but firm dialogue.[26] In August 1817 the sentences of Michael Hoare and James Gilchrist were remitted by Macquarie, and Hoare became, as he told another magistrate later that year, 'as much at liberty as any other convict in the colony'.[27]

Frederick Garling, who was acting judge advocate after Ellis Bent died in office, claimed that the severe sentences of Gilchrist, Hoare and others were tailored to the savagery of the crime, but also handed down in hope of reformation. Solitary imprisonment, which worked Enlightenment and theological principles into an increasingly elaborate penal theory, had gained increasing traction since the 1770s.[28] Prisoners were to dwell on their histories and, between a dawning awareness of God's gracious but exacting forgiveness and the arithmetic of personal cost and benefit, would willingly align themselves with moral society.[29] Prisoners, that is, were compelled to reform themselves. Garling put it this way: 'leisure for contemplation' would afford the prisoners 'a due sense of their evil and depraved habits and induce a resolution to reform their lives'. In this event, 'it would always be in the power of the executive authority in this colony to mitigate further their sentence' and Macquarie, as the good judge noted, was 'always forward' in exercising this prerogative.[30] If prisoners came to harm – as Garling tacitly admitted was possible – gaol doctors were available to tend to them. It was an idealistic and inefficient scheme: the courts handing down extreme sentences to force repentance; gaolers overseeing the manufacture of despair; a governor descending in mercy with his robust executive power; and doctors in attendance, to preserve life.

Garling's penal philosophy was somewhat confused. His main contention was that the convicts in question were practically irredeemable. Hoare and Gilchrist, especially, had arrived as convicts for life, and had 'persisted in their evil ways', joining up with 'a banditti, who marauded about in the woods' – bushrangers.[31] They were 'men of the most alarming and dangerous description, who, lost to all sense of moral or social duties, live by plundering the honest settler of the property he may have acquired by his industry'. In a penal colony, bushrangers were not merry men.[32] But this line was rather undercut by the fact that two others, also convicts for life but without such magnificent recalcitrance, had been handed the same sentences three months prior, for breaking, entering and taking away their plunder in a cart. It was simply 'difficult', wrote Garling, 'to inflict any additional punishment on men, situated as these prisoners were'. They had earned execution and even madness, perhaps, was a mercy. Besides, sentencing was by majority of the bench, Garling added as a plaintive postscript, of at least 5-2 in capital crimes. The judge advocate had no particular sway over the six military officers who joined him on the bench. His chief responsibility was to advise on points of law, and even these were subject to the decision of the bench.[33] In his audit of court records during the Commission of Inquiry, some years later, commissioner Bigge found that sentences under Garling's short tenure as acting judge advocate strayed from the court's characteristic 'humanity and tenderness'. In addition to the sentences in question, four prisoners received twelve months in solitary, a fifth received two years, and four others were handed the absurd, fatal sentences of three years in solitary confinement.[34] There was some reformist desire in the members of the court, Bigge noted quietly, to replace flogging and transportation with solitary imprisonment.

Macquarie did eventually intervene in the sentences of Michael Hoare and the others, ensuring they were only 'partially and very leniently executed'. The majority were 'mitigated, or entirely remitted, by my authority', he explained to London. This was not on account of the men's repentance but because Macquarie had no faith in the means of grace. The sentences were simply so very '*severe*'. He never 'sanctioned or allowed sanguinary or cruel punishments', and had 'frequently interposed my authority, either in mitigation or total suspension of sentences, when I conceived I could with propriety do so, and that the circumstances of the case merited humane consideration'.[35] Macquarie issued 366 absolute pardons, 1365 conditional pardons and 2319 tickets-of-leave in his eleven years, while William Bligh, in his eighteen months as governor, had granted only two pardons.[36] Even corrected for time in office, Macquarie had a different algorithm for, in his turn of phrase, the 'mingling of mercy with justice'.

IT WAS A TIME OF CONSIDERABLE STRAIN. MACQUARIE WAS aware of the growing stream of letters being written to London about him by disaffected colonists. On 1 December 1817, he wrote his own, warning the Colonial Office about 'discontented and seditious' individuals. Marsden, whom he had cleared of everything in Hoare's case except being the 'dupe of a schemer', was nevertheless the first name on the list: 'discontented, intriguing, vindictive'. There were eleven others on the list; Bayly was third. All twelve had 'long been in the habit of writing *home* the most gross misrepresentations'.[37]

Macquarie had clashed with Marsden shortly after arriving in the colony, after the magistrate objected to serving with two former convicts on the Parramatta road turnpike board of trustees.[38] Both felt strongly about crime and emancipation. Their feud likely made Macquarie unreceptive to Marsden's sentencing advice, and when he read the anonymised extracts, he assumed that Marsden was the author; Ellis Bent sought in vain to convince him that Marsden wrote in a different style. The feud reached a climax in January 1818, only weeks after Macquarie sent the documents he had compiled on Hoare to London, when he learned that Marsden had taken depositions from the men he had (illegally) had flogged for trespassing in the Government

Domain. In a moment of rhetorical fury he banished Marsden, the head of a 'seditious low cabal', from his presence.[39]

These charges were vitally important to the Colonial Office. It was in 1817, as British criticism of the cost and management of convict transportation mounted, that Earl Bathurst moved to appoint a formal Commission of Inquiry into convict transportation and the colony of New South Wales.[40] His instructions noted the 'ill considered compassion for convicts' preventing the penal colony from performing its function – imperial terror – but the commission also became an opportunity for a thorough investigation of the colony's progress.[41] During the course of his inquiries, commissioner Bigge inquired yet further into the treatment of Michael Hoare. But madness is difficult to pin down, not least after the passage of several years, and Bigge found nothing new about Hoare himself. He did, however, learn more about the confrontational relationships between gaol, court, medicine, magistrate and government, which the prospect of madness had brought into focus. Bigge tacitly rebuked Marsden's reliance on the medical opinion of Ravenscroft, who had since been caught embezzling patients' bedclothes and sent to the penal settlement at Newcastle.[42] Brushing aside the point of West's availability, he concluded: 'It seems somewhat extraordinary, that Mr. Marsden should have taken upon himself to decide upon his insanity without a previous reference to Mr. West'. For it was not an isolated incident; Marsden and other magistrates had moved prisoners to the asylum 'upon their own view' and 'whenever their custody in the gaol became a cause of annoyance and disturbance to the other prisoners, or to the neighbourhood'. Such cavalier usage presented a real risk since, as Bigge had seen for himself, the asylum was even more dilapidated than the gaol. Marsden should have consulted properly with the surgeon, and consulted with Macquarie, who in turn should have sought instruction from the Court of Criminal Jurisdiction and the judge advocate and relayed their decision back to Marsden and the staff of the gaol and asylum.[43] The commissioner was describing a complex theoretical bureaucracy in a place of practical disarray.

It is surprising that Bigge should find any of this extraordinary. In England, magistrates were the main gateway to the asylums. The County Asylums Act 1808 made local, amateur magistrates responsible for arranging funds, land and building contracts; they administered the poor law and were empowered to send people to the asylums.[44] This diffusion of responsibility was perfectly in keeping with the popular desire for local decision-making.[45] It was only in 1819, while Bigge was in New South Wales, that a new English Act required the signatures of two justices of the peace and a doctor before a pauper could be committed.[46] Notwithstanding Bigge's alarm, this law did not work its way into colonial legislation until the Dangerous Lunatics Act 1843, which will feature in the final chapter. Bigge was generally critical of both magistrates at Parramatta, Hannibal Macarthur and Samuel Marsden, which may have coloured his assessment, but he was working to demonstrate that the colonial magistracy was out of control.[47]

HOARE'S CASE OFFERS A REVEALING VISION OF THE POWER of the colonial magistrates at the turn of the 19th century. Magisterial power 'had always been the lynchpin of the convict system', as Lauren Benton and Lisa Ford write in their study of the place of magistrates in empire, but there was little capacity to control it.[48] By the 1810s, colonial magistrates enjoyed enormous authority, much of which was inconsistent with the tenor, and occasionally the letter, of English law.[49] Untrained, and selected precisely for their investment in local industry and politics, magistrates were regularly found to be working for private gain or, more alarmingly, for political ends. Under Macquarie there was conflict over the power of governor and magistrates to interfere with the situation of convicts, particularly in so drastic a manner as re-transportation to one of the harsh penal settlements.[50] So crucial to the spread of the rule of law throughout the empire, magistrates were beginning to threaten it, and to compromise whatever integrity and system there had been in convict labour and punishment.[51]

This realisation led to a series of colonial and imperial measures which were designed, as Benton and Ford show, not to reduce the power of the magistrates so much as to draw that power closer into the control of government. In New South Wales a balance had to be found between the effective discipline of convicts and their abuse by a self-interested class of wealthy landholders. Macquarie issued a circular in 1820 regulating magistrates' role in assignment and tickets-of-leave and limiting their authority to re-transport convicts, a particularly contentious plank in their raft of powers (and in his own).[52] Thomas Brisbane, Macquarie's successor, appointed new police magistrates who were easily controlled because they received stipends from their office as well as prestige. The New South Wales Act of 1823 implemented a number of Bigge's recommendations, so that the powers of magistrates acting alone were limited, but when two or more assembled as the Court of Quarter Sessions, they enjoyed summary power over all convict non-capital offences.[53] The Act also created a Supreme Court and gave it oversight over magisterial judgements, which the magistrates, who frequently strayed beyond what one called 'legal technicalities', resented.[54] A weak legislature was also created, and one of its first acts was to enumerate and standardise magisterial powers, so that single magistrates could punish with ten days at the treadmill; fifty lashes;

seven days in solitary on bread and water; or hard labour for seven months.[55]

In July 1824, after Bigge had come and gone, and Macquarie, too, Henry Fulton, another chaplain–magistrate, found and arrested 'a man, who calls himself Michael Hoar', who had been able to produce 'neither free pardon, certificate, emancipation or ticket of leave'. Few convicts shared Hoare's surname in these years, and the description seems to fit. The man said 'he came home a prisoner from the Isle of France' (Mauritius) and was punished for cow stealing in the colony, Fulton wrote to the colonial secretary. 'As he gives various contradictory accounts of himself I have thought it advisable to send him to Sydney that you may dispose of him.'[56] It has proven difficult to trace this man further, and to know, finally, whether he was a madman who needed treatment, or, as Macquarie called him, 'a schemer'.

COMMISSIONER BIGGE DECIDED THAT IT WAS REGRETTABLE that the governor had not listened to the magistrate, Samuel Marsden, 'and interposed the authority which he derived from his commission, for the purpose of mitigating punishments that it was plainly impossible or highly improper to execute'. The tussle between the jurisdictions of New South Wales is implied, but so too is the clear authority of the governor over sentencing. It was not so straightforward in practice, and Michael Hoare's case had revealed the practical and political difficulties of such interventions. The commissions gave similar authority over madness, entrusting governors with the care and custody of the insane, but this, too, was subject to practical limits. These often devolved from the formal authorities to those who were closest to the insane.

Settler colonies were places of exaggerated fixedness and

mobility, isolation and reworked community, and these themes shaped the life of their asylums.[57] These characteristics were even more pronounced in the penal colony of New South Wales, where family faltered at first; where ties were abruptly cut by transportation. It was a colony of actual or effective singleness. Those who sought to 'settle' in the midst of these exiles were even more isolated than settlers elsewhere. The new families which formed between convicts, soldiers, officers, merchants and whalers – and importantly, with Aboriginal people – were not what they had been. Families elsewhere tended to come together in at least a semi-secure environment. Here they gathered together against a storm of isolation, alienation and exile, of depression and derangement. Madness tested and strained family bonds; it might overflow in wretchedness and violence, but it could also prove the strength of love in difficult places. Madness reveals families in crisis, at their most intimate and stripped back.

The Leveys were a remarkable family. Several of the children of Deborah and Moses Lyon Levey, of Whitechapel, London, migrated to New South Wales, but not together. Some came as transported convicts, some as free migrants, but even those who were convicted seemed almost to be seeking a passage. The first to arrive in New South Wales was Solomon Levey, transported in 1813, aged nineteen, as an accessory to the theft of 90 pounds of tea in a wooden chest. He fared spectacularly well, buying a property in George Street for £400, a house in Kent Street and a piece of land, all before he received his free pardon on 8 February 1819. Three days later, he married Ann Jane Roberts, daughter of another wealthy emancipist, the proprietor of the King's Arms on Hunter and Castlereagh streets. Solomon continued to prosper as a storekeeper, shipbroker and agent.[58] Barnett Levey arrived in 1821, as probably the first free Jewish migrant to the Australian colonies. He was a successful businessman and banker, and is hailed as the 'father of the Australian theatre'.[59] Other siblings also migrated, including Isaac, who became a leader of the early Jewish community.

Several biographical pieces have been written about the Leveys but none about the eldest child, Samuel. He was convicted in 1821 of stealing a bundle of gowns, aprons, handkerchiefs, caps and a petticoat from a widow, while walking along Houndsditch in London's East End.[60] He had already served four years of a previous sentence on the hulk *Bellerophon*, and was sentenced to transportation. He arrived in Van Diemen's Land in December 1821, aged thirty.[61] Six months later, Solomon appears to have contrived to have his brother assigned to himself, and Samuel went to live with him and Ann in Sydney. They were in some strife, however. Solomon had advertised in August 1821 that he would no longer be liable for any debts Ann might incur.[62] (We can only wonder what might have precipitated this.) Still, Ann continued living with her husband and brother-in-law, but within a year, Samuel exacerbated things by assaulting Ann. Perhaps there was more than one incident, since Ann is reported as 'reluctant' to see Samuel punished, 'under the consideration that he was Insane'.

In 1817, John Thomas Campbell, colonial secretary, libelled the chaplain Samuel Marsden in an anonymous letter. Marsden won £200 in a civil suit but his London connections also worked behind the scenes, so that when Macquarie suggested Campbell might take on the vacant role (and salary) of provost marshal, the Colonial Office agreed, and appointed someone else to the senior position of colonial secretary.[63] The provost marshal had charge over the bodies of prisoners either awaiting trial or recently sentenced, and was responsible for carrying out the sentences of the courts. In this capacity, the keeper of Sydney Gaol wrote to Campbell about a prisoner awaiting trial who was proving difficult – Samuel Levey. Campbell passed the information to Frederick Goulburn, who had replaced him as colonial secretary. Levey had been 'a madman' for several months, he offered, and 'it appears to me, from all that I know and have heard of this man, that he is a much fitter inmate for the asylum at Castle Hill than for the jail.' Whereas a magistrate, like Samuel Marsden, had authority to admit and discharge patients from the asylum under his remit, the provost marshal had no such power. He could only make recommendations, to be acted on by the man who had replaced him.

Levey 'is a prisoner of the crown', wrote Campbell, 'and of course is disposable at His Excellency the Governor's discretion. If a question should arise in regard to the fact of his being lunatic, a medical survey and consultation (if ordered by government) would ascertain the fact.'[64] This discretionary power was displayed in a brief letter from Goulburn to the chief constable at Sydney about the convict John Macklin at the Carters' Barracks, which housed brickmakers and carters and was located where Central Station now stands.[65] 'The lunatic named in the margin you will take into your charge and convey with the accompanying letter to Parramatta, for the purpose of being forwarded to the Castle Hill Asylum.'[66] The colonial secretary wrote with the governor's authority, so confident in it that he felt no need to cite it. Nor was there any reference to any magistrate, court or doctor – merely a note to Marsden (who is everywhere in this history) about the logistics.

Samuel Levey either never made it to the asylum, or came and went: the records, again, fail us. Campbell had written to Goulburn in March; on 6 November Solomon Levey wrote to Goulburn for assistance, 'unfortunately having a brother who is a prisoner of the crown & a lunatic'. 'Of late,' wrote Solomon, 'his malady has got to that pitch I very much fear he will do himself or some other person an injury.' Whatever had happened earlier in the year, he now saw that institutional care was necessary, and clothed his request in official language, requesting 'an order for the lunatics reception at the Castle Hill's Asylum'.

For all their past and present criminality, the Leveys retained plenty of agency, and it was a delicate letter, asking for government help but avoiding the discretionary mechanisms of the 'disposal' of convicts. That the Leveys were established in the colony among respectable people was perfectly clear from the witness Solomon called on to substantiate his brother's illness, William Cowper. An evangelical chaplain, Cowper was tireless in his pastoral visits, especially to children and prisoners, and when he died in 1858 a third of the people of New South Wales turned out to farewell him.[67] The good chaplain had been recently 'disturbed at unseasonable hours on mad applications'. Although the governor had the authority to dispose of Levey as he wished, Solomon was invoking the respectable trappings of the commission of lunacy, without going so far as to give the formal information requesting one. His letter, though it was riddled with spelling errors, showed that he had both money and connections – the real currency in an aspirational penal society. 'I have tried all means medical advice would allow at the suggestion of William Bowman Esquire, principal surgeon,' he wrote. 'I tried a private apartments & had a proper person to attend him with medical advice but all to no effect. As my own premessis does not allow the conveniency sufficient to keep him closely confined I am willing to pay all expences to the Government as to his victualling, medical attendance, cloathing and any other charge that may be required for the care of my brother at the Castle Hill Mad House.'[68]

Transportation was 'a sort of lottery', just as Jeremy Bentham said.[69] When convicts showed signs of madness, the response depended significantly on whether they were assigned to a settler or to the government, and according to the character and capabilities of masters, commandants and colonial secretaries, doctors and magistrates – and even families. Some convicts were assigned to their wives or husbands; Samuel Levey was assigned to his brother. This meant that Solomon was perfectly, if rather oddly, placed to liaise with the government on Samuel's behalf, and also that, unlike most masters, he was willing to pay his way.

It transpired that the governor's powers over convict madness, supposedly comprehensive and discretionary, were limited. In December 1823, a month after Solomon had requested help, Goulburn wrote to William Bennett, superintendent of Castle Hill. When was Levey 'received at your establishment', he wanted to know, 'together with the date and reason of his subsequent discharge'.[70] The governor and the colonial secretary were chasing down a convict patient. This game of tag was not as uncommon as we might imagine. Only a matter of weeks later, Goulburn wrote to Bennett about another patient and discovered that he had been discharged three years earlier and assigned to a master tailor in Parramatta called Dickson. On the reverse of his letter the governor scribbled, for Goulburn's attention: 'transmit to me every particular you are able to collect respecting Patrick Logan a Convict.' A month later, they were still corresponding about him.[71] At one point, in 1826, the superintendent of convicts wrote to the governor asking 'who lives in the lunatic asylum and has the immediate charge of the convicts?'[72]

With Levey, too, it was something of an ordeal. Wherever he had been, on whatever authority, Levey was admitted to Castle Hill in January 1824.[73] On 1 April, however, Bennett reported that Levey had run away. He had been 'informed' that Levey was 'now taken care of by his friends in Sydney'.[74] Runaways were, in the normal course of events, followed by keepers and constables, and recaptured. Had Levey been permitted to leave? Assisted? By what means was Bennett informed about Levey's new living arrangements in Sydney, and in what tone? Bennett's letter did not mention any action to recover his runaway patient. It is not clear how long Samuel Levey stayed with his family (assuming the information was good, and referred to them), or whether there was further violence, but he was admitted to the asylum again eight months later, 'much deranged'. This time he stayed in the asylum a year and a half before he was discharged, by order of the principal surgeon, 'quiet & inoffensive'.[75] A month later, in May 1826, Solomon left with his son to pursue business in London. His 'bustling activity' and success with prestigious Indian merchants drew praise from *The Australian* the following year.[76]

Samuel's family seem to have been reluctant to admit him to the asylum. There are many possible explanations, from the traditional distrust of institutions for the insane, common through the 18th century in England and elsewhere, to fear of social stigma or the cost of maintenance.[77] It could be that Solomon, after working his way into the ranks of the respectable and wealthy, preferred not to appear to need assistance. Or perhaps it was simply that Samuel was family, and they wanted to care for him at home.[78] In established societies, families played a crucial role in managing mental illness well into the 19th century. Asylums tended to be used by families for respite care: temporary relief for what were often long-term illnesses.[79] Poorer families, who likely had less capacity to adapt and less time available to care for each other, used asylums more readily.[80] Families like the Leveys might institutionalise 'those whose demeanour, behaviour, antagonism, resistance or withdrawal failed to fit their immediate context', in the words of legal historian Mark Finnane – and take them back, and repeat.[81] Or perhaps it was a sadder story. Ann left Solomon, but she died in February 1824 after a savage beating by her lover. Before she died she had an emotional reconciliation with her husband, to whom she left valuable properties at Bulli, Bondi and Coogee.[82] Asylums offered families relief from the exhaustion, chaos, and sometimes the violence, of the mad, but also from their own troubles.

In three 1830s musters Samuel was listed, simply, as 'missing'.[83] He died in Sydney on 18 August 1872. Between the support of his family and his own resources, he appears to have established some form of regular life beyond the power of government. Solomon died in 1833, long before his brother, in London. A large investment connected with the colonisation of West Australia had gone poorly, but he still had wealth to bequeath to his son and to various relatives, including £100 each to Samuel and others in New South Wales. Bequests to a range of benevolent institutions suggest a certain integrity, which likely underwrote the communications he had with the government about his brother's care.[84] 'He was a great lover of New South Wales,' the *Gazette* eulogised, 'and strove, according to his views of its prosperity, to promote its welfare.'[85]

Families also asserted themselves in other ways. The Commission of Lunacy, which had been deployed by Macquarie in 1812 to deal with mobility and disorder, was in time resorted to by families for more traditional purposes. Wives, particularly, arranged for commissions to secure their access to the income and assets of their insane husbands. James Birnie, a merchant who had arrived in Sydney in 1806 and contributed to the early growth of commerce in the colony, was declared insane in 1828, at the age of sixty-six or sixty-seven. Birnie's wife testified that he was frequently intoxicated 'for several weeks together', and whether he was drunk or sober showed 'such imbecility and wandering of mind' that he was incapable of managing his affairs – and hers. The estate was valued at over £5000, and Birnie was placed in the care of Richard Jones, another merchant, with a yearly allowance of £120 for him and his wife. The Birnies remained at their house in O'Connell Street, Sydney, until James died sixteen years later.[86] Families who used such means might still have to live with their relatives – or rather, might still be able to care for them in their illness.

The Commission of Lunacy could also protect the insane from their family, or from those who would use marriage to take advantage of them. Joseph Inch had arrived in the colony in 1790 after stealing three gowns, a muslin apron and a handkerchief, but made his way as a merchant. He prospered, becoming the owner of a boat and a member of the Commercial Society of Sydney, a kind of private bank for Sydney merchants, and when he died in 1836 he left his wife Eliza and fifteen-year-old daughter Jane six houses in Sydney, a farm to the south-west, and eight shares each in the Bank of New South Wales and the Bank of Australia, which together yielded £500 per annum.[87] When Eliza also died, Joseph Wyatt, the executor of her husband's will, arranged a Commission of Lunacy to be held on Jane.[88] It established that she had for a decade 'manifested extreme imbecility of mind without any prospect of improvement'. She was at times very violent, and had been physically restrained. William Bland was one of the certifying doctors, and had known Jane from birth.[89] 'The formation of her head,' he explained, 'would not convey the idea that she was an idiot, but, from her general manner, it would appear that her faculties were in abeyance.' And her father had 'had very little more sense than she'.[90]

In Jane's case there was a literal test of her capacity to manage her estate. It was proved that she could not distinguish between coins of different value, and 'had no idea of what property meant'.[91] One commissioner asked 'if she had not a good deal of property? She laughed. He said he heard that the Courthouse belonged to her. She said it did.' Wyatt worried that 'some designing person, by marrying her, might obtain possession of her property'. Or, perhaps, designing family members – Jane had two cousins in Bungonia, south of Sydney. Both were convicts; neither was 'born in wedlock'. The jury 'without any hesitation, unanimously' found Jane of unsound mind and incapable of managing her affairs.[92] Wyatt was appointed trustee, and Jane lived in his house, but her estate fared poorly, especially after the Bank of Australia collapsed in 1843. Four years later Wyatt sought permission to reduce Jane's allowance from £400 to £250, and the attorney-general, when it was granted, said that Wyatt might congratulate himself on not having to make up the difference, since the estate was diminished from 'his own imprudence'.[93]

By another twist of fate, the constable who had once had charge of Michael Hoare became mad towards the end of his rather remarkable life. Francis Oakes, a shoemaker from Warwickshire, joined the ill-fated first voyage of the London Missionary Society in 1796. In Tahiti, the missionaries fell apart socially and theologically. Some lost their faith. Oakes and another missionary requested permission to marry Tahitian women, but were refused. A contingent fled to New South Wales (for fear of their lives) in 1798, including Oakes, who, after resigning his membership, worked as a shopkeeper, baker, contractor and as superintendent of the 'female factory'.[94] J. D. Lang called him 'a settler, a chief constable, an auctioneer and a scoundrel', and a fellow missionary described him as 'a bold rough creature'.[95] In 1840 Oakes's wife and two sons requested a Commission of Lunacy, where two doctors and two clerics testified to his sometimes 'very violent' insanity. A second solicitor argued that Oakes was sane, but the seventeen jurors disagreed, and the court found that he had been insane, with lucid intervals, fully nine years – another story of forbearance and stamina.[96]

THOUGH MADNESS WAS AN IMPORTANT ISSUE IN METROpolitan politics from the beginning of the 19th century, this concern rarely encompassed the colonies before the 1860s, when British colonial asylums became a matter of significant embarrassment after a Jamaican scandal.[97] In a penal colony, however, liberty was at a premium, and legal declarations of insanity entailed a total loss of liberty and control over property. It was therefore an especially charged arena in the aftermath of a rebellion which had challenged the moral and legal basis of colonial government, drawing attention particularly to its arbitrary truncation of property and liberty.

Empires depended on the delegation of authority, argues Lauren Benton, but 'tangles of jurisdiction' formed as power was passed around. Geographical distance from London, even from Sydney, translated into temporal delay which nurtured confusion. Magistrates and other officials might define their own jurisdictional boundaries, deploying the power of the sovereign as they saw fit, until they were checked by a governor, a statute or a public inquiry.[98] When colonial officials overreached, it was not only a threat to their own standing, but to the integrity of the empire which depended on them to maintain the rule of law. This was why the news of men raving and wasting away in Parramatta Gaol was treated so seriously by Earl Bathurst. There were also the bills Macquarie was drawing on the imperial treasury with seeming abandon, the enemies he made in the colony, and the countless insinuations and accusations that filled reams of letters carried in the holds of ships which circled the globe.

Macquarie defended himself as best he could, but madness tested the limits of his authority. Asylum staff, magistrates and family members acted more freely than we might expect in a place where government theoretically enjoyed a wide and robust range of powers. The size and singularity of the penal colony threw everyone together into a sometimes uncomfortable proximity – it was a 'prickly society', in the words of historian David Neal.[99] But this also meant that there was something of a village feel to the treatment of madness. Colonists, government ministers, gaolers, magistrates and medical administrators had access to each other. A principal surgeon could be a family doctor and the one who signed for an asylum discharge on behalf of government; the recommendation of a provost marshal might be shaped by a conversation with the brother of a prisoner, but also by long experience in the role of colonial secretary, who, regardless of organisational hierarchy and formal regulations, might know how things actually functioned.

In such an environment a governor might struggle to keep the mad in sight, under his authority – to know who was making decisions about the mad, and how they were making them. The governor's commission gave him responsibility for madness, and the authority to act upon it, but in practice this authority was broken down into various evaluations, assumptions, delegations and decisions, which were often at cross-purposes. Madness was not neatly arranged within a formal hierarchy – and the imperial hierarchy was, in any case, in flux. Commissioner Bigge's read of the treatment of Michael Hoare provided material for a comprehensive review of the executive and judicial power stretched across the globe. Servile populations, like the convicts, presented London with a 'constitutional challenge', and the magistracy was the crux. Rampant amateurism and overt class interests compromised the rule of law throughout the empire, and created a 'permanent threat' to the good functioning of imperial authority.[100] This means that magistrates and malingerers in Parramatta helped bring on what Benton and Ford call the 'rage for order', the coming tide of international law.[101] The politics of madness in a penal colony were clearly convoluted.

6

DARLING'S SUICIDES

Commissioner Bigge and Governor Lachlan Macquarie had talked of converting Parramatta Gaol into a new building for the colony's insane, but Macquarie's successor, Thomas Brisbane, entertained a grander vision. He allocated 50 acres for a new lunatic asylum at Elizabeth Bay, east from Sydney along the southern shore of the Harbour. The image of a new building with such 'commanding views' over the water suggests a place of real therapy, with resources and rhythms to match the splendour of the site.[1] Private, luxurious madhouses often presented patients with a pleasant outlook, which helped calm and restore patients.[2]

Bigge had underscored the need for parsimony even more pointedly than he had the need for new infrastructure, and Brisbane's parsimony, not a pretty harbourside asylum, would be his main legacy.[3] The bulk of convicts were assigned to private settlers, which saved the cost of housing and feeding them but also meant that they were unavailable for public works. Brisbane pursued a far more modest construction program, and the asylum at Castle Hill was allowed to continue deteriorating. By the end of Brisbane's administration, it was barely capable of keeping its forty patients, still less treating them.[4]

This made the asylum an unpalatable prospect for free patients, and Brisbane experimented with repatriation. The surgeon Daniel MacDonnell was treated for mental symptoms at Parramatta General Hospital for most of the year in 1824, and by January 1825 he was convalescent, but despondent. Brisbane convened a medical board of three surgeons to examine his state of mind, and they advised 'restoring him to his family' – back home – because he had twice attempted suicide.[5] A second board examined John Duncan, a Royal Navy purser, six months later, and found that he had been 'labouring under mental derangement' for eighteen months, including eleven 'under medical treatment in Sydney' – note the respectable aversion to the words 'lunatic asylum'. By the time of his examination Duncan was in 'a complete state of mental derangement, approaching to idiotism', and the board recommended him to be sent home 'by the first favourable opportunity' because there was little chance of recovery.[6] For quite different reasons, both boards were explicit on the need to send the men away.[7] Both sailed away the very day after Duncan's examination, on the *Phoenix*, as if the idea had presented itself to Brisbane when he saw the ship entering the Harbour out of the corner of his eye.

The two free men had 'remained here' and 'been a burden to the government' for too long, wrote Brisbane, while their recovery was anticipated, but this was now highly unlikely. 'I am induced,' he wrote, 'under the authority of my commission which especially invests me with the care and keeping of individuals under mental derangement, to send them home to England by the present opportunity of the ship Phoenix.' He trusted London would pay £240 for their passage.[8]

Earl Bathurst, secretary of state for the colonies, was furious. His reply, addressed to Ralph Darling, who succeeded Brisbane, pointed out that the governor's commission 'vests him with the *care* and *keeping* of individuals under mental derangement'. The former governor had clearly sent the men home 'to rid the Colony of the expense', and it had placed the Colonial Office in an 'awkward predicament' – an empire which stretched around the world startled by two of its agents arriving by sea, and 'not knowing in what manner to dispose of them'.[9] It rendered the home government liable for significant costs, and, obviously, great vexation. That parsimony, so eagerly embraced in Sydney, had not after all been for the sake of the colonial coffers, but to spare the British treasury. No persons 'labouring under the same calamity', Bathurst made clear, should be returned to England without 'the fullest information' preceding them. The colonies were to deal with whatever madness they encountered. Darling apparently took the hint, and there are no records of other repatriations, no further ships of fools.[10]

The course of madness among the free population of the colony was, like that of the madness of convicts, shaped by the peculiar situation of the colony. The free navigated the same legal and political structures, with judges and administrators working to apply English precepts to meet the specific situations that arose around them. Where convict insanity emerged from barracks and labour gangs and the shadow of the gallows, however, the madness of free men and women came upon them as they set about their colonial lives, especially where they clashed with the law, or with the core business of government. After Bigge, the colony was to be both a site of effective discipline and a place of progress, developed by the industry of free emigrants: a place of 'punishment and profit', the phrase used by John Ritchie in his history of the commission.[11] The free mad, who fell between these two poles, were neglected: settler madness tended to be subterranean, to travel beneath the gaze of government. It was often treated informally, outside government structures, to avoid the stigma engendered by the legal system and the asylum, a convict institution.

We see this madness in fleeting episodes, whenever its sufferers jostled with government, with its record keeping, or with private persons who kept journals or wrote for the newspapers – but we encounter it vividly when suffering led to complete unravelling; when lives became unbearable, and men and women killed themselves. When otherwise respectable, upstanding persons killed themselves, coroners typically concluded that they were temporarily insane. In some cases this seems to have been a convenient fiction. In others, the coronial courts heard ample evidence of pressure, loss and despair, and a range of mental symptoms which were linked with those experiences. After a string of suicides from 1825, the radical colonial newspapers used the insanity of suicide not to neatly close off discussion, but to attack the culture of terror which they saw as spilling out from metropolitan troubles and the convict system, casting a pall over the entire colony.

THE COMMISSION WHICH WAS ESTABLISHED EARLY IN 1819 to inquire into the functions and qualities of New South Wales was far from open-ended. The coffers were empty, and the home government was struggling to deal with a rising tide of crime and vagrancy after the Napoleonic Wars, as demobilised soldiers found themselves unemployed and desperate. Bigge was to discover how the colony could be made to serve again what Earl Bathurst understood to be its original 'peculiar cause': to act as an 'object of real terror'. It did not matter that that object had been far from clear at the time. 'Botany Bay' was now to produce a terror which stretched around the globe to deter crime in Britain – and do so on a shoestring.[12] The day after issuing this instruction, however, Bathurst issued another which anticipated a future for the colony free of convicts altogether.[13]

A key concern was to encourage the emigration of people of good character and capital. At the 1819 Committee on Gaols, in London, prominent colonists had already called for incentives for those with some capital to emigrate to New South Wales. The Colonial Office had been wary of such schemes, given its continuing stake in the transportation of convicts, but in that same year the firebrand colonial-born William Wentworth looked out from London and saw the 'vast tide of emigration' sweeping through North America beginning to turn towards New South Wales. Shipping between the colony and metropole was growing strongly, and more and more people responded to the Colonial Office's modest advertisement calling for emigrants.[14]

New South Wales entered a sort of limbo. It was to be both more terrifying and more free than it had been at the outset; a place of state savagery and private prosperity.[15] In response to Bigge's reports, the discipline of convicts in New South Wales was made harsher.[16] Floggings and executions increased, the pillory and treadmill were introduced, and new penal settlements created what the historian Raymond Evans calls a '*cordon sanitaire*' ringing the Australian colonies. A parallel set of reforms which anticipated the end of convict transportation was also introduced – measures which sought to protect and promote industry and prosperity. 'The influx of private capital on a grand scale' was encouraged, writes Evans; land policy shifted to favour the wealthy, increasing the dominance of the colonial elite.[17] Class, stressed the reformers, had to be protected in such a place. An April 1827 Colonial Office memorandum clarified that settlers desiring to procure land by a grant would be assessed according to moral as well as capital worth, and the capacity to raise sufficient livestock and tools.[18] Darling thought the first-mentioned was most important. 'Whenever I am asked as to people going out as settlers,' he wrote to his brother-in-law, 'I invariably say, it depends entirely on the character of the individual – and that one man would do more with one thousand pounds than another would with £5000.'[19]

Terror also rapidly became a strategy for establishing control over the Aboriginal population which surrounded the colony. This had far-reaching effects also on the European population, as historian Mick Warren demonstrates in his research on the emotional history of the colony.[20] Evans demonstrates a 'culture of terror', born in England amidst the unrest which culminated in 1819 in the Peterloo Massacre, and finding colonial form in Bathurst's instructions. The commission itself, with its directive to instil terror, was read to the assembled people of Sydney shortly after Bigge arrived, and printed in the *Gazette*. Terror loomed over Bigge's investigations, with hundreds of interviews held over sixteen months, and underlay the voluminous reports published in their wake. It then found tangible form in the reforms which followed, for convicts, first, arriving in ever greater numbers through the 1820s and 1830s, and then for the free.[21] English historian Douglas Hay, exploring the terror which engulfed protesters at Peterloo, wrote that 'the ideology of justice could be used by gentlemen to quiet a mob, and with success', but 'words sometimes lost their magic. Then the discretion embodied in the law allowed the authorities to use terror with great flexibility'.[22] This discretion extended across the seas, and found special purchase in New South Wales.

Ralph Darling appears in our histories, still, as a martinet, glowering at colonial society through his brief reign from Government House in the Domain. It is not that historians have not tried to reclaim him. Brian Fletcher's biography has him as 'a governor maligned' by the disciplinary bent of modern historians towards liberalism, and the great historian A. G. L. Shaw pointed this out explicitly.[23] Darling did not enjoy more power than his predecessors; indeed, he had rather less power than those who governed before the New South Wales Act of 1823. He followed much the same reform program as his predecessor, Thomas Brisbane, who is not maligned – is not, indeed, very well remembered.[24] Darling nevertheless wielded his (still-extensive) gubernatorial powers to intimidate and humiliate colonists.[25] The measures he employed against his opponents stretched the flexibility built into the structures of colonial government, straying in places into outright illegality. Darling's positive contributions were therefore overlooked, not least because he fell into an egregious war with the radical press and other liberal elements of society, who made their claims with an eloquence that later generations have found increasingly compelling.

The mad were caught between the two arms of Bathurst's instructions. The prospect of a new, therapeutic asylum at Elizabeth Bay fit poorly with both of the agendas of the commission. Such an asylum might function as a bastion of hope or a chance for escape, and allay whatever terror the colony could muster. It was equally liable to compromise the image of sobriety and industry the Colonial Office was seeking to encourage for prospective emigrants. Impressive asylums in Europe and, later and more modestly, in the colonies might bespeak the power of rationality to impose order upon madness, but in the absence of that imposing architecture, asylums were more likely to conjure images of breakdown, disorder and despair. Certainly few could have been moved to marvel at modern science after visiting the asylums of the penal colony. Together with the need for economy, these reasons may explain why a new asylum was not forthcoming. Instead, Darling passed off the luxurious Elizabeth Bay site to his colonial secretary, Alexander Macleay, shortly after he arrived.[26] It was valued a decade later at over £27 000, and the house built there by the Macleays, at great cost and with surpassing taste, now houses a museum and 'gleams like a Greek temple' by the water.[27]

Still, something had to be done with the insane. In April 1826 a grand jury toured the asylum at Castle Hill and found it 'highly unfit, in every point, for its present occupation'.[28] Two months later Brisbane was on his way home, and Darling and his brother-in-law and special adviser, Henry Dumaresq, paid a surprise visit to Liverpool. They toured the various gaols and watch houses, but their 'principal object' was to 'appropriate some place for the reception of the lunatics about to be removed from Castle Hill'. They decided that the Anglican parsonage, then serving as a temporary courthouse, was 'well adapted', and gave instructions for a hasty renovation.[29] 'A neat commodious brick-built parsonage house, two stories high and stuccoed in imitation of stone', early admirers compared it favourably with Castle Hill.[30] But clean, orderly, safe and even comfortable as it may initially have been, it was hardly a purpose-built asylum.[31] Designed for a large clerical family, by 1834 it housed seventy-three patients, and the following year the new governor, Richard Bourke, found it a 'wretched hired building without outlet of any kind'.[32]

When James Holland became mad in 1827, therefore, he was placed in the general hospital rather than the asylum, as MacDonnell and Duncan had been before him. Holland, who had been attorney-general in Bermuda, was appointed solicitor-general for New South Wales in 1826. When he arrived in Sydney the following February, however, Chief Justice Francis Forbes refused to swear him in.[33] 'The fact is too obvious that Mr Holland is unfit for the situation,' Darling complained, and was liable to expose the government to embarrassment.[34] Holland was nevertheless offered the lesser role of commissioner of the court of requests.

In that capacity he quickly displayed an alarming 'singularity' and a high 'capacity for error in his court duties'. These gave 'just cause of complaint to many'; one man threatened to horsewhip him.[35] After a 'very serious attack' with 'strong symptoms of an aberration of mind', *The Australian* suggested that the stresses of court work mixed with Holland's 'naturally vehement temperament' to produce 'delusive feelings'. Struggling to keep him calm in his bed, his carers sent for 'an old school-fellow', but when he arrived he found Holland physically restrained and incoherent, with the curtains lowered and the lamps dimmed. There was no improvement, and Holland was placed in the general hospital. *The Australian* suggested a less arduous role, but a fortnight later, Holland's life was 'in a very precarious state', and a further three weeks saw Darling, Forbes and other senior military and civil officers following his hearse down Macquarie Street.[36]

Increasingly through the 19th century, experts warned that neglecting madness could have serious consequences. Medical treatises explored the links between insanity and suicide and emphasised the importance of early intervention; typically, institutionalisation. Institutions provided medical attention, but also a variety of preventative measures securing the person while the mind recovered: handcuffs and straitjackets, at first, but later specially equipped rooms with bedding that could not be torn and tied into nooses. They also allowed close surveillance of at-risk patients, though it was pointed out that such 'shadowing' could sometimes aggravate the problem.[37]

But during Europeans' first half century in Australia, there was no asylum for the free men and women of social standing. Castle Hill and Liverpool asylums were intended for convicts, and mostly populated by them. They offered little in the way of therapy. Convict madness revealed the jurisdictional and ethical tensions of a penal colony. The madness of free men and women, similarly, gives us access to the way that the subtler characteristics of the society which developed around the convicts produced strain and despair. Because these people rarely crossed the threshold of an asylum there are few institutional records capable of reconstructing this strain. Except where private records survive, or where there was some special public clash with the branches of government, this madness threatens to elude our histories altogether.

Suicide, however, was more likely to leave records, since at death, as at birth and marriage, the government asserted itself in the private lives of its charges. When authorities suspected that a person had been killed by others or by themselves, coronial inquests worked to open up their death, and their life. Suicide is hardly synonymous with madness, of course, but according to prevailing philosophies and theologies, it was a crime, a sin, even something like an act of insanity – a definitive renunciation of selfhood. Confronted with suicide, coroners and coronial juries frequently resorted to the legal category of temporary insanity, a highly versatile formulation which meant that they could do justice to the suffering of the deceased as well as abjure the act itself. Evidence was gathered which at once identified the pressures likely to have inspired a desire for self-destruction, suggested likely causes and sometimes culprits, and absolved that desire by declaring it a moment of madness, brought on by those pressures. This allowed suicide and madness to be drawn up together into the politics of colonial society, into discussions of terror and industry.

The early colonial newspapers show limited interest in suicide. The *Sydney Gazette*, the only paper in the colony until 1824 and censored by the colonial secretary, reported the suicides of sailors, soldiers and convicts tersely. Coroners' reports almost invariably delivered verdicts of temporary lunacy. Sometimes reportage included details of disappointment or shame. Andrew Kenelly, a New South Wales Corps private, left a confession that he had made a false accusation against the deputy commissary before he stabbed himself, twice, and then hanged himself. Two soldiers testified to his 'mental derangement', but given that the man he accused was Garnham Blaxcell, whom the next chapter will reveal as a man of little integrity, it is possible Kenelly's injuries were not self-inflicted. The coroner's conclusion, however, was 'lunacy'.[38] Others cases showed depressive symptoms. A coroner found that Mr Brown, a midshipman, 'shot himself through the head in a fit of insanity' late in 1807, while his ship was in port, and noted the 'unhappy' state of mind of 'the young gentleman'.[39] In 1816, Henry Hackett, another private, shot himself while standing watch in George Street. He had previously showed symptoms of insanity as well as a marked 'gloom'. The verdict was, again, lunacy.[40]

Sometimes a lunacy verdict was based on nothing more than the absence of other explanations, or those that could be offered publicly. In late 1804, Mary Nicholls's behaviour had been 'extravagant' when she visited a friend, leaving 'no doubt of a mental derangement'. Nicholls went home, but stepped out again at two o'clock in the morning. At noon a pair of grass-cutters found her body floating near Goat Island. 'Accidental death,' the inquest concluded, 'by insanity.'[41] In 1809, 'a Portuguese mulatto, who was servant to Captain Dundas, put a period to his existence with a pistol, the contents of which were lodged in the stomach, after which he lived about half an hour.' Again, the verdict was lunacy.[42]

But were those who were declared insane after killing themselves necessarily insane? Across the 18th century, English coroners increasingly declared suicides *non compos mentis*. In Ireland, in the year 1841, no less than eighty-four of eighty-five recorded suicides were attributed to temporary insanity.[43] These verdicts often had more to do with money and delicacy than with madness.[44] A finding of insanity allowed the family to inherit the deceased estate, which was otherwise confiscated by the crown. It could also help work around religious condemnations of self-murder and the stigma which could accompany a finding of considered, rational suicide. Until 1823, indeed, the law allowed for those who killed themselves while sane to be buried at a crossroad with a stake through their heart.[45] Insanity verdicts tended to be handed to the elite; the poor were more likely to be simply found to have killed themselves.[46] A similar pattern has been found in 20th century English criminal trials; though temporary insanity plays a different function in a criminal courtroom, the main differentiator between 'crimes of passion' and temporary insanity verdicts was 'financial standing'.[47]

When more prominent and more permanent colonists killed themselves, the press took more interest. At the turn of the 19th century, Edward Riley was taken with the possibilities of colonial trade. When he was seventeen he had obtained an apprenticeship as a merchant and auctioneer in Calcutta and was soon trading energetically between India, Canton and New South Wales.[48] His fortunes rose and fell, which was common enough, but when his wife died in 1810, he became deeply depressed. His brother and business partner, Alexander, recommended that he migrate to New South Wales and start afresh. He remarried and migrated in 1816. The Rileys rented Ultimo House, the grandest and most conspicuously expensive house in the colony. They advertised for cooks, butlers and servants, and lived a luxury life highly uncommon in that society, contributing greatly 'to the conviviality of Sydney'.[49] One night no fewer than 175 guests danced at one of the Rileys' 'grand balls'.[50]

The business continued to wax and wane, however, and

after a dramatic downturn, Ultimo House was sold, and Edward sank again into a profound melancholy. Though he gathered his strength for a trip into the interior, finding good land around Goulburn to graze the merino sheep he and his brother planned to raise, his moods were swinging wildly. 'His lowness of spirits' grew more pronounced and more obvious to others. Someone noticed how depressed Riley appeared one day as he sat in judgement in a magistrate court (he, like other people of wealth and standing, acted as an amateur judge).[51] A week later, two clergymen had breakfast with Riley and thought him very depressed and 'irregular' to the point even of mental derangement. Later that morning, Edward placed his pistol beneath his chin and shot himself. An inquest found that he had been insane; that he had been for two or three months afflicted by 'severe indisposition, attended with hypochondriac symptoms, that induced mental derangement'.[52] The historian Jill Conway suggests that Riley's depression was exacerbated by gout and by 'the limitations of colonial life'.[53]

There were different ways to talk about suicide. It could be recalled sadly, in the wake of Edward Riley's entertainments; it could also be draped in Romanticism. A florid benediction was written for Patrick Shennan, an overseer on a farm at Bathurst who shot himself in July 1826. Shennan had emigrated from a wealthy family that had lost its wealth, a common colonial story. He adapted well, excelling in agriculture and grazing sheep; he was 'a successful and popular colonist of New South Wales'. But he fell ill, and was treated for insanity for some time, his main symptom 'an incessant inclination to suicide'. Shennan had eagerly anticipated the arrival of his wife and child from England, but this acute happiness, his doctor suggested, had exacerbated his madness. Following an evening of 'festive hospitality' soon after their arrival, he retired to his chamber, had 'a few minutes' affectionate and mirthful conversation' with his wife, 'snatched a pistol from his dressing table, applied it to his breast, and pulled the trigger'. His public success rendered 'the catastrophe singularly awful' – enough to make him another Caesar, for the *Gazette*: 'nature might stand up,/And say to all the world, "this was a man!"'[54] An original poem appeared in the next edition, tracing the fine line between grief and valorisation.

The following year, *The Australian* reported that an unnamed convict had hanged himself with a handkerchief, and that it was not on account of his master's treatment.[55] The suffering suggested by such an act was brushed aside, just as it was for the metropolitan poor, while elites were forgiven their sins after their passing and even celebrated for their classical virtues and the intense human interest of their stories.[56]

THE *ALFRED* SAILED INTO SYDNEY IN APRIL 1824. ON BOARD was William Wentworth, returning to his birthplace from London. There he had published a highly popular account of the colony's early history laying out a reform program: trial by jury, representative government, and free institutions. He was accompanied by Dr Robert Wardell, who proceeded to sue the ship's owner for the 'wet and comfortless cabin' and for the lack of refreshments on the voyage out, winning £200 damages.[57] John Mackaness, the newly appointed sheriff, travelled with them, and in the hold there was, of all things, a newspaper plant. Wardell, who had edited the *Statesman* in London, recruited Wentworth to help him found a newspaper in the colony. Their paper, *The Australian*, began publication in October 1824, championing small settlers, emancipated convicts and free institutions. Both Wardell and Wentworth also continued to practise as barristers and frustrated Darling enormously as they kept 'the Court and the Bar, by their effrontery and talent equally in subjection'.[58]

The Australian would be a key voice for the more liberal elements of colonial society as Ralph Darling set about governing the colony as he would a military establishment, and pursuing reforms that favoured the elite. The *Gazette*, edited by Robert Howe, continued its conservative stance even after censorship ceased, and tended to support Darling's administration, but Wardell and Wentworth were joined by Edward Smith Hall, a restless, deeply religious man who had brushed up against Macquarie, worked as a coroner, as secretary of the Bank of New South Wales, and at Jones and Riley after Edward Riley's demise.[59] Hall had clashed briefly with Macquarie, but in May 1826 he and Arthur Hill founded the *Monitor*, which quickly became a special thorn in Darling's side.[60] It was Hall who criticised Darling's reallocation of the Elizabeth Bay site and his negligence of both its Aboriginal residents and the insane. Like *The Australian*, the *Monitor* advocated trial by jury and representative government. It defended the rights of convicts as discipline and terror constricted them.[61] Within six months of publication Darling singled out the *Monitor* as a seditious rag. He would have Hall gaoled multiple times for libel, making him, in time, a martyr.[62]

John Macarthur junior, a conservative, complained that the Supeme Court, under Chief Justice Francis Forbes, offered the liberals a 'sympathetic forum' – that, for all his talents, Forbes had 'theoretical views concerning liberty'. Wentworth left *The Australian* to further disrupt the colonial courts, realising their full potential as political theatres in the absence of a colonial parliament. He decried government policies as 'diabolical and damnable', wrote Macarthur, and 'repeatedly left political opponents, like Governor Darling, spluttering with frustration'.[63] Wardell was just as brazen, calling Darling a 'tyrant, a monster and a scoundrel'.[64] Like Macarthur, the governor began to suspect that Forbes was giving them free rein in court. The judge was '*greedy* of power, almost beyond example', he wrote to London.[65] But Darling himself had 'the instincts of an autocrat', as legal historian Bruce Kercher writes, and grew ever more 'paranoid, defensive and intolerant of criticism'.[66]

It was not only convicts who found their colonial lives unpalatable. In late 1826, Joseph Sudds and Patrick Thompson committed trivial crimes in order to be relieved from military service. They expected a light punishment followed by discharge, but were instead sentenced to seven years' transportation to a penal settlement. Even this was not enough for Darling, who felt that a public example was necessary.[67] He personally had Sudds and Thompson stripped of their uniforms on the parade ground, dressed as convicts, and placed in iron collars with long horizontal arms. Though only slightly heavier than standard irons, they were far more cumbersome and degrading.[68] Intended to demonstrate government power, the spectacle rather cheapened and weakened it, but there was worse to come.[69] Sudds was ill and died after only five days of working in a chain gang. *The Australian* went into overdrive, even though it had previously called for double irons for bushrangers, 'and even neck-collars' in place of the standard, 'toy-like chain' (as the *Gazette* recalled with glee).[70] The *Monitor* joined in. William Wentworth sought to impeach Darling in the British Parliament, and sent a petition to London.[71] A Select Committee eventually exonerated Darling of blame for Sudds's death, but law officers in both Sydney and London concluded that he had acted illegally. The governor brushed aside such 'legal niceties' and sent another defendant to the Moreton Bay penal settlement against the orders of the Supreme Court.[72] These were the first glimpses of an autocratic style which would become more and more pronounced.[73]

Two months after Sudds's death, the *Monitor* published an

expansive critique of Darling's government, a year in, with its '[abhorrent] system of excise-duties, with all its detestable consequences of informations, stealth, gamblings, trickings, perjuries, fines, imprisonments, suicides, disgrace, wretchedness, and degradation'.[74]

In this environment, George Galway Mills, registrar of the Supreme Court and secretary of the Turf Club, a social group which revolved around horse racing, began to be very anxious about his job. Like others, he had arrived in the colony in roundabout fashion. Born in 1765 into a West Indies plantation family, his inheritance was reduced by war and the declining slave trade. Mills failed to also reduce his lifestyle, and in 1807 the King's Bench sent him to gaol for magnificent debts, more than £43 000. He managed to free himself by obtaining a seat in parliament, much to the outrage of creditors and his fellow MPs. Mills promptly fled the country to work as a small-time diplomat and spy in Europe. He was elected to parliament again in 1818, from Paris; his wife died in January 1820; he was not re-elected, and instead accepted the unlikely post of registrar of the Supreme Court of New South Wales, which came with £800 a year.[75] Forbes thought the appointment could only be a sinecure, 'a provision for past Services; it were impossible to suppose that he could have been expected to perform the duties of his office'.[76]

There was no colony where the 'selection of individuals' was so important, Darling warned during his first year in New South Wales. 'Not only the character of the Government, but the moral improvement of the people' depended on the careful moral curation of the administration.[77] In a society composed of former convicts and fortune-seekers, it was incumbent on government to give moral guidance and discipline. The selection process, both for emigrants and government positions, had clearly been lacking. Darling's 'autocratic tendencies' came into full swing, and he set about a general purge of the government of New South Wales.

It began with Mills's friend, sheriff John Mackaness, whom Darling saw associating with 'the Wentworths and the Wardells'.[78] Mackaness was secretary of the Turf Club. At a meeting in January 1827, celebratory toasts were made to Thomas Brisbane, its founding patron, before a toast was proposed for Darling. People jeered, and the band offered a jovial rendering of 'Over the Hills and Far Away'. Darling reported the evening's entertainments to the new secretary of state, Viscount Goderich (one of Hall's 'informations') and that November, with his approval, Darling dismissed Mackaness for his association with 'certain factious individuals' and 'the common defamers of the Government'.[79]

It was merely the opening volley. 'The dismissal of all other persons, who have given these individuals their countenance,' Darling wrote a fortnight later, 'is necessary to the due support of the Government.'[80] 'There is not a man of character or consequence amongst them.'[81] He dismissed Henry Douglass from the Court of Requests – something the Colonial Office queried – suspended W. H. Moore, crown solicitor, and intended to do the same to his brother, C. D. Moore, all for Turf Club indiscretions.[82] To be fair to Darling, the Moore brothers had been included on Macquarie's list in 1819, as 'seditious, intriguing, & discontented'.[83] The policy 'has had the best effect', Darling effused. 'A few more such examples ... will tend to the peace and happiness of society and render the conduct of the Government comparatively easy.'[84]

But Mills pre-empted the governor. On Monday 11 February 1828, he called upon Dr William Bland, who had briefly been the surgeon at the lunatic asylum, to ask about the easiest method of self-destruction. He would not be diverted by Bland. Was not a certain dose of laudanum almost immediately fatal, he asked. A constable, seeing Mills in town two days later, was 'struck by his altered appearance'. He muttered as he walked in the evening, sticking his umbrella into the ground, 'it must be that – that must be it.' Early the next morning Mills visited the gunsmith W. M. Macdonald and selected a pair of pistols. He was going 'up the country'. Macdonald suggested a better pair, but Mills said they were for his servant. Bland met him later that morning in the street and found him 'calm and composed'. That afternoon he shot himself; there was a pistol ball in his coat when he was found, and a bottle of laudanum in his desk.

'George Galway Mills, Esq, committed suicide whilst labouring under a temporary fit of insanity', concluded the coroner's inquest. Where some inquests used insanity as a convenient fiction, here plenty of evidence was presented of a longer and deeper disturbance. Bland had frequently seen Mills 'in fits of momentary insanity', he said, and thought his intellect had been deranged for several weeks. Mills's servant Charles Horton spoke, guardedly, of recent oscillations in his moods. Mackaness thought that his friend 'laboured under a considerable aberration and depression of mind', and that 'this mania' had been present 'some weeks'.[85] Two theories were suggested. Horton thought that although he often talked about those 'who had been suspended from their situations', he had been driven to suicide by the surety he was liable for – a debt of Mackaness's, some three or four thousand pounds. Mackaness put Mills's death squarely down to Darling's culture of terror. He 'laboured under an apprehension that he would be dismissed from his office', he said, and had lately 'become quite secluded, and never mixed in society'. 'In a strong mind certainly, this would not produce insanity', admitted Mackaness – but Mills never did have a strong mind.

Though he did not testify, chief justice Francis Forbes agreed with Mackaness. Mills had been terrified that Darling's conflict with Wentworth, and especially Wardell, would spread to himself, wrote Forbes in a letter to the Colonial Office. Despite his failings as a clerk (and as a businessman), Mills had at least read some of the classics and Forbes counted him as a friend and ally. 'I cannot get rid of the belief,' he wrote, 'that he has been cruelly sacrificed.'[86] *The Australian* set down in print what Forbes would not allow himself to write even in private, that Darling was directly to blame for the loss of Mills. 'Buoyant', 'vivacious' Mills. The 'gradual sinking' and 'mental disquietude', that 'mental alienation' that had 'terminated in self-destruction', had an obvious source. Mills had followed Darling's purge closely; the apprehension that he would lose his office had taken 'possession of his mind' and 'sat heavily on his heart' until at last he 'sunk under the impression they produced'.[87] If anything could restrain the authorities in Sydney and London, concluded *The Australian*, 'it must be this event, which, while it is the most disastrous, is also the most instructive that could have happened.' 'These sort of dismissals,' wrote Edward Hall bluntly in the *Monitor*, 'make gentlemen blow out their brains.'[88]

On Saturday morning, 22 February 1828, John Mackaness accosted Robert Howe – editor of the *Sydney Gazette*, which supported the government – in the street, calling him a 'scoundrel' and a 'vile slave to the Government'. Howe simply presented his 'hard-headed horsewhip', he wrote with relish in his next editorial, and rode the torrent out. Better to be a slave to the government, '*a slave to his duty*', than enslaved like Mackaness '*to his passions*', and 'ranked with those who seem to lose sight of what is due to themselves, as well as what is owing to society'. In the same issue, Howe wrote of his shock that the *Monitor* had not 'merely insinuated, but broadly asserted' that Mills had committed suicide 'on account of certain treatment he had experienced at the hands of the Colonial Government!' The *Gazette* appealed 'to the inhabitants of New South Wales' (or to the better sort among them who patronised its pages) asking 'whether, directly or indirectly, the Government could possibly have prompted the unhappy gentleman to have committed suicide?'[89]

We do not know how the people of New South Wales would have answered, but Darling protested rather too much. In the afternoon or evening after Mills shot himself, Darling wrote to London. He felt the need to give an account. Mills 'was a man of profligate character and dissolute habits', he wrote, callously, and heavily indebted – he had even provided security for that reprobate, Mackaness. 'He appears to have been driven to desperation,' Darling explained, by some distressing news from England 'coupled with the impossibility of extricating himself from the difficulties which immediately surrounded him'.

Just as much as *The Australian* and the *Monitor*, Darling sought to draw Mills's suicide, and Mackaness's disgrace, into the bitter politics of the colony. Their 'want of principle and profligate course of life' were to blame for what Mills had done. 'Whatever degree of commiseration the frailties of human nature may excite' – little, apparently – the governor hoped their fates would 'not be without effect'. 'There are persons here,' wrote Darling, 'and of no inconsiderable station', who would use Mills's suicide to indicate the 'unhappy state of the colony', but no society, he wrote blithely, could 'exhibit more satisfactory proofs of tranquility and prosperity'. There was still work to be done; 'a few indeed of the immediate associates of Mr. Mills and Mr. Mackaness may feel their perilous situation', but the colony was not as they were. 'Few indeed,' he ended caustically, 'have expressed or felt surprize' at these events: the tranquil colony barely blinked as natural justice played out. Mills had, in a sense, simply hastened and extended the purge.

But New South Wales was not so easily aphorised, and when the patently respectable colonist Charles Throsby shot himself some six weeks later there was widespread 'surprize'. Throsby, a surgeon and landowner, was an excellent example of that class of emigrant the government encouraged. He was firm with his convict labourers, and built great wealth through what the *Gazette* deemed the 'extraordinary and patriotic attention to the rearing of stock of a very superior quality'.[90] The New South Wales Act had established an advisory Legislative Council, a concession to Wentworth and other advocates for political reform which had been recommended by Bigge. When the council grew from five to seven members in 1825, Darling chose Throsby to sit on it. He was one of those few upon whom the face of the governor shone.

Despite the governor's talk of tranquillity, the colony was in the grip of a punishing drought, which ruined harvests and dwindled fortunes between 1826 and 1829.[91] The same *Gazette* which reported Throsby's suicide also ran an address by John Jamison, president of the Agricultural and Horticultural Society of New South Wales, on the drought, one 'of very unusual duration'.[92] 'We have had the most surprising continuance of dry weather,' wrote Elizabeth Macarthur in March 1827. 'Thousands of acres of grass have been destroyed by fire, so that the country wears a melancholy aspect.'[93] Throsby had lost some forty head of cattle earlier in the year at Boong Boong, in the Southern Highlands; the price of wool was falling, and Throsby had been ill.[94] But he still had 20 000 acres in two 'fine estates' together with 'large and valuable herds of cattle', Darling wrote home, bemused.[95] Throsby was not the sort of man Darling expected to 'destroy himself with a pistol-ball'.[96]

Some twenty years prior, Throsby had become a surety for £5000 loaned to his friend Garnham Blaxcell. Blaxcell had been a flamboyant and opportunistic participant in the rebellion; he appropriated two French burrs belonging to the government to grind his grain. In 1817 Blaxcell fled the colony to escape his debt and for this debt, a decade later, the Supreme Court had found Throsby liable.[97] This knowledge was 'supposed to have operated so powerfully on his mind, as to have originated occasional mental aberrations', and it was in one such that Throsby had 'terminated his existence by means of a gun, at his country residence!'

News reached Sydney just as people were reeling from some other unnamed 'catastrophe' that morning – perhaps the duel on Garden Island that dawn, in which the third mate shot and killed the chief officer of the *Elizabeth*.[98] The 'melancholy intelligence' of Throsby's death 'seemed to produce general petrifaction'.[99] That debt might drive men mad was common enough. Two years later John Cullen was in debtor's prison and the *Monitor* made a public service announcement that he was quite mad, lacking all judgement, incoherent, and going about the gaol in the night. Cullen's madness was attributed to his imprisonment, 'misfortunes' and 'a certain infirmity' whenever he found himself with some money.[100] But the scale of the enterprise of a 'very large grazier' like Throsby was expected to buttress him against drought and debt and the mental pressures that attended catastrophe; agricultural and commercial success was taken as an indicator of moral fibre. In 1832, another member of the Legislative Council, John Macarthur, fell apart, as we'll see in the next chapter. His insanity was more permanent and its source more apparent, and he died in its grip, but not by his own hand.

Darling set about trying to replace Throsby, but found the task challenging.[101] There were precious few people in the colony who met his character standards, for all the Colonial Office's efforts to induce respectable emigrants. His preferred nominee was William Browne, a colonist worth some £12 000 when he emigrated from Bengal on account of his asthma in 1816, and a founding director of the Bank of Australia.[102] But as the governor began to place the wheels in motion to appoint him, barely a month after Throsby's suicide Browne also tried to kill himself and was placed in hospital. It was enough to make Darling break away from the conventional sobriety of official correspondence. 'I may be permitted to observe,' he wrote, 'that persons, who have suffered from any temporary aberration of mind, should not be sent to this Colony.' It might be fatal. 'If there is nothing in the climate which induces colonists absolute derangement, there is undoubtedly something peculiar, which affects the spirits and produces extraordinary depression.'[103] It could be the weather, he thought, the 'sudden transitions from heat to cold and vice versa' common in the colony. This was not far out of step with the science of the time. That same year, the English physician George Man Burrows concluded that although climate was not 'an exciting cause of insanity', environmental factors, including high temperature, could certainly dispose people to mental derangement.[104] And no doubt to depression, and suicidal thoughts.

The year 1829 was brutal. On 24 January the *Gazette* carried a 'dreadful suicide' from the English *Liverpool Advertiser*: a man stabbed himself and bled out, saying, 'Trouble, I cannot bear my troubles.' The verdict was temporary derangement.[105] On 31 March 1829 the *Gazette* was shocked that 'there were no less than three instances of attempt at suicide' in the colony the week prior. One man had been in service to a doctor. Caught out in an act of fraud, he grabbed a razor and cut his throat, but his master sewed the wound, sent him to hospital, and likely thence to the bench of magistrates.[106] Six weeks later, *The Australian* bemoaned that its last issue 'presents an unusual number of melancholy cases – murder – attempted murders – suicide, &c. &c.'[107] There had been a string of robberies near Parramatta, an atrocious murder, and the suicide of the comb-maker Benjamin Smith, who threatened violence when drunk and was dejected when sober, exhibiting 'symptoms of melancholy frenzy'. He was found at the Talbot, on George Street, with his head nearly severed by a razor. It was 'a most awful and appalling spectacle', and very good copy.[108] There was also a 'curious piece of statistics' collected by the French police, which detailed the manner and cause of suicides in the 'dear lively land of mirth and social ease'.[109] On 15 August, finally, young Patrick Brodie was found lying in his blood, his right hand clenching a pistol. *The Australian* broke into verse, again.[110] The *Gazette* was matter of fact: 'the deceased had *destroyed himself with a pistol ball in a momentary aberration of mind*'.[111] The *Monitor*, however, saw dots that might be joined. 'This is the third suicide which has occurred in the present administration,' Hall declared, 'by gentlemen connected with the Government, namely, Mr. Throsby, Col. Mills, and now Mr. Brodie.'[112] He also called up again from the dead Joseph Sudds, who 'died indeed of severity of treatment'.

The year 1830 brought some respite, but the following year, the final year of Darling's administration, was punctuated by a string of suicides. On 11 April, the convict Philip Richards hanged himself in his master's stable. He had indulged in the 'baleful practice' of over-drinking while his master had been gone for two days, and told his punishment would be not receiving new slops – clothes; he had said he would shoot himself if he had a pistol, and did. He clearly had no great love of his colonial life. It was noted that the jury listened 'patiently' – patronisingly? – to the evidence before returning the verdict 'insanity'.[113]

In August, the *Gazette* ran two articles one after the other – 'Distressing Suicide' and 'Another Suicide'. The respectable Mrs Crampton, after asking her servants what the active ingredient of rat poison was, had them procure two ounces from separate druggists. The chemists, ironically, demanded a note from a respectable person before they handed over the poison. Alerted to her action, doctors made Crampton drink warm milk and then applied 'the stomach-pump', but they were too late. The verdict, again, was insanity. Her husband, with two infant children, was himself left 'in a state of mind nearly bordering on distraction'. Crampton was 'an exemplary wife and mother' and 'by no means a person of violent passions', and the *Gazette* found it 'somewhat difficult to account for her tragical end'. The second article was a complication of the first. A police officer named Collins, after attending the scene of Crampton's suicide, left his beat to buy half an ounce of arsenic and apparently in perfect equanimity went to a pub and drank it with gin. The publican is recorded as saying: 'I hope you have not been doing as poor Mrs. Crampton did!' Despite 'copious amounts of lime-water', this time, and the stomach pump, and 'every other means that medical science could devise', Collins died. Was it a pact; was it an affair?[114]

Far away, George Man Burrows published his *Commentaries on Insanity* while Darling governed New South Wales. He blamed the 'teeming and cheap press' for promoting suicide with its reckless, even sympathetic, accounts of suicides. When they ran out of domestic cases, he wrote bitterly, they scoured foreign papers, searching for stories of self-murder.[115] And indeed, the next issue of the *Gazette* reported that these last suicides had incited further 'acts of rashness'; the following week there were more still. 'We hinted in our last that four efforts at self-destruction took place in various parts of the town the same week,' ran a piece which seemed to be enjoying the recounting altogether too much, 'and on Monday last, no less than four more raised their suicidal hand to rush uncalled for into the presence of their Maker.' There had been doubts about the 'mental health' of the innkeeper of a respectable establishment for two or three days but, escaping those who were watching him in consequence, he went out to the yard, found 'an old reaping-hook', and 'lacerated his throat in a dreadful manner'. Another young man, 'respectably connected', became 'much dejected' and tried to kill himself with a razor after those connections displayed 'some coolness of deameanour' to him. A third was caught in the act of killing himself, and a fourth had laudanum pumped from her stomach. All survived. 'This horrid mania,' wrote the *Gazette*, 'like an infectious disorder, has passed from street to street through our metropolis, plunging family after family into anguish and distress, and creating a feeling of intense interest and excitement in the minds of the public generally.'[116]

THE EDITORS OF THE *MONITOR* AND *THE AUSTRALIAN* SAW more than imitation in the spate of suicides in 1827–31. This self-destruction, and the madness bound up in it, were easy to account for. These were Darling's suicides. He had become 'a scourge and a nuisance' to the colonists, *The Australian* declared, and at his departure they 'testified their extreme joy, by bonfires, illuminations, fetes, and fire-works; and their contempt and hatred, by burning and hanging him in effigy all over the town!!!'[117]

The *Gazette* described suicide as a 'horrid mania' looking to break out like an epidemic. Suicide is traditionally not seen as a collective madness, however, but as a private act. It reflects despair and, perhaps, a kind of insanity. Indeed, being a danger to oneself, like presenting danger to others, was a key indicator of insanity and rationale for institutionalisation. A 1924 *Lancet* report warned that it was crucial not to neglect early signs of mental illness, which had been discovered in two-thirds of the suicides documented in a Royal Commission.[118] A late 20th-century survey found that more than 90 per cent of suicides studied were either diagnosed with psychiatric disorders before their death, or could be afterwards without controversy.[119] Madness and suicide are intricately related; suicide is one jagged edge of madness; a point of no return which community, medicine and state were responsible for guarding.

But if families, doctors, and judges are tasked with preventing suicide directly, others have taken up suicide as the expression of some social disturbance, an indication of a different kind of problem on a different order of magnitude. The 1924 *Lancet* study linked suicide to unemployment, family breakdown, war and social disruption. This perspective is heir to the work of Emile Durkheim, who argued in the late 19th century that psychology did not have the best instruments for understanding a complex societal problem like suicide. He developed social scientific methods to show that suicide, which seemed so private, in fact conformed to social patterns, and therefore could be analysed and learned from at the level of the social body.[120]

By the early 20th century, the connection between suicide and insanity was prevalent. English coroners objected to the conflation of insanity and suicide, and to the legal framework which bound them to pronounce the deceased as either *felo de se*, literally 'felon of one's self', or *non compos mentis*, or not of sound mind. Juries felt pressured to return verdicts of temporary insanity where there was no indication of it.[121] A quarter century later coroners argued that there should be no obligatory inquiry into state of mind in cases of suicide, and no reference to it in the verdict.[122]

English coroners applied law in an 'inchoate' fashion, writes R. A. Houston, compared with the other courts; the regular resort to insanity to explain suicide is one example.[123] In criminal cases, temporary insanity is used to allow consideration of more diverse evidence than the law typically allows. It makes room around doctrine and precedent, argues Russell Covey, for juries' 'intuitive, or commonsense, assessments of culpability'.[124] Derided by some as a 'perfect defence' for crime, temporary insanity in fact may open trials up to such alternative reasoning, yielding sentences which better adhere to 'moral intuitions about fairness and justice'.[125] In colonial New South Wales, however, the concept of temporary insanity allowed the friends, families, colleagues and subordinates of those who suicided to talk about their suffering. It was a thin veneer, provided by medical vocabulary, which allowed the representatives of society gathered in a coroner's court to hear grievances, offer sympathy, and absolve the deceased of moral failing and legal liability. Madness, or the fiction of it, separated the deceased from the consequences of their actions, and societies from the moral implications of their deaths.

Darling's autocratic reputation is well-founded, but it was exaggerated by the relentless pens and tongues of the 'Wentworths and Wardells', and of Edward Hall from his prison cell. Darling attempted to purge the colony of immorality, and to discipline convicts into obedience. His efforts only aided the reformers, led by William Wentworth, who lobbied, sued and spoke out against the despotic power of colonial government and the weak institutions and threadbare liberties in the colony. They were conducting a purge of their own, and in time it proved far more successful.

Earl Bathurst, by reiterating that the governor of New South Wales was invested with the care of those who became mad there, drew the boundaries of the problem: madness was to be dealt with in the colony. But Darling, like Brisbane before him, could not find a way to accommodate and treat the madness of free men and women in the colony which Bigge, and the Colonial Office, had divided between criminality and respectability, terror and piety. It was filled with people trying, and sometimes failing, to make or remake themselves in a place where they did not belong. It was delicate and precarious work, and in such a place it was dangerous not to cater for madness, but Darling went further, by deliberately increasing colonial anxiety. His relentless discrimination between fit and unfit colonists, soldiers and civil officers exposed free society to that terror in which the Colonial Office sought to steep the penal establishment. This terror could break people, ending in a final collision of interior world and exterior reality, the private erupting into the public.

7

AFTER THE REBELLION

In the colony, inner crises which began with the failure of a crop, the spurning of a hand or the sinking of a ship might lengthen into depression, or erupt in mania, or end in a momentary, destructive insanity. This private suffering and chaos spilled into the public realm, in courts and newspapers and government correspondence. But how might a public crisis, like a rebellion, bleed into the private? This chapter reaches back to the uprising known for many years as the 'rum rebellion'. It excavates carefully around the protagonists, seeking access to the inner world of this set of soldiers and merchants who overthrew a governor and then had the temerity to hold court themselves. It does so on advice, from the settler and sometime asylum superintendent George Suttor, that two of the three central leaders of the rebellion went mad, and the third killed himself. It maps the lives of those who witnessed and participated in the rebellion, and asks how this crisis, which reverberated throughout the empire, might have scarred its protagonists, and their families, and the colony.

JOSEPH BANKS, HAVING TRAVELLED THE PACIFIC WITH James Cook in the *Endeavour*, became an advocate of a colony at Botany Bay, in 'New Holland'. He maintained an active interest in the colony as it grew, and, in 1805, was able to secure its governorship for his protégé, William Bligh, who had demonstrated a remarkable sense of duty and leadership capacity in navigating an open boat from near Tahiti to Timor, almost 6000 kilometres, with eighteen loyal members of his crew.[1] Banks explained to Bligh the requirements of the role as he understood them: 'integrity unimpeached, a mind capable of providing its own resources in difficulties without leaning on others for advice, firm in discipline, civil in deportment and not subject to whimper and whine when severity of discipline is wanted'.[2] He thought Bligh an ideal candidate, but outside the higher London circles the famous captain's deportment was not so civil. His 'bad language' at sea was the subject of some scandal, and some wonderful historical musing centuries later.[3] After just eighteen months in Sydney, on 26 January 1808, Bligh was deposed and arrested amidst a 'phrensy of party bigotry which blazed forth', as the botanist George Caley bore witness, 'in the illuminations, bonfires, burning effigies, roasting sheep, and in all manner of riotous dissipation'.[4]

The first histories of the rebellion continued in this vein, drawing the personalities on either side starkly, siding with Bligh,[5] despite his bad language and dictatorial mannerisms, or John Macarthur,[6] leader of the rebellion, whose bravura, charisma and belligerence tend to eclipse lesser characters. Historian A. G. L. Shaw drew attention to the tendency in Australian historical writing to make 'heroes and villains' of historical subjects. 'In biography,' he warned, 'there are special dangers.' He himself navigated delicately between the two.[7] After two centuries, however, John Macarthur has emerged as the hero of the rebellion. His reputation has been shielded in perpetuity by the long shadow of the patronage network he built in his lifetime, and by the affinity between his ambitions for the colony and the nation's growing sense of its own significance. Bligh, by contrast, strove to ensure that colonial society remained subordinate to the empire and to the needs of the British justice system, adhering to an imperial order which was passing away.

Rum, a core commodity and sometime currency in New South Wales, was once considered the impetus of the rebellion, but a generation of historians have revealed a structural discontent which went far beyond rum. By the time of Bligh's administration, the Corps officers had moved beyond monopolising traders to become landlords and employers, taking on and calling in debts; they were at the centre of the colony's economy. Wealthy businessmen outside the Corps also began to feel an imminent and fundamental threat to person and property. These officers and settlers appear to have been taking rational and defensible measures to protect their economic interests, and taking up the language of legal and political rights to so do.[8] At least some of the officers believed firmly in the justice of their cause, and so historian Alan Atkinson has styled the crisis Sydney's 'little revolution'.[9]

Bligh arrived in Sydney in August 1806 with instructions to continue the program of his predecessors, especially in the regulation of spirits.[10] He quickly outlawed the barter of spirits and banned private distillation, again. For the officer Joseph Foveaux, this simply forced every gentleman 'who would blush at being detected in an illicit transaction' to join cause with smugglers and distillers.[11] Bligh made few real innovations. He adhered strictly to his notion of the colony's calling as a quiet society of yeoman farmers which was to incorporate emancipated convicts.[12] Unlike his predecessors, Bligh would not give out land grants, even when the Colonial Office had explicitly instructed him to, as in the case of surgeon Robert Townson. Townson understood Bligh's refusal as evidence of his 'bad heart, his malicious disposition'.[13] This land policy contributed to Bligh's progressive alienation from different sections of colonial society. Bligh planned to implement Arthur Phillip's plans for Sydney Cove with little regard for those whose homes and businesses stood in the way. As he set about cancelling leases and demolishing buildings, John Macarthur publicly refused to be evicted, and this was one of the sparks leading to the conflagration.[14] Bligh also fined and jailed the three most prominent emancipist traders, Simeon Lord, Henry Kable and James Underwood, for a letter 'couched in improper terms'.[15] 'The Governor is behaving so very arbitrary,' wrote the free settler John Blaxland, 'that I do not consider either my person or property safe a single hour; indeed, I think it will not be long before I am sent to gaol.'[16] 'All Bligh did seemingly he did alone,' writes historian and biographer of Macarthur, Malcolm Ellis.[17]

Among his other failings, William Bligh waded unwelcome into the management of medicine in the colony. The surgeons of the Colonial Medical Service baulked at being forced to treat free settlers without recompense, and between courts-martial, suspensions and resignations, and deaths, their numbers were fast dwindling. When principal surgeon Thomas Jamison requested permission to return to England to bring his family out to the colony in early 1806, Bligh refused. He also moved the medical store into the general store so that Jamison had to request supplies from the commissary, a cause of great frustration. Surgeons arriving on convict transports refused to serve in the colony under such conditions; there were now only two physicians providing medical care to Sydney and its surrounding districts, and Jamison warned the Colonial Office that he would resign if Bligh remained governor.[18] Jamison supported Macarthur – a business partner in the sandalwood trade – in his skirmishes against the governor. When Major George Johnston visited the governor to protest his interference in the New South Wales Corps, Jamison accompanied him to protest the obstruction in the Colonial Medical Service. After the meeting Bligh dismissed Jamison from his position as magistrate, on the grounds that he was 'not an upright Man, and inimical to Government', but as surgeons were in short supply Jamison kept his medical post.[19]

Tensions escalated. Late in 1807 Bligh had D'Arcy Wentworth court-martialled for having sick convicts work for him for free. He was found guilty, but Bligh, thinking the sentence too light, suspended Wentworth from his duties (a measure the Colonial Office would later find 'highly irregular') and publicly humiliated him.[20] Jamison supported his surgeon. On 25 January, Macarthur defended himself against a charge of sedition by challenging the right of Richard Atkins, judge advocate, to try him. The officers sitting alongside Atkins supported Macarthur, and the court adjourned. On 26 January, John Macarthur was arrested, but the officers again supported him; Bligh, furious, summoned them to appear before him the next day, but Macarthur outplayed him. Suspecting that a new and far more serious charge was being made out, he had penned a petition to Major Johnston requesting he arrest the governor. Although the bulk of the 151 signatures of officers and colonists appear to have been added after the deposal, it was a powerful statement of the colonists' right to hold land, protect their property and pursue profit, in Botany Bay as in Birmingham. Johnston ordered Macarthur's release, proclaimed martial law, and marched on Government House to arrest the governor.

Doctors were prominent in the move against him. Principal surgeon Thomas Jamison, D'Arcy Wentworth and the good doctor Robert Townson all sided with the rebels. Jamison assisted in the deposal and served on the key committees which sought to establish Bligh's despotism. Townson was reported to be one of the inner circle, though he complained about the grant he was offered at Botany Bay in the aftermath, and soon turned against the rebels. The following decade found him living frugally on his farm in social isolation, described as 'singular', eccentric, and developing a 'psychopathic personality'. Macquarie would later identify him as a chief, 'discontented' opponent of his administration.[21]

ONE YEAR AFTER THE DEPOSAL OF THE GOVERNOR, ALMOST to the day, Cadwallader Draffin was struck with madness. He had, by coincidence, travelled from England on the *Coromandel* with John Grant. The two had become friends and Draffin, a 'very amiable pleasant fellow', introduced Grant to George Johnston.[22] In a long account of the rebellion, Bligh wrote that 'on 1 February at an early hour, Lieutenant Draffin, who had been at the seizing of my person on the 26th of January last year, and was very active among the officers, was attacked with violent insanity'.[23] Draffin in fact led the march on Government House together with another lieutenant, William Minchin, was part of the group who sifted through Bligh's documents looking for incriminating evidence, and sat in judgement in several key legal trials, including the trial of provost marshal William Gore for perjury.[24]

This is all the more remarkable because Draffin had been mad for years. When the commandant of Newcastle penal settlement, Charles Menzies, requested a transfer somewhere his military career might advance, Governor King offered his position to Draffin, then an ensign, who had been part of the small force which established a settlement at Port Dalrymple in Van Diemen's Land the previous year. Charles Throsby, who we met in the previous chapter, was also appointed to Newcastle, but the ship which carried him wrecked off the coast, and when he at length clambered ashore and made his way to the settlement, he found acting Commandant Draffin 'perfectly insane'.[25] 'He is much debilitated,' Throsby wrote to the governor, 'and is perfectly incapable of even assisting himself with the common necessaries of life, so much so that his servant is obliged to put every morcel of his food in his mouth. He never speaks, except when asked a question he sometimes answers yes or no, and when placed in any particular position he remains so until removed.' He must be sent to Sydney immediately, or 'very shortly pay the debt of Nature'.[26] Draffin was placed on the sick list, and treated, but according to his fellow officer Minchin, 'the greater part of the time that he was in New South Wales he was mad', and it 'rendered him almost unfit for any service'.[27] It did not, however, impede his promotion to lieutenant the following year.

The striking place of madness in the higher ranks of the rebels suggests a desperation which diverges from the ways in which the rebellion has been written about, and remembered, for despite his madness, Cadwallader Draffin was one of the lead actors in the rebellion. It was a challenge to find officers who could be trusted with mutiny and the consequent responsibilities of governing. 'If I exempt Kemp, Lawson and Draffin,' Macarthur wrote to his friend John Piper, commandant at Norfolk Island, 'there is not a man that affords Johnston the least support.'[28] Draffin was needed to maintain the order of revolutionary New South Wales, which underscores the disintegration of the party that deposed the governor, splintering into incompatible interests, concerns and fears; it points to the deep divisions of New South Wales.

One division was between the wealthy, who talked loudly about liberty and property, and the small settlers, who struggled to make a living. Twelve Hawkesbury colonists wrote to William Paterson, anticipating his arrival in Sydney to restore order. 'We have embarked our all,' they wrote, and wanted to see their children inherit the proceeds of their colonial labour. 'With pleasure we saw the colony reviving from the most melancholy calamity, the streams of justice purified, crimes of the deepest dye prevented, discipline established, a system of monopoly and extortion in some measure suppressed.' Just as their 'hopes were beginning to revive, and prospects heighten', the officers arrested the governor who was transforming the colony.[29] One author was John Lewin, a close friend of John Grant, who like others had been pressured to sign the petition to arrest Bligh.[30] On Bligh's arrival, Macarthur had taken it upon himself to welcome him to the colony on behalf of 'the free inhabitants', but in a series of petititions 369 settlers from Sydney and the Hawkesbury disavowed him, an 'unfit person to step forward on such an occasion'.[31] After the deposal, settlers wrote to Johnston that they had no confidence in Macarthur, who, assuming the role of colonial secretary, claimed again to represent the colonists. He was 'the last man we would depute to represent us in any case whatever', they wrote. 'We believe John McArthur has been the scourge of this colony by fomenting quarrels between His Majesty's officers, servants, and subjects.'[32] A similar address to William Paterson begging him to put down the coup denounced 'the turbulent and troublesome Macarthur', who was clearly 'the principal agitator and promoter of the present alarming and calamitous state of the colony'.[33]

George Suttor, who would later take on the role of supervisor at the Castle Hill asylum, was furious at the deposal. Loyal to the king and the governor, Suttor gave his full support to a series of petitions against Johnston and the other officers. He refused to attend a general muster announced by Joseph Foveaux, who relieved Johnston as acting lieutenant-governor in July, in memorable, colourful terms. Bligh applauded his 'very particular and strong terms'; the rebels called them 'contumelious expressions' and prosecuted him.[34] At trial, Suttor would not enter a plea. 'Every drop of blood within my veins,' he likely enjoyed declaring, 'prevents me from ever acknowledging the legality of this court.'[35] For his trouble he was fined a shilling and gaoled for six months. While he was in prison, or on his release, his wife Sarah gave birth to her sixth child, who was named John Bligh.

Bligh took Suttor to London to testify on his behalf. He was away two years, and returned in some anxiety about the welfare of his family. Suttor took the position Macquarie gave him as superintendent at the 'lunatic asylum', it seems, on account of the portion of the former Government Farm that came with it, but both land and job were thorough disappointments. He benefited from the western expedition across the Blue Mountains in 1813, eventually achieving prosperity on freshly dispossessed land at Bathurst. When he came to write his memoirs, however, it was clear that he still bridled at the actions of the New South Wales Corps – a set of self-interested mutineers who ruled the colony 'with tyrannical insolence'.

While some of the negotiations that produced the rebellion remain secret, no one doubts that John Macarthur, former paymaster in the Corps and now a grazier and wool merchant, was the driver of the rebellion, and, for a time, the effective governor. In his memoirs Suttor claimed that Macarthur plotted with Edward Abbott, Johnston's second-in-command, and Nicholas Bayly, a disgruntled former officer and farmer. Johnston was nothing more than the 'dupe' and 'catspaw' of this 'triumvirate'. He later 'pined to death', wrote Suttor, while the ambition of the three leaders ended in 'evil consequences'. Two 'went mad, and the third shot himself in Sydney'.[36] The preceding chapters have shown how the tensions which coursed through the penal colony, and came to a head in the rebellion, played out in madness. Looking more closely, we find that the intensity of the rebellion spilled not only into the minds of the rebels but visited their families.

EDWARD ABBOTT HAD BEEN PROMOTED TO OFFICER BY merit, not purchase. He had a significant hand in the rebellion, as Suttor thought, but after Johnston declared himself governor in Bligh's stead he steered away from the rebels.[37] Abbott refused to serve as judge advocate, and offered his resignation from the army after Johnston's court-martial. Perhaps these actions helped him retain his good credit with the Colonial Office, and he was appointed judge advocate in Van Diemen's Land in 1815 and then commandant at Port Dalrymple, developing a reputation for generosity and justice.[38] Little is known of his inner life, but he clashed with George Arthur, lieutenant-governor of Van Diemen's Land, who was building his own culture of surveillance and terror. The report of his death in 1832 makes only vague reference to anxieties, infirmities and dissolution – words which might, or might not, refer to madness.[39]

Nicholas Bayly had strongly supported his former comrades in the Corps against Bligh, and fared well in the aftermath of the deposal, but later fell out with Macquarie. Unsuccessful as a farmer, he asked for a government appointment, but did not manage to find anything until he became cashier and secretary of the Bank of New South Wales in 1820. On 16 May 1823, Bayly shot himself at the bank, a fact which is recorded in the burial registry at St John's Cemetery, Parramatta. The ink is heavier along the strokes of the word 'shot', a departure from the register's usual probity.[40] He 'had for some time past been in a declining state of health', the *Gazette* reported discreetly, 'and on that day, and the day preceding, had manifested symptoms of delusion in the mind'.[41] The family vault listing is similarly circumspect.

Lesser characters also fell apart, like Garnham Blaxcell, whom commissary John Palmer derided as a grain man who had never grown 'a single grain'. A business partner of John Macarthur, the deposal placed Blaxcell in an excellent position to profit, and he daily siphoned from the public stores: two pairs of valuable millstones, thirty guns, rope, iron, canvas, sailcloth and clothing. 'The prisoners were left almost naked,' wrote Palmer.[42] Despite this prodigious profiteering, and the spirits monopoly and £10 000 which he, Alexander Riley and D'Arcy Wentworth each received in exchange for the grand hospital they built on Macquarie Street, Blaxcell's businesses eventually failed.[43] In 1817 he had the forthrightly criminal Lieutenant Charles Jeffreys smuggle him out of Sydney on his ship, the *Kangaroo*, with several convicts. On the Derwent outside Hobart, Jeffreys boarded a patrol ship, assaulted the captain, and took him and others hostage to ensure their departure. Blaxcell drank himself to death during the voyage, in Batavia.[44]

Gregory and John Blaxland were two of the earliest settlers of significant means. From the first they expected support from the government in land, convict labour, livestock and free passage. They were frustrated in their expectations, and the governors were frustrated by them. Bligh thought them 'so speculative as to care for nothing but making money'.[45] The Blaxlands were among the civilian leaders of the rebellion, and their names figure prominently on Macarthur's petition for Bligh's deposal. Gregory Blaxland clashed with Macquarie and then with

Darling, despite a moment of honourable respite for his celebrated crossing of the Blue Mountains. He made important advances in viticulture, but his interests suffered from drought and depression in the late 1820s.[46] John died in 1849. Gregory retreated from the public gaze, to re-enter only momentarily when he hanged himself, aged seventy-four, on 'an unusually hot' day with some symbolism, 1 January 1853. He had been in the habit of reading 'abstruse works'; he 'was accustomed to be affected in the head, and a little delirious' in hot weather; he 'had not had his clothes on for a week past'. He had had medical attention for six months, lately for 'pains in the head'. He was found, as others were, to have been temporarily deranged.[47]

As tensions escalated, George Johnston had found himself in an awkward position, caught between an autocratic and inflexible governor and the charismatic and manipulative John Macarthur, who retained a great deal of popular support in the Corps despite his resigning, like Bayly, in 1803.[48] Macarthur successfully undermined Johnston's authority among the soldiers, and when he brought him a petition with the signatures of prominent colonists and officers, Johnston perhaps felt he had little option but to depose the governor (he later explained that if he had not, there would have been riots in the streets). 'Even in the act of arrest,' write historians Ross Fitzgerald and Mark Hearn, 'Johnston deferred to Macarthur.'[49]

Johnston lost rather than gained authority by deposing Bligh. Macarthur was appointed a magistrate and 'secretary to the colony', but it was clear to all that Macarthur 'was in possession of the command', as George Caley wrote in a scathing open letter to Johnston, 'and that you were a tool in the business to answer his ambitious views'.[50] 'Captain McArthur, under the title of colonial secretary, does everything,' wrote surgeon Robert Townson, who had been one of the lead conspirators, and it would not 'be productive of good'. Those who had 'had the honour of governing this colony' were well acquainted with his character.[51] 'I really am extremely sorry for Johnston,' Edward Abbott wrote to former governor Philip King, 'for having suffered himself, to the astonishment of everybody, to be led.'[52] (If Suttor was correct, Abbott was one of those leading.)

For all its drama, the rebellion did not address the underlying divisions in New South Wales, and neither Johnston nor Macarthur were able to stop the Corps from disintegrating, as the most powerful officers and settlers proved just as quarrelsome as they had been with previous governors.[53] Johnston was relieved by his superior, Joseph Foveaux, and Foveaux by his, William Paterson. None of them wanted power. Johnston and Macarthur sailed for England, to prepare a case against Bligh and to defend Johnston against an inevitable court-martial. Macarthur's impressive network of patrons and supporters ensured that the charge against Johnston was downgraded from high treason to mutiny.[54]

On 7 May 1811, under the cavernous ceilings of the Great Hall of the Royal Hospital in Chelsea, aristocrats, officers and journalists assembled to see the famed William Bligh and the enactment of high colonial drama (Bligh's first mutiny, on the *Bounty*, had featured in West End plays).[55] Their theatre, the hospital, had been established to treat soldiers unfit for duty, which did not bode well for Johnston – but the trial, which ran a full month, almost seemed to be not of him but of the former governor. Bligh complained that rumours and vague reports had been dredged up from his entire life in order to exonerate the rebels.[56] Still, Johnston fretted, awaiting the result after the tribunal wound up with 'uneasiness and distress of mind' and the 'greatest anxiety', as he wrote to his own powerful connection, the private secretary to the Prince Regent.[57]

The verdict, when it arrived, was a compromise between

sovereign power and the power of imperial networks. It was surely a disappointment to the spectators and to those following at home, but more disappointing still to George Johnston. He was cashiered – cast out of the army without the refund of his commission. He was without friends, without prospects, and broke. His barrister was good enough to provide his services *pro bono*, since the rebels had not followed through on their promises of support.[58] He had to beg the government not only for permission to return to the colony, where he had established a family, but for the price of the passage out.[59] It was all 'particularly severe' and 'uncommonly vindictive', he complained to his former commander and patron, the Duke of Northumberland. The others had avoided censure, and even been promoted or allowed to retire in peace. 'I alone am the Sufferer,' he complained, 'and they seem determined to persecute me to the utmost.'[60]

On Johnston's return to the colony in 1813, Macquarie, the new governor, treated him like 'any other ordinary Settler', as he was instructed to do by the Colonial Office. Johnston was pressured by Macquarie to marry his lover, Esther Julian, as part of the new campaign for marriage and morality. In time the Johnstons dined at Government House with the Macquaries, and were favoured with land grants and other privileges. Although Johnston's biographers see him retiring to a model agrarian life, historians of the rebellion see him living in quiet ignominy, and drinking himself to death. In the midst of this supposed idyll, in 1820, he could still complain that everyone who had promised to support him had 'risen upon my ruin'.[61] These were wounds which still festered. According to Suttor, before Johnston died in 1823, Samuel Marsden heard his deathbed confession, replete with regret.[62]

The subsequent history of the Johnston family supports the bleaker version.[63] Six years after her husband's death, the

Supreme Court found Esther Johnston insane. She had built up the family estate significantly, to which the reiterations of their name throughout the pleasant, forested streets of Annandale and Glebe in Sydney's Inner West bear witness. Esther suspected that the commission of lunacy initiated by her family in March 1829 was a conspiracy to take control of the estate. She told the court of their 'violent and oppressive acts'. They said it was she, not them, who had been abusive. Esther had apparently been drinking excessively and 'driving furiously through the streets', like some shattered Dostoyevsky widow. William Bland, by now a specialist in mental illness, found it difficult to say 'whether her insanity is the effect of drinking, or whether a habit of drinking has been induced by insanity'.

Esther, for her part, 'declared her determination to bear it no longer, but to quit the Colony altogether'.[64] After the court ruled her insane, of course, she could not. To escape from her sons she moved into the Fox and Hounds on Castlereagh Street, where the publican, Isaac Moss, 'acted more like a son to her than a creditor'. Moss, who had known Esther was legally insane, was not able to recover the money for her lodging in legal proceedings in 1830, though a friend who had known her for decades said she was perfectly 'collected'. She was, it seems, returned to her estate and to her own sons.[65] It is little wonder, after her husband's years of pressure and anxiety, his betrayal by the officers and colonists, and his drinking and possible domestic violence, that Esther was finished with New South Wales.

WHEN JOHNSTON LEFT LONDON IN LATE 1812, HE DID NOT say goodbye to John Macarthur, who was beginning to question his decisions. He had been exhilarated at the outset. 'I have been deeply engaged all this day in contending for the liberties of this unhappy colony,' he wrote to his wife Elizabeth on the eve of 26 January 1808, 'and I am happy to say I have succeeded beyond what I expected.'[66] At a celebratory gathering, Nicholas Bayly, Garnham Blaxcell, John Blaxland, William Wentworth and others lauded Macarthur's 'manly and spirited conduct', and his 'wise and salutary measures' that had brought about 'the happy change'. They voted to send him to London with a sword worth a hundred guineas, to give their side of the 'ever-memorable' day. Macarthur rose to the occasion with a comic rendition of the evils of that 'parcel of assassins', Bligh and the magistrates, those 'villains who wanted to drink his blood'.[67] 'The tyrant is now gnashing his team with vexation at his overthrow,' he wrote to Elizabeth. 'May he often have cause to do the like.'[68]

Alan Atkinson has written much about John Macarthur and the rum rebellion. He sketches Macarthur as a 'marginal man' from the periphery of British society, the Scottish highlands. His people, the lower gentry, stood alongside the lairds but could not join their ranks, and as Scotland was opened to the world, they embraced a range of professions, administering the empire and trading across its breadth. John, whose father became a mercer and draper who traded across the Atlantic, grew into adulthood in Plymouth Dock. His family purchased him a commission in the army, and he married Elizabeth Veale, a Cornishwoman whose family thought him 'too proud and haughty for our humble fortune'.[69]

Macarthur's pride cloaked deep anxiety. Heavily in debt, he was trying to avoid being sent to Gibraltar, a 'notorious cul-de-sac', and Elizabeth had just given birth to their first child, Edward. Macarthur tried three times to resign his commission without forfeiting its value. His anxiety shifted towards dejection with each refusal. Eventually, however, he managed to transfer his commission to New South Wales, and the Macarthurs sailed in 1790, bent on success.[70] Near the Cape of Good Hope, Macarthur became ill after overexerting himself in the blinding ocean sun. He was diagnosed with lumbago. 'A violent and very alarming fever', wrote Elizabeth, 'continued to rage till every sense was lost and every faculty but life' in danger.[71] It left a profound impression on mind and body; Macarthur traced the gout and depression that plagued him to this sickness.[72] If it originated in this severe attack, the 'mental malady' was nevertheless intimately connected with the colonial politics of New South Wales, which so engaged his energies and ambitions over the next four decades.

Unlike Gregory and John Blaxland, Macarthur had little capital when he arrived in the colony, and unlike Garnham Blaxcell, he did not primarily build wealth by trade.[73] He raised sheep on the increasingly large grants of appropriated land which were the fruit of his prodigious talent for developing patronage networks, and plied those networks to develop a lucrative wool trade between the colony and England. His wealth was, according to his biographer, 'solid and material', where that of the merchants was 'mainly ephemeral paper riches, born of speculation and dissipated in speculation'. His estate was, indeed, largely free from the ravages that hurt others, and managed to weather even the periods of drought.

Macarthur seems to have had ambitions and drives far beyond wool and wealth. He was often led by his temper, which was incendiary. His frequent conflicts with others, including his superior officers, conformed to a pattern of rapid escalation, a sort of shock and awe, deployed on multiple fronts. His tactics were manifold: intimidation, litigation, the rhetoric of honour, barracks humour and even, perhaps, the language of rights and liberties, were used to conquer his opponents.[74] Failing to manoeuvre his superior William Paterson against Governor

King, Macarthur challenged him to a duel. He won, and though Paterson's wound was not fatal, it plagued him for the rest of his tenure in the colony. King sent Macarthur home to be court-martialled, with a sharp warning: 'There are no resources which art, cunning, impudence and a pair of basilisk eyes can afford that he does not put in practice to obtain any point he undertakes.' He was 'the master worker of the puppetts he has set in motion'. The creative invective to which the governors resorted is a testimony to the height of Macarthur's ambitions and the force with which he pursued them. 'Scarcely anything short of the full power of the Governor,' wrote Governor Hunter, when Macarthur was merely inspector of public works, 'wou'd be consider'd by this person as sufficient for conducting the dutys of his office.' 'If Captain Macarthur returns here in any official character it should be that of Governor,' wrote King. 'One-half the colony already belongs to him, and it will not be long before he gets the other half.'[75]

Legal historian Lauren Benton argues that mutineers who acted against 'despots' tended to have specific grievances rather than ideological objections to just authority.[76] On the surface, this seems to fit the 'little revolution': the rebels arrested Bligh, aired his tyrannies in the courts and streets and planned a delegation to London to argue their case. It was not, as a recent book has it, *Captain Bligh's Other Mutiny*; unlike those Tahiti-bound *Bounty* sailors, they stayed put, fully expecting to be vindicated in England.

English legal theorist and reformer Jeremy Bentham lobbied tirelessly for his model panopticon penitentiary in preference to the 'lottery' of convict transportation. In his 1803 pamphlet 'A Plea for the Constitution', he suggested that the governors of New South Wales had at no point enjoyed legislative power and that the colonial government was without foundation.[77] Fully aware of the volatility of his arguments, Bentham printed only a handful of his pamphlets and distributed the copies carefully. He sent one to David Collins, former judge advocate in Sydney then preparing to establish a colony at Hobart, and the two met and talked extensively. Collins may in turn have discussed these ideas with Macarthur, currently in London in exile.[78] In any case, Macarthur became convinced that Bligh's personal tyrannies and bad language were not anomalies, but crude renderings of the basic despotism of his position.[79] Hardly a radical, he did not brandish Bentham's arguments publicly, but merely hinted, in his stoushes with various authorities, that they may not be on as sure ground as they thought.[80]

Together with his former comrades and far-flung patrons, Macarthur rewrote the rebellion so compellingly that, leaving Sydney with his sword, he thought there would be no repercussions at all. 'In two months I hope to be in England,' he wrote to Elizabeth from Rio de Janeiro, 'and in three months after on my way back.'[81] He expected the empire to not only approve of the overthrow of Bligh, but also to restructure the colony according to his vision. In May 1809, under the name of his London agent, Macarthur sent a letter which echoed Bentham's arguments to Lachlan Macquarie, as the new governor prepared to depart for New South Wales. Macarthur was brilliant, writes Atkinson, but 'remarkably naïve in his self-confidence and his understanding of British high politics'.[82]

Macarthur saw the tide shift when Johnston was suddenly called for court-martial. During the trial, Johnston's defence made no mention of Bentham or the illegitimacy of colonial government. Rather than building a case for Bligh's despotism or for colonial reform, it deflected responsibility; if Johnston had not intervened, there would have been riots and massacres in the streets.[83] Macarthur, taking the witness stand, also avoided constitutional theories, and simply cast everything back on Johnston, and Bligh. He would not be led into confessing his role in the rebellion, and the closest the court came to his culpability was the following exchange, that might have been written by Samuel Beckett:

> *A Member.* What was Mr. McArthur tried for?
>
> *Another Member.* We have never understood, though he seems to have been the main-spring of everything.
>
> *The former Member.* It would be a satisfaction to know what was the cause of so great a revolution.[84]

Macarthur anticipated the 'unfortunate and inevitable' result of the trial; when Johnston was at length cashiered it became clear that he had overplayed his hand. His schemes ground to a halt.[85] After helping defend the charges against Captain Kent, who had refused Bligh's order to fire upon Sydney, Macarthur was 'plunged into a state of mental despondency' which he found difficult to explain. His life was a 'complete burden', he wrote to Elizabeth. He was 'without a ray of hope for a favourable change'. He slipped into a 'mental despondency' and would 'often pass weeks, without one cheerful moment'. His gout became an ally: 'I am seldom relieved from this dreadful gloom, except by the return of an acute pain.'[86]

Macarthur entered a period of frustrated ignominy, afraid to return to the colony for fear of prosecution. As a civilian, Macarthur had to be tried in the jurisdiction in which he had broken the law, and so opted to remain in England until was confident he would not be prosecuted.[87] It would be an eight-year exile. He tried his hand at speculation, and barely a year after the court-martial wrote to Elizabeth that he had lost the capital they had raised in the colony. Macarthur was still in partnership with Blaxcell, whose business was rapidly failing. He wrote home comparing the 'plenty and affluence' of their colonial life with the 'pinching penury' they could expect should Elizabeth wind up the estate and bring their children to England.[88]

The government first intended to charge Macarthur with high treason, but this was in time downgraded to conspiracy and high misdemeanour. Macarthur knew nothing firm; he heard only rumours.[89] After five years in exile, a friend confirmed that he was considered 'the leading promoter and instigator of the mutinous measures' of 1808, and that there were standing orders to prosecute him as soon as he set foot in New South Wales. 'All the ill success of my labours here,' wrote Macarthur, 'have produced a depression of spirits.' He continued to wait and to nurse his 'wounded mind'.[90]

Lachlan Macquarie arrived in New South Wales to impose imperial order, together with the 73rd Regiment and Judge Ellis Bent, who would establish legal order, including over madness. Macarthur, from afar, felt colonial opinion was turning against him (many, of course, had been against him for a long time). The Macarthurs had been optimistic about Macquarie, but he publicly promoted the interests of emancipated convicts, placed them in positions of honour, and even had them to dine at Government House. John was shocked at his wife's reports.[91] 'Every paragraph increases my amazement, and every circumstance you relate adds to the perplexity of my mind. God alone knows how such a state of things as you describe may terminate, or how operate on our affairs.'[92] Macarthur's biographer, Malcolm Ellis, attributes his growing inner distress to these developments: his legal situation, financial situation and political machinations were twisting together into a mental malaise he could not conquer.

Macarthur finally received permission to return to Sydney

in 1817 – on the condition that he not interfere in public affairs. This prohibition may have contributed to the fact that, despite his relief at being reunited with his family after eight years, his depression did not lift. He confided in his friend Walter Davidson the following September about a recent conversation with a good friend 'blest with the cheerfullest temper, with excellent health', and £50 000 acquired in the East Indies over thirty years. He had returned to England to enjoy his wealth, but the novelty of opulence wore off and he began to feel that he 'had no business left except the pursuit of pleasure or amusement'. He would have given up all he had if he could only return to the colony. It reads like a parable. 'Words cannot convey to you,' Macarthur's friend told him bleakly, 'how heavily my time hangs and how thankful I feel when the day is at an end.'[93]

Macarthur did not return to the centre of colonial society, though the Macarthurs continued as one of the leading families. They continued to shape the colony's politics, but chiefly through the lobbying of the younger Macarthurs in London.[94] It was partly due to the family's efforts that Macquarie returned to England in 1821 in some disrepute. His successor, Thomas Brisbane, was initially well-disposed to Macarthur. He had served in the army with Edward, and thought to appoint his father to the magistracy, as a favour but also because of Macarthur's long experience. Judges John Wylde and Barron Field dissuaded him; for all his talents, Macarthur had precipitated a rebellion, and he was likely to divide the magistracy.[95] Frederick Goulburn, colonial secretary, did not favour the Macarthurs with appointments and favours, and the Macarthurs, including John's nephew Hannibal, led the resistance to Goulburn and Brisbane which ended in the removal of both.[96] It was a matter of some pride to the family; John Macarthur junior reported his laughter, with under-secretary Robert Wilmot Horton in London, over 'poor Sir

Thomas Brisbane – his probable surprise at being superseded – his vanity – weakness of character'.[97]

The quality and value of the Macarthurs' wool increased, the estate grew enormously, and the Australian Agricultural Company the Macarthurs helped found in 1824 looked promising: a million acres purchased with a million pounds. Macarthur's connections ensured his appointment to the colony's first, unelected Legislative Council in 1825, against the better judgement of the secretary of state.[98] 'It certainly was a wise measure,' wrote daughter of the colonial secretary Fanny Macleay sarcastically: 'He is a sad wicked being.'[99] John junior had helped shape the new constitution, which created the council.[100] Much of this influence was exercised behind closed doors, and mostly across the seas, rather than in Sydney, where John senior became increasingly isolated.

Ralph Darling replaced Brisbane, as the Macarthurs desired, in December 1825. In mid-1826, Macarthur complained to Darling of the *Gazette*'s libellous writings about him, and demanded that the government defend him, as a council member. When the two met, Macarthur mentioned to him 'very significantly' that 'he had never yet failed in ruining a Man, who had become obnoxious to him'. 'I understand,' Darling wrote to London, 'when speaking to others, he does not except even *Governors*.' Darling was struck by Macarthur's energy and simmering violence: 'He is a man of strong passions and observes no medium in anything. He is equally ardent in his exertions to serve as he is to injure. Naturally factious and turbulent, he considers the accomplishment of his plans as secondary to the subjugation of his opponents.' These traits had left a long wake in the colony, and Darling concluded that 'his intemperance and violence' rendered his talent and knowledge 'unavailable'. To work with Macarthur would be to 'embroil myself with the community, to whom he has rendered himself extremely obnoxious'.[101] Perhaps noting the fate of his four predecessors, Darling simply suggested to Macarthur that 'another line of conduct' might have placed him at 'the head of this society'. He 'would soon know the people [he] had to deal with,' Macarthur replied, and proceeded to avoid both the sessions of the Legislative Council and the Darlings at Government House.[102]

By the mid-1820s, Macarthur's 'party' was reduced, by his own biographer's count, to 'himself and four quaint followers': Archdeacon Thomas Scott, who lived rent-free in Macarthur's garden cottage; the humanitarian attorney-general Saxe Bannister, whom the chief justice and governor thought slightly mad; Surveyor-General John Oxley, who had been engaged to Elizabeth Macarthur junior until her father discovered Oxley's considerable debts; and James Bowman, inspector of colonial hospitals, who had married Mary Macarthur. All had benefited from Macarthur's influence.[103] Beyond this circle his reputation continued to deteriorate. 'Old King John is of all men the most disagreeable,' wrote Fanny Macleay. 'He quarrels with every one, who does not yield implicit obedience to his opinions whatever they may be. The very look of the man would make you shudder.'[104] Even those who agreed with Macarthur's politics found him difficult to negotiate: he was a 'man of the most violent passions', wrote Robert Scott, 'his friendship strong and his hatred invincible'.[105]

FOR MORE THAN A DECADE MACARTHUR HAD SHOWN A private despondency, but it began to break into his public life in a flurry of eccentricities. The governor referred to a former letter from Macarthur, with details of 'some of the thousand projects he had in view for the aggrandisement of the Australian Agricultural Company'. By this point, 'they *all* seem to have vanished, as the excitement, in which they were engendered, subsided'. In May 1826 Macarthur had planned to take his daughter to England, even chartering the *Lady Rowena* and sending an agent ahead to make arrangements. He mentioned his trip '*formally*' three times to Darling, reading the details from a book, but 'he is still here', wrote Darling in September. Each time the itinerary had changed, from England to China and Bengal, and finally to South America, for the 'more practicable scheme' of introducing a 'breed of asses!' Darling apologised for wasting the time of the undersecretary with these details, but thought it would not be entirely wasted because they indicated the '*soundness*, if I may so term it, of the projector'. Macarthur no longer deserved 'that deference' which had been 'too generally and without due consideration conceded to him', suggested Darling. 'He is now like a wayward child, and remains at home brooding, but I expect is not altogether *idle*.'[106]

Others noticed Macarthur's decline. News of his departure was 'too good to be true' for Fanny Macleay. He had been 'very wretched', she wrote, because he could find no-one to gossip with about the dire state of the colony.[107] The trip may have been an attempt to escape a situation that was becoming untenable. Macarthur was physically ill, and grew increasingly depressed. 'Altogether hypochondriac,' wrote his wife, but she was deeply concerned, and wrote often to John and Edward about their father's poor spirits.[108]

In April 1831, in London, the younger John Macarthur collapsed and died from 'an effusion of water on the brain'.[109] The Macarthurs learned of their son's death five months later.[110] A letter to Edward soon after maps his father's grief in the rhythms of his life. He slept from midnight to four, then dwelt upon 'important affairs both public and private' until daylight, when he went to inspect the improvements on his house. Evenings were spent in conversation with his doctor, Matthew Anderson, who moved into the house so he could attend Macarthur closely. 'By these means I keep in subjection many melancholy thoughts,' he wrote, 'which in spite of all my philosophy at times bear very heavily upon me. Poor dear John. How often do I suffer when alone I undergo a bitterness of grief which no language can describe.' Writing plunged him into a fresh 'burst of grief which the world will never suspect me of giving'. He slept, woke again at four, and concluded his letter.[111]

Macarthur hid his grief from his wife. Elizabeth had only just written a parallel letter, which probably travelled in the hold of the same ship and confused their eldest son, saying that his father had been in good health and kept active, although 'we who know him observe the occasional pang that comes across his mind when anything recalls the image of him whom he dearly loved'.[112] Two months later, she wrote again to Edward. Macarthur had born his son's death with 'becoming fortitude'. His efforts to 'conquer his feelings' came at the expense of theirs, as he talked aloud '*continually*' of John. He 'became more and more restless' and was anxious 'to talk any where, and with every person, who came in his way'. It was something more than sadness. 'He labours under a partial derangement of mind and views many objects through a distorted medium,' she wrote. 'May God grant that these mists of the mind may soon disappear.'[113]

The Macarthurs' cottage at Parramatta felt the assault of Macarthur's energies. '*The steam engine power,*' wrote Elizabeth, 'is applied to the veriest trifle when in this excited state of mind.'[114] He worked almost feverishly, building, painting and digging, making plans and changing them often.[115] It was the same vigour which had led him to cast himself at the government in successive waves, like ocean breakers. The stonework and timbers, in their manicured grounds, were the resting place of Macarthur's ambitions.[116] This house, which John would never inherit, would be a 'valuable inheritance' for Edward.[117]

Macarthur went to Port Stephens to replace the managing agent of the Australian Agricultural Company after he and the other colonial directors turned against him.[118] He ran it nearly into the ground.[119] 'If the object of the Committee had been to bring the enterprise to utter ruin, I do not know what more effectual steps could have been devised,' a superintendent of the Company wrote eighty years later.[120] Macarthur attended a Legislative Council meeting in May 1832, and visited Elizabeth and his children. He was better, wrote Elizabeth, but still 'restless'.[121] On 5 June he took his grandson to the King's School, Parramatta, and wrote to a correspondent, in a faltering hand, that the new governor Richard Bourke agreed with his view of the colony.[122] Later that month he accused James Bowman of being a 'conspirator' who was plying him with poison; sent his daughters away from the house, thinking that they had robbed him; and 'made the most fearful accusations' even of Elizabeth. His family placed 'a wholesome restraint' on him to prevent 'greater violence', and entrusted him to John Moore, their 'old faithful servant', and two or three others 'who attend to his personal comforts in every respect and administer to his wishes'. 'Still, be not alarmed,' wrote Elizabeth to Edward. 'His fine mind may yet right itself.'[123] In the meantime, writes Elizabeth's biographer Michelle Scott Tucker, 'she bore her husband's capricious demands with calm resignation'.[124]

The family requested a commission of lunacy, which would protect the estate, contain Macarthur's violence, and minimise social damage. The commission assembled on 17 July 1832, at Hambledon Cottage, the second house on the Elizabeth Farm estate, Parramatta. The attorney-general attended, with a 50-guinea fee.[125] Arthur Hamilton, surgeon of the 39th Regiment, related Macarthur's delusions (assassination attempts, poisoning, 'that a number of persons were concealed about his house with hostile intentions') and gave his medical opinion that Macarthur was 'disordered in his reason'. A letter he received from Macarthur was presented as evidence: 'The wretch who administered the dose is I think fled. Is it not melancholy that we have no magistrate in the town except an implicated person?' Macarthur's suspicion engulfed even his physician. 'I have a bottle of charcoal prepared by Mr Anderson which from some peculiarities in his remarks when he saw it I suspect is highly medicated,' Macarthur wrote. 'Would it be possible to analyse it.' He asked Hamilton to breakfast with him in the morning, and signed off. 'P.S. I am very drowsy is that favorable or not. Saturday night.' Then, perpendicularly across the letter, 'I hear nothing of the soldiers'. He had written to Parramatta for 'a party of soldiers' to guard him.[126]

Macarthur drafted a desperate letter to Richard Bourke, reading it to his officer friends Patrick Lindsay and Donald Macpherson, who retold it to the commission.[127] Poison was flowing through his veins, having 'the most grievous effect' to his body and causing a 'sore on his head'. His sons had been poisoned too, so that 'their intellects were deranged and their loyalties perverted'. With 'a formidable band of adherents' they had 'taken possession of a strong position in some remote part of the Colony' – James and William grazed sheep on James's farm at Sutton Forest, in the Southern Highlands – and must be dislodged 'by force of Arms'. Macarthur's own intellect 'was fortunately preserved intact'. In fact, Lindsay said, Macarthur was 'so wild and incoherent' the night he and Macpherson visited that they thought him 'completely deranged'.[128] A lifetime of boasts, threats and schemes were concentrated in these delusions, in which sons became enemies and helpers assassins, and

Macarthur looked to the government, at last, for refuge. He was restaging the trauma of revolution.

The commission agreed with the various witnesses that John Macarthur was mad, and had been 'for some months past'. 'He is now mad in law,' reported *The Australian* '– tho' not more crackbrained probably now than he was thought to be years ago.' He had been 'a fit subject for it' three years prior, offered the *Tasmanian*.[129] Concluding that Macarthur was unlikely to recover, Bourke declared his seat on the Legislative Council vacant.[130]

The Macarthurs' education and social background mean that they wrote extensively to each other and to their friends; their standing meant that these letters were preserved. They wrote often about John's 'excitement', 'disordered mind' and 'excessive nervousness'.[131] It has been called later a 'crippling depression'.[132] These letters, and the rich sources of Macarthur's colonial accomplishments, offer the rare chance to view his inner drama against the colonial drama he helped to orchestrate. His madness was embedded in his schemes and dreams, for though his illness appeared from an early age, his mental energies coiled around the 'little revolution' he engineered in Sydney, and appear to unfold over the rest of his reverberant colonial life. There is a certain fatalism to be found in the discussion of his faculties. 'We cannot attribute this excitement to any *one* particular cause,' Elizabeth wrote, as John slipped into mania.[133] As it developed further into incoherence and violence, Elizabeth could not say 'the blow – severe as it is – had come upon them without long previous apprehension'. 'Sooner or later,' she had thought for long years, 'the mighty mind would break down and give way.'[134] George Suttor may have relished the thought that Macarthur's madness, especially, was a punishment for the rebellion he had engineered, but the many words written about him show that his illness threaded through his colonial career, as he negotiated and manipulated, flouting all policies and ruining all persons who stood in his way. It preceded the rebellion, but then wrapped around it, and rose fitfully in its wake.

A book like H. V. Evatt's *Rum Rebellion* shows how in New South Wales men like John Macarthur and William Bligh became caricatures of themselves, or of who they might have been in settled societies. It may be delicacy that has kept historians from drawing these threads of anxiety and despair together, but they are all too clearly bound up in the rebellion, or revolution, and the colony which produced it. Madness lies beneath the surface of even the most celebrated of our national narratives. The 1808–09 rebellion stripped away many of the pretences of civilised, orderly colonial life. For two years, a coup prevailed in the belly of the empire, attended by rampant cronyism and a judicial vindictiveness which made a mockery of the rule of law. As the empire reasserted itself over the following decades, the drama of the rebellion continued to play out in the lives of its protagonists in regret, alcoholism, madness and suicide. These glimpses of unravelling reveal the longer and deeper confrontation between private property, theories of liberty, and the strong power of government in a penal colony.

8

WRONGFUL CONFINEMENT AND IRRESPONSIBLE POWER

Tarban Creek Lunatic Asylum opened at Gladesville, on the Parramatta River, in 1838, as the transportation of convicts to New South Wales approached its end. It was the first real asylum in the colony. Its expensive sandstone had been raised from the cream skimmed off the colony's growing wealth, from the fruit of free enterprise, and it was intended to house the madness of free men and women. But first it became an arena for the final convulsions of penal society. The core dynamic of a penal colony as a place where prisoners were worked and punished and where others lived freely alongside them played itself out here, under the shadow of the new Legislative Council. A purely advisory and unelected body when it was first installed, the council was expanded and empowered in 1843, with half of its members now elected by the colonists. Still, New South Wales lacked self-government. Its government answered to London. Tarban Creek was a perfect analogy for such a society since, as reformers pointed out, its power over patients was like that of the empire over the colonists: immense, arbitrary and irresponsible.

Shortly after the first elections for the Legislative Council in

1843, a suit for wrongful confinement was taken up by a set of lawyers and new council members in their continuing attack on the colonial government. These were members of the 'Australian party', an informal group gathered around William Charles Wentworth and the newspaper he had helped to found, *The Australian*, campaigning for free political institutions and responsible government.[1] Their success in the courtroom very quickly produced the first lunacy legislation passed in Australia, an Act which protected society from 'dangerous lunatics' and the government from their lawyers.[2] A minor amendment to that Act precipitated a barrage of editorials and public letters roiling around an inquiry. As the reformers interrogated and wrote and conspired to overhaul the management of the asylum, they worked to cleanse both it and the colony itself of their history.

TARBAN CREEK LUNATIC ASYLUM EMERGED FROM THE vision of Richard Bourke, governor of New South Wales 1831–37. As a liberal and urbane man, Bourke had been reluctant to take up a remote post ruling the empire's criminals, but his concerns were assuaged by Robert W. Hay, undersecretary of state. The Australian colonies were the 'most thriving' in the empire, Hay wrote in 1828, 'every day increasing in importance'.[3] Bourke was under the impression that the flow of convicts would soon end when he left for New South Wales, but it did not, and indeed increased during his administration. Some 30 000 convicts arrived in the colony in the 1830s, more than a third of the total received across the course of transportation. But the free population was also growing strongly, so that by the end of the decade the colony was its most divided: a receptacle for British criminals but also a flourishing colonial society with a free population increasing in its sense of entitlement as well as in number.[4]

'This Colony,' wrote Bourke, 'is like a healthy child outgrowing its clothes.'[5]

Large profits from wool and whaling fed into a land revenue windfall, which colonists wanted to invest in local infrastructure – a new set of clothes.[6] The governor agreed, and planned a suite of new schools, gaols, courthouses, roads and bridges, an expanded Government House, and a semi-circular quay at Sydney Cove. These were not for Britain or for its convicts, who had a limited tenure in the colony, but for the coming free society. Even the new gaol planned for Sydney was to be of a 'permanent character', wrote Bourke, servicing the colony 'long after the mother country shall have ceased to send out convicts'. The asylum, too, was to be a 'permanent building' designed to 'outlive the arrangements that now throw so large a proportion of the expences of the colony upon the mother country', wrote Bourke. It was intended to outlive transportation.[7]

Tarban Creek quickly entered the colonial consciousness, embraced by the newspapers even while it was under construction. 'We always thought [the editor of *The Australian*] a little *touched*,' the proprietor of the *Gazette* wrote in November 1836, 'but, after his last production, we consider him but one step short of being "stark staring mad." His friends, if they act advisedly, will immediately apply for his admission into the new assylum at Tarban Creek.'[8] A year later, the asylum was nearing completion. It would soon be open, noted the *Gazette*, 'for the accommodation of some of our literary friends' and later Edward Hall, editor of the *Monitor*.[9] He was mad to think he had any, *The Australian* shot back.[10] Under this tongue-in-cheek barrage, readers grew more aware of the coming asylum, which quickly achieved a presence that Castle Hill and Liverpool never had. There was genuine interest in the impressive construction, which involved no less than sixty-nine mechanics (skilled labourers), including painters, glaziers, plumbers, diggers, carpenters, joiners, shinglers, smiths, plasterers and fifteen masons.[11]

The expense and design of the building indicated that it was not for convicts. So did the site, chosen by Bourke and the principal surgeon – Bedlam Point, on the Parramatta River, in present-day Gladesville. It was a place of tranquil beauty, an echo of Brisbane's planned asylum at Elizabeth Bay.[12] As the colonists had already discovered, however, the attractive image of colonial society dealing with madness in a permanent asylum of which it could be proud had to be followed through with funding – and George Gipps, who replaced Bourke early in 1838, was slightly preceded by a severe drought. Depression followed, with deflation, bankruptcies, bank failures and unemployment, all on a drastic scale.[13] Gipps's consequent parsimony would mean a far more frugal asylum than the one envisioned by Bourke, and lead to difficult relations with the staff.[14] Bourke had requested the secretary of state to find a superintendent and matron in England, ideally a married couple, since there was no one 'well qualified' in the colony.[15] It was later claimed that the earlier asylums had descended into 'a deplorable state' for precisely this reason.[16] Joseph Digby was appointed from a London asylum, with a reference from Dr Sutherland of St Luke's Hospital. His wife Susannah was appointed matron. On their arrival in Sydney in early July 1838, they were alarmed to find the asylum still incomplete. Gipps would not pay them the half-salary promised by the Colonial Office for the voyage out and expected them to proceed to the unfinished building to save on lodgings and expedite construction.[17]

There were further disappointments in store. Gipps flatly denied Digby's request for furnishings for their on-site residence – they would have to find their own furniture. He forwarded another request for English mortise locks and the special sashes used at the Retreat, a famed English asylum, to the colonial architect Mortimer Lewis, with a warning to avoid unnecessary cost.[18] He was reluctant to approve requisitions for clothes and equipment, would not replace convict staff with free men and women, and vacillated on whether an ox or horse could be provided to carry goods, messages and water from the creek (it was not clear whether Sydney or London should pay). 'Let him begin with an ox,' Gipps decided, but the animal, when it arrived, was 'worked down so much as not to be able of drawing the smallest load without falling down continually'.[19] Four years later, Gipps was unmoved when the old mare that had replaced it fell ill: 'considering the number of able-bodied men who are at all times in the asylum I am disposed to think that if due exertion were made a horse would not be required'.[20] The buildings and grounds were only kept in good condition by the patients' labour, which included, in the first eight years, clearing and stumping a two-acre garden and cutting and installing two miles of timber fencing. The asylum 'scarcely cost the Government anything,' Digby said.[21]

There were costs for staff and supplies, however, and these were divided between colonial and imperial governments according to the ratio of free and convict patients in the asylum. Colonial funds had been used to build the asylum, and it was decided that the home government should pay for the ongoing expenses, with the colony to reimburse the cost of treating free colonists. Despite Bourke's plans, Tarban Creek primarily catered to convicts when it opened.[22] This arrangement would be neatly reversed when transportation ended in 1840.[23]

These funds were the site of various skirmishes. John Blaxland, that early settler capitalist who with his brother had pained successive governors, had been appointed to the Legislative Council by Darling in 1829, and remained there as the 'defender of the public purse'. He argued that the paupers supported by the colonial government were the remnants of the transportation system. When the budget estimates were presented to the council for 1839, he opposed the £500 for final construction work, £2625 for the support of free paupers there, and £3000 for free pauper patients in other hospitals. London had sent '*aged infirm* convicts to the colony', he argued, 'whose labours in their youth and prime of life were expended in England'. A decade later, a transport ship surgeon agreed, after an especially trying voyage to Hobart. After seventy years of transportation, mentally and physically ill convicts were still being sent to the colonies, and there were 'too many of this and the old and useless class there already'. The United Kingdom had used transportation to remove 'a large portion of her criminal population', Blaxland concluded, and should pay the continuing costs of their care. The estimates were approved.[24]

WILLIAM CHARLES WENTWORTH WAS BORN *EN ROUTE* TO Norfolk Island on the *Neptune*, to Catherine Crowley, a convict. His father, D'Arcy Wentworth, was a serial highway robber connected with the illustrious Fitzwilliam family who had chosen exile in New South Wales during his fourth criminal trial. D'Arcy Wentworth, as we have seen, served as principal surgeon, chief police magistrate, and in a range of other roles. William was educated in England and became an outspoken and political colonist. He was shaped by the history of the colony, especially the rebellion, though he was in England while it unfolded. In his history of the colony, written and published in London in 1819, Wentworth argued for government by elected representatives, trial by jury, and free emigration. William Bligh's authoritarianism – including the humiliation of his father – pointed, he said, to 'the impropriety of confiding unlimited power' to the governor. 'The mere possession, indeed, of such vast authority, is calculated to vitiate the heart, and to engender tyranny.'[25]

On his return to the colony in 1824, Wentworth pursued this reform program through public meetings, petitions and formal addresses, as well as the legal and editorial grandstanding with Robert Wardell that featured in Chapter 6. Other prominent colonists joined him, including John Jamison, and William Cox and Gregory Blaxland, whose crossing of the Blue Mountains with Wentworth was celebrated among Europeans for 'opening' a way to the Bathurst plains (Wiradjuri country). Their activity crystallised in 1835 into the Australian Patriotic Association, which aimed to more effectively lobby the British Parliament for political rights in Australia, cutting through the competing voices which clamoured from across the seas. Key members included secretary William Bland, who had been surgeon at Castle Hill two decades prior, now a recognised specialist on madness and an inveterate dueller, as well as Edward Hall, and John Mackaness, Darling's 'reprobate'.[26] It transpired that the association was, like the rest of colonial society, divided between large landholders, small landholders and professionals.[27] Nor is it surprising that those who advocated the rights of colonists refused them to Aboriginal people. Wentworth supported the perpetrators of the Myall Creek massacre in 1838, and was furious with attorney-general John Plunkett for pressing for their execution, which amounted, he said, to judicial murder. Richard Windeyer, 'a barrister of superior abilities' in J. D. Lang's estimation, and later elected to the new Legislative Council, was lead counsel in the perpetrators' defence.[28]

Self-government did not preclude convict labour. The members of the association were shocked at the workings of the Select Committee on Transportation in 1837–38, and by its conclusion that New South Wales had been corrupted by convicts (which appears to have been decided before hearings began by advocates of Wakefield's theory of systematic colonisation, and ensured by the careful selection of witnesses and questions).[29] They advocated vigorously but unsuccessfully for the continuation of transportation, and against systematic colonisation and other efforts to engineer colonial societies. William Bland argued that the assignment of convicts to private families did not corrupt the families, but reformed the convicts.[30] He would be remembered in his old age as 'struggling, sometimes against imperial, and at other times against local tyranny' for half a century.[31] But as the association's friends in London tried to make clear, representative government would never be introduced while transportation continued.[32]

The transportation of convicts to New South Wales ended in 1840, and within two years the British parliament agreed to allow elected representatives into the legislature of New South Wales. It had become 'expedient that further provision be made for the government of New South Wales', as the New South Wales Constitutions Act explained drily.[33] It drew from the many proposals and petitions of the association, as well as those of former chief justice Francis Forbes and James Macarthur. The Legislative Council was expanded to thirty-six, with one-third appointed by the governor and the remainder elected by the landholding and householding men of the colony. Although the council's powers were still limited, the new constitution looked toward the future.[34] The new asylum, the new council and the Australian party were about to be thrown together in a legal suit for false imprisonment and assault.

EARLY IN 1840, AN IRRITABLE MAN ATTACKED A WAITER called Murray at the Royal Hotel in Sydney, while playing billiards. Charles Hyndman had asked two or three times for a piece of welsh rarebit, and called Murray a 'damned careless rascal' for ignoring him. Murray said he had not heard; Hyndman said, 'You can neither hear nor see properly.' 'I will get a pair of spectacles,' replied Murray, 'and then I shall see better.' Hyndman, who wore glasses, 'immediately reversed the cue with which he was playing, and holding it with both hands, struck the witness as forcibly as he could with the butt end of it, on the right side of the head close to the temple, inflicting a severe wound, from which the blood streamed copiously.' The next morning he returned to the hotel and sought out Murray. 'I lost a breast pin last night,' he said. 'If you find it I will give you a pound.' Murray refused, and Hyndman threatened to kick him. Hyndman was charged with assault, but shortly before his trial he returned again to the Royal. 'I hear that you are going to bring an action against me,' he told Murray. 'I don't care a curse, if I go to the police office they can only fine me £5.' He snapped his fingers. 'Five pounds are nothing to me, and after I have paid it, I will come here again, and give you another d—d good thrashing.' The judge called Hyndman's conduct degrading and 'unmanly', and fined him £30, suggesting he might also pay £5 to poor Murray.[35]

Hyndman was an energetic, eccentric citizen who seems to have enjoyed listening to himself at public meetings.[36] His family had settled at Port Macquarie after he retired from the dragoons. They were rumoured to be in financial trouble, but were still able to feed, house and clothe a convict baker. Hyndman was actively engaged in local politics, giving 'a very excellent speech' in favour of a new Presbyterian Church in early 1841.[37]

In June 1842, Hyndman accosted a young man in the street who had, as agreed, fashioned a canoe from one of Hyndman's cedar slabs. A surveyor who was passing by tried to intervene, and Hyndman lost his temper, accusing him of making a 'gratuitous assertion'. The surveyor, who was clearly a gentleman, took offense, and 'the whip was immediately applied to the delinquent's back', as he would later declare on oath. 'That person very wisely concluding "discretion to be the best part of valour" darted off at a tangent along the streets of the town, collecting lawful witnesses of the assault, in reserve for a "day of retribution".'[38]

The papers came to view the old dragoon as an entertainment, and took his violence in stride. When Hyndman proposed to start a theatre company at Port Macquarie, *The Australian* responded: 'We fear that the gallant captain will find that producing plays, sans actors, sans orchestra, sans scenery, and indeed sans theatre, will be a rather puzzling speculation.'[39] Three years later, after Hyndman had spent two days 'amusing the lieges, and occupying the time of the bench' trying to make a perjury charge in an impounding case stick, the case was dismissed, and *The Australian* hoped that he would 'at length, take a hint and keep his eccentricities in the back ground'.[40] This was the sort of language used in depositions, trials, columns and editorials to describe those with borderline mental symptoms, sometimes suggesting to their readers the existence of more serious disorders. Here they give the impression of an eccentric, litigious and violent man living at the edge of madness.

From March until July 1843, elections were held to fill the elected seats of the new council. Charles Hyndman did not stand for election, but he spoke at several public meetings during the campaigns, thrusting himself into the centre of things.[41] On 31 July, soon after the Cumberland election, he gave a speech before a large crowd at the Sydney racecourse in which he called Gipps 'a miscreant' and threatened to put him on a gridiron.[42] He had earlier tried to warn the governor of a conspiracy among the mechanics to burn down Sydney. When the governor refused to see him, Hyndman drew up a handbill depicting him as Nero, playing his fiddle while Rome burned. He was also seen driving wildly around the streets of Sydney, an image often used to evoke mania, as it had for Esther Johnston.

Constables interrupted Hyndman's racecourse speech and arrested him. The charge was minor – creating a disturbance – but Hyndman refused to pay a surety for good behaviour and was taken to Darlinghurst Gaol. There he showed signs of madness, telling the gaoler 'a great many improbable and conflicting stories' – that he was the head of 'the cabbage-tree mob, a secretly organised force of 7000 men, whom he had with difficulty prevented from burning Sydney'; that after saving the Queen's life, an 'intimacy' had 'sprung up between himself, Prince Albert, and Lord Combermere' (Her Majesty's former commander-in-chief in Ireland and India). The governor had 'ruined the colony', and Hyndman would lead the mob with 'sword in hand' to 'drive him from' it. The cabbage-tree mob, in Sydney parlance, were ne'er-do-wells who wore cabbage-palm hats and were known for knocking the hats off gentlemen outside the theatre; 'loafers', noted the visiting aristocrat Godfrey Mundy with distaste, 'an unruly set of young fellows, native born generally, who, not being able, perhaps, to muster coin enough to enter the house, amuse themselves by molesting those who can afford that luxury'.[43] (Mundy, incidentally, had been aide-de-camp to Lord Combermere.) It was not an organised gang, as Hyndman claimed, but a term men like Mundy used for the boisterous, unruly youth of the colony.[44] The term seems to have been used as a joke in the election campaigns, although, said magistrate Henry Weston, the mechanics really were 'very clamorous'.

Two days before he was due for routine discharge, Hyndman was moved to Tarban Creek Lunatic Asylum. No formal medical certificate was made out. When he requested writing materials, he was told there were none available by Susannah Digby, the matron. It seems like cruelty, but paper, quills and ink were expensive, and had to be requisitioned from the government. In any case, Henry Weston and his cousin Robert Johnstone, another magistrate, found out about Hyndman's admission 'by some good fortune' and went to Tarban Creek to visit him. When they arrived, however, they were told they had not come on the appointed visiting days – and, as superintendent Joseph Digby later explained, 'it was necessary on all occasions to abide by the regulations'.[45] George Robert Nichols, a lawyer who had represented Hyndman in the billiard cue incident, next went to Tarban Creek, demanding to see the warrant for Hyndman's admission and threatening a writ of *habeas corpus*. The script, which could prise a body from any illegal grasp, had been used by innovative jurists since the 18th century to challenge the confinement of those whose insanity was doubtful, especially where statutory law was seen as inadequate.[46] The threat was enough, and Hyndman was discharged.

Hyndman swiftly brought a suit against Joseph Digby and Joseph Innes for assault and false imprisonment, which appears to have been a scheme of the Australian party. Nichols was prominent in the Australian Patriotic Association and closely associated with Wentworth. The son of a wealthy emancipist, he bought *The Australian* in 1833 and used its platform to argue against government tyranny and to call for the end of convict transportation and for self-government.[47] The lawyer who represented Hyndman in his suit was Richard Windeyer, a key player in the Australian party.[48] Both Windeyer and Nichols had given speeches at a public meeting in March 1842 calling for a petition to the British parliament for representative government in New South Wales, and Nichols was elected to a committee established to continue the campaign.[49] Windeyer attacked the colonial government in council and court, arguing for reform of land revenue and trial by jury.[50]

In a theatrical opening speech, Windeyer exaggerated Hyndman's political activities, which clearly 'did not please some of the persons in power', to make his treatment out as a form of censorship. He spoke against against Hyndman's admission to Tarban Creek without a medical examination, and under the 'pretended authority' of a warrant he said had never been produced. In fact Nichols had seen the warrant, and there had been some medical examination, but the documents used Hyndman's talk of conspiracy, and his speaking 'disrespectfully of the Governor', as evidence of his insanity. It was just what Windeyer needed to conjure a dark image of the asylum, 'this prison – this Bastile [sic] for such persons as were hardy enough to use disrespectful language against the Governor'. A free man had been 'deprived by arbitrary power of his liberty', he thundered. His allusions to the French *ancien regime*, and its fate, were none too subtle. Bastilles were bound to be broken.

Hyndman won his suit and £100 damages, because 'due caution and care had not been exercised in order to ascertain the state of plaintiff's mind'. It was a striking result, especially since the evidence seems to show him in control throughout this saga of supposed despotism. In gaol he had boasted that he 'could get plenty of bail if he wished it; but it did not suit his purpose, as he was desirous of punishing those who had confined him'. Weston, the magistrate, said that Hyndman was perfectly sane and had a political program. 'I believe he said,' Weston told the court, 'that a good case of oppression was one of the best things he could have to go home with.'

When the suit ended on 16 November, the government acted with alacrity, sending the Dangerous Lunatics Bill to the council just twelve days later. It was intended to make provision for the detention of the 'dangerously insane' and those of unsound mind.[51] Criminal lunacy would be dealt with by criminal courts; in other cases, supposed lunatics were to be brought before two magistrates and two doctors and could then be placed in a gaol, house of correction or hospital. The governor's order was required for entry to an asylum. If families wanted to avoid this process they could approach a judge of the Supreme Court with a certificate from two doctors, and arrange committal through the Commission of Lunacy process.[52]

In George Gipps's message accompanying the bill to the Legislative Council, he referred directly to the Hyndman case. The transfer to Tarban Creek 'was performed under the authority of government', he reiterated, and the officials in question had only rendered themselves liable to litigation because the legislation was inadequate. After the provisions for the legal treatment of the insane, then, the ninth clause 'indemnified all persons concerned in the confinement of the insane persons in the lunatic asylum from any legal proceedings'.[53] This was not a rhetorical or a theoretical move. Other parties had been 'emboldened' by the suit, attorney-general John Hubert Plunkett told the council, and 'were contemplating proceedings against the authorities'. Without the bill there was nothing to prevent them proceeding, 'as long as solicitors were found willing to incur the hazard, for the remuneration and notoriety the business afforded'.[54]

Politics spilled directly from the courtroom into the new council, and the elected members pounced at the second reading of the bill. Wentworth was at a loss 'why the Governor should be thrust forward in so odious a measure'. The authority for the admission and discharge of the insane from the asylum rightfully belonged to magistrates, who were drawn from the people. Delegating this power to the head of executive government was 'unconstitutional and unsafe, as it gave a power to incarcerate for life any one whose principles or politics were opposed to the constitution'. While some law was necessary to govern madness it should 'not be a Bastile Law but an English Law'.[55] Such power was 'too onerous' to be held by a single person, '*especially one whose situation was an irresponsible one*'.[56] Richard Windeyer, unsurprisingly, agreed. The attorney-general replied that the bill was taken almost verbatim from its English counterpart, and diverged only on the power of the governor in admission and discharge. This section was modelled on the Irish Criminal Lunatics Act of 1838, since the lord lieutenant of Ireland enjoyed similar powers to the governor of New South Wales.[57] For the Australian party, this was precisely the point.[58]

Two months after the trial Hyndman's wife and five children sailed for England with a servant, perhaps using some of the damages for their fare.[59] Twenty years later, Hyndman was admitted to Tarban Creek, where a new superintendent found him delusional, 'egotistical and troublesome', and talking of conspiracies. He concluded that it was 'extremely doubtful' that Hyndman had been 'perfectly sane' at any time in the intervening years.[60] This time his solicitor was less motivated. After a brief, tense visit to the asylum he told the superintendent, 'Why, he is madder than I thought him.'[61] Some years ago a psychiatrist historian diagnosed Hyndman (from the asylum records) with 'affective psychosis', a condition which manifests in 'excessive states of depression or elation with resultant disturbances of thought and behavior'.[62]

The Dangerous Lunatics Act did little to address the concerns which had surfaced during the Hyndman trial about the relationship between the asylum and the government. Although it was supposed to protect society from the physical violence of the insane, the Act served rather more effectively to protect the government from the insanity of free men and women; these were its 'dangerous lunatics'. Convict insanity had never posed a legal problem, since the governor had custody of those who were serving their sentences. Free insanity had been a liability from the start, and not least when a royal pretender nearly wrested Port Dalrymple from an equally insane commandant (see Chapter 2). He, too, had threatened legal proceedings. Now, with the colony poised on the edge of self-government, free lunatics were far more dangerous.

THE VISITING MAGISTRATE OF TARBAN CREEK LUNATIC Asylum, Joseph Innes, wrote to the colonial secretary in March 1846 warning of the conditions at the asylum.[63] Soon afterwards he gave a tour of the asylum to Joseph Phelps 'Humanity' Robinson, a Quaker banker lauded for his social work and a member of the Legislative Council. They found it so crowded as to make proper classification of patients impossible.[64] On 6 May, the colonial secretary received a second, anonymous complaint along the same lines: the lack of patient classification and their general discomfort; uncleanliness; and poor ventilation.[65] The governor, who was preparing to leave the colony, referred the complaint to the council, and nine days later, sent a second short amendment to the Dangerous Lunatics Act to the council. It merely clarified the formal requirements for certifying doctors and authorised the governor to remove patients from the asylum in the case of overcrowding or discharge them to their families insane, on the condition that a bond was entered into for those committed as dangerous lunatics or idiots.[66]

Before the first reading of the amendment, Charles Cowper, who was also known for his humanitarian zeal, called for an inquiry into the asylum. Robinson voted in favour, and the colonial secretary, on behalf of the government, agreed to a Select Committee on Tarban Creek.[67] Three days later, a lettrist called

'Iatros' submitted a lengthy commentary on the 'lunacy bill' to the *Sydney Morning Herald*. It was a strident, learned call for the reform of Tarban Creek, its author either unaware that the bill was a negligible amendment, or pretending to be. Over the next four months, in nine long letters to the *Herald* which ran to almost 16 000 words, 'Iatros' pointed to the fundamental flaws of Tarban Creek and dwelt on the qualities of a modern, European, medical lunatic asylum. Even in 'highly civilised, rich, and beneficent England', the mad were still to be found in 'a state of misery, oppression, filth, neglect, and heartless tyranny'. Readers were left to reflect on their plight in New South Wales.[68]

'Iatros' outlined the glorious recent advances in asylum design and therapeutic regimes, including the eradication of physical restraint. He wrote at length about the crowning promise of the medical asylum and the cure of madness – and he found an audience.[69] The Select Committee interviewed several witnesses in early June, the week after it was appointed, and then fell silent even though it was supposed to report after a month. The *Herald* threw its support behind 'Iatros' with two forthright editorials published on 9 June and 4 September, and when the committee resumed its interviews in mid-September, its agenda closely resembled his.[70]

The fifty pages of transcribed interviews published with the Select Committee's report show its members seeking evidence of physical abuse and physical restraint, but finding little evidence of either. The only glimpse came from James Eckford, surgeon at Liverpool Hospital, who seems to have been angling for a job at Tarban Creek. Several of the patients arriving at Liverpool from Tarban Creek 'had never had the belt taken off them while they were at Tarban Creek', he testified: in one case fully six years. 'As a professional man,' he told the committee, 'I highly disapprove of that.' Eckford released them 'immediately on arrival' at

Liverpool, where he rarely resorted to restraint, and then for no 'more than a day or two' (by the ankle, to a log).[71] Physical restraint was avoided where possible in moral therapy, but its total elimination had emerged in the late 1830s as a signature element of moral therapy led by medicine.[72]

Joseph Innes, visiting magistrate, who had written his own complaint in March, asked to testify to the committee again after the *Herald*'s September editorial. He wanted to refute its 'innuendoes'. Asked how much of the restraint at Tarban Creek might be dispensed with, he replied sharply, 'I cannot say "much of the restraint" because there is not *much* used in the Asylum now'. Eleven of the 131 patients of the asylum were under restraint, generally only by one hand. The committee pushed back: was there a record of restraint kept? No. How could he tell which patients were under restraint? By personal inspection. Might not many of the patients be restrained between visits? It was possible. Did the staff know when he was likely to visit? His visits were highly irregular. 'If they saw you coming,' pressed one member, 'might they not take the restraint off? I think that is hardly likely,' replied Innes curtly, and the committee moved on.

The main accusation of physical abuse took the form of a complaint which surfaced during the course of the inquiry. A woman identified as Mrs P—— had given birth to a child on the passage out, with no one to attend her, and developed puerperal insanity. The committee members asked many questions about Mrs P——, but did not find what they were looking for. George Turner, rector of St Anne's Ryde and the only one of the official visitors to the asylum to show any real interest, described how she was in an almost continual 'state of raving mania … constantly jumping about'. Her restraints were removed during one lucid interval, and 'immediately the door was opened, she struck the female keeper in the face, and threw her back against the wall'.[73] She sometimes injured herself in these paroxysms, at one point wounding her left arm, damaging the brachial nerve, and paralysing her hand.[74] This was why she was restrained, generally with a leather belt and handcuffs at the waist.

The committee's report, printed on 21 October, was accordingly quiet on violence, restraint, and Mrs P——, but the *Herald* was less cautious. In a review nearly double the length of the report, replete with gratuitous italics and punctuation, George Turner was derided as 'an advocate of chains, fetters, *comfortable* iron belts and collars, hand-cuffs, and leather muzzles', and Mrs. P—— elevated as a free woman 'nightly strapped and chained down to her bedstead, in a room within hearing of the horrible language of the female convict lunatics'.[75]

The chains and collars were important. The *Herald*'s image of Mrs P—— had great disruptive power, evoking the horrors of insanity – the loss of control, dignity, personhood – but also the horrors of convictism. The flow of convicts had only just stopped, and the cries from the convict prison on Cockatoo Island still carried across the water.[76] The link was made by frequent association; sometimes it was made explicitly. 'A more deplorable state of things,' the *Herald* bemoaned, 'has seldom been exposed, not even, probably, in the very worst days of convict misrule' – and the attendants were still-serving convicts, 'selected from the very refuse of the worst penal settlements'.[77] Despite its elaborate design, significant cost and the expertise of its senior staff, Tarban Creek could efficiently summon all kinds of horrors.

'Iatros' argued, relentlessly, that a medical doctor should be at the head of a lunatic asylum. James Eckford had a similar agenda. Madness, he argued, was proven to flow from organic disease. A man with a liver disease, said Eckford, might slip into a 'mental aberration' on losing his wife, but if he recovered from liver disease, his mind might also recover. In every mental patient who had died in his care, autopsies had found 'organized disease either of the brain, heart, or liver'. A layperson could could hardly be expected to follow these advances in medical knowledge.[78] The patients at Tarban Creek, Eckford added with a condescension which was surely calculated, 'were treated, as far as I could ascertain, as well as a non-professional man would be inclined to treat them'.[79] The instructions Eckford circulated at Liverpool asylum, and presented to the Select Committee, made his views very clear. Authority was concentrated in the surgeon; the attendants answered to the 'keeper', who was responsible chiefly for administering physical restraint, but on this and all matters the keeper was to 'receive his orders immediately from the surgeon in charge of the insane.'[80] It is by no means clear how authority was actually configured at Liverpool.[81]

Eckford, and likely 'Iatros', as well as the shortcomings of the elderly doctor at Tarban Creek, persuaded the Select Committee that 'the chief authority of the institution should be vested in a duly qualified medical man', and that the 'moral as well as medical' treatment of madness was 'the distinct province of a physician'. At the start of the century The Retreat, that exemplary and famous Quaker institution at York, had demonstrated the effectiveness of a deliberately lay regime.[82] By deploying increasingly sophisticated and authoritative medical discourse, however, professionalising doctors displaced lay therapies by the mid-century, just as they had earlier established their profession over untrained 'barbers', and would later denigrate the work of nurses.[83]

One aspect of the medicalisation of Tarban Creek was the insistence that it should keep proper paperwork – admission registers, casebooks and transparent records of all use of physical restraint. Transparency, in fact, was the key, since the asylum doctor Thomas Lee and especially Digby did take notes and keep them in private diaries. Modern medicine, however, required clear, public books. This insistence was both a nod towards the introduction of a proper medical regime at the asylum and a means of facilitating remote visitation; it was William Dawson, inspector of hospitals, who had first brought up the lack of books, and who was particularly frustrated by it. He had no means of judging the management of the asylum, he told the committee, because there were no written records. The work of the asylum, which by all accounts was exemplary, was eclipsed by its paperwork failures.[84]

But there was more at play here than medicine. George Turner remained sceptical about the conduct of the inquiry, and particularly the provenance of Mrs P——'s statement. When the report appeared, he wrote to the *Herald* to complain that the committee members had tried to lead their interviewees towards the answers they wanted.[85] In another letter he mentioned 'Iatros's letters, and noted that a medical superintendent was 'now made a paramount condition of future reformation. On this point I will simply ask a question. Is it true that the writer of those papers has alread sought his Excellency's patronage for the appointment?'[86] He grew more sure as time passed. A medical superintendent had been 'the obvious end for which almost all persons connected with the enquiry have been working together', he wrote in June 1847.[87] Thomas Lee, too, complained of the 'hostile and interested persons' who had been 'interesting themselves' in his removal through the course of the inquiry.[88]

The lettrist 'Iatros' was a doctor named Francis Campbell.[89] Those reservations expressed in the Legislative Council at the conduct of the inquiry and the contents of the report were overcome by a supplementary inquiry in 1847, and Campbell was appointed medical superintendent of Tarban Creek, which brought the *Herald* 'very much pleasure'.[90] Campbell suggested that his title, 'Superintendent and Resident Physician', might be profitably amended to 'Medical Superintendent', to avoid the impression that there was some other superintendent.[91] Joseph Digby was demoted to the role of steward, but in 1850, after two years of conflict, he was dismissed in disgrace.[92]

Campbell's motives, like those of Eckford, seem clear enough, but why were members of the Legislative Council and the *Herald* so supportive of his cause? None of his reforms would come cheaply, after all. The expansion or even rebuilding of Tarban Creek Lunatic Asylum, had his plans been acted upon, would have come at enormous cost, and the report warned that 'the council should also be prepared to provide liberally for a duly qualified person'; £400 should do the trick, one (medical) lettrist suggested.[93] Blaxland died in 1845, and who would defend the public purse now?

The matter did not escape notice. 'Many consider the [Select Committee] to be a well-managed scheme to oust one surgeon in order to make room for another at a much higher stipend', the editor of the *Freeman's Journal* wrote in 1851.[94] Others attacked the empty reformism of the *Herald*, which had been so incensed at the 'abuses' at Tarban Creek, and of its 'own particular pet', Charles Cowper.[95] Cowper 'gave no impression of believing in the reforms which he effected', writes historian John Hirst.[96] He was also aligned with the interests of the Australian party, which may have inflected his efforts at Tarban Creek. According to the *Freeman's Journal*, Cowper's ardour had achieved nothing, and the 'repeated and unsatisfactory "investigations"' in the five short years since the enquiry left a sour impression of that 'expensive and badly managed Institution', Tarban Creek, and of the integrity of the reformers.[97]

WHILE DEFENDING THE ASYLUM OFFICERS, GEORGE Turner had quoted an 1838 treatise by Sir William Ellis, superintendent of Hanwell Lunatic Asylum and an early proponent of occupational therapy and puerperal insanity.[98] He might not have, suggested the *Herald*, if he had read further. 'No one except a medical man, and a benevolent one' should be entrusted with managing an asylum,' wrote Ellis. He had met Digby at Hanwell, and considered him of good character, but 'the only knowledge of the disease possessed by himself and his wife, the matron,' he wrote, 'has been derived from their being keepers in a private asylum'.[99] Bourke and Lord Glenelg, Secretary of State, had placed the insane of New South Wales '*under the control of a class of persons entirely unqualified for their management*', the *Herald* italicised, and there were profound implications.[100]

Ellis saw a colony clawing out of convictism, a coming 'mighty empire of the south' which would surpass Europe in significance as it already did in size. Medicine was needed to treat the madness to which 'the habits and characters of its inhabitants' would 'render peculiarly liable'. Ellis, like 'Iatros', cited the recent revelations of abuse in England, 'in the midst of medical knowledge, and with a population advanced in morals, intellect, and benevolence' and he, too, left readers to draw conclusions about New South Wales. Asylums without medicine were nothing more than places of 'safe custody', and for Ellis, the appointment of the Digbys showed that 'in the opinion of Government, insanity is not a curable disease'.[101]

Now that the transportation of criminals had ceased, and a Legislative Council had been installed, social institutions had to be made to support this image, rather than undermine it – they had to be free, transparent and curative. Medicine held out the promise of cure, especially with early intervention.[102]

The Legislative Council had from its first year applied

itself to the question of madness, and trod a fine line between legislative oversight and executive functions. Considering the Dangerous Lunatics Act in 1843, the Legislative Council had proposed a small amendment: as well as the five official visitors to be appointed by the governor, two should be appointed by the council. It proceeded to appoint the prominent Australian party member William Bland, and another doctor, Charles Nicholson, who also advocated responsible government.[103] Both had spoken at the March 1842 meeting, with Windeyer and Wentworth.[104] The governor referred controversial legislation to the Colonial Office, however, and when he saw the amendment the secretary of state, Lord Stanley, decided that it was a dangerous 'usurpation' of executive government by the legislature. Liberties like these tended 'to multiply themselves', he wrote, as he struck the offending legislation down.[105] But the brief amendment remedying the usurpation in 1845 gave William Wentworth an opportunity to add a further provision giving the Supreme Court the power of review.[106] A judge could issue a warrant for any patient to be brought to the court and order their discharge immediately if satisfied they were sane.[107] The *Herald* noted with approval this 'safeguard against one of the most dreadful species of oppression to which human beings can be subject'.[108]

Henry Hothersell Browne, the first visiting magistrate to Tarban Creek, quarrelled with Joseph Digby about their relative responsibilities, which had never been made clear. 'Having been left so many years to himself,' he wrote later, Digby 'fancied himself supreme, and did not like any interference'.[109] The superintendent sought clarification from the governor, but there was none, and Brown's successor, Joseph Innes, was also annoyed that Digby seemed to think he was 'independent of the supervision of the visiting magistrate'.[110] Innes perhaps expected the asylum to function like Darlinghurst Gaol, where as visiting magistrate he was closely involved, signing requisitions, laying down rules and managing staff. The Select Committee was willing to accept the image presented of Digby as a petty tyrant, jealous of his small measure of power, but the *Herald* went a step further. 'The irresponsible Digby' derived his inflated sense of power because he had been appointed in England, by the Secretary of State. '*Neither Superintendent nor medical man*' – the author grew irate – '*has anything binding upon him; it is left to his own discretion!!!*' Joseph Digby was nothing less than the '*ne plus ultra* of irresponsible power'.[111] The journalist Samuel Sidney had never been to the colonies, but that was not a prerequisite for writing an account like *The Three Colonies of Australia*, which was published in 1853. Sidney was well informed, offering a thorough critique of convict transportation and a strong case for self-government. In a section ominously headed 'official responsibility', Sidney summarised the findings of the Select Committee on Tarban Creek. He took special interest in the Digbys, who having been appointed by the secretary of state 'habitually resisted all attempts to control, or even investigate the performance of their duties, by the visiting magistrates or colonially-appointed physician'. This destructive 'independence and irresponsibility' flourished in the absence of a locally elected legislature. Tarban Creek, indeed, presented a perfect analogy for the colony. Digby, he said, 'ought to have been a colonial governor or a colonial secretary'. The colonists were 'treated like the Tarban Creek lunatics: they do not know what is good for them neither do their representatives. The governor is the man; he is responsible to no one; and although the Legislative Council, like the doctor, may recommend removing restraint, he knows better.'[112]

Over five decades, restless colonists had used the courts and the colonial newspapers, to press for trial by jury, freedom of expression, and responsible government. They organised in formal groups like the Australian Patriotic Association and informal ones like the Australian party. In 1843, the creation of a Legislative Council with a majority of elected members concentrated these energies. Tarban Creek Lunatic Asylum immediately became a site of special significance for the new members, not because of its failings, but because madness offered them a powerful metaphor for colonial politics. In the year the council was established, several members used Charles Hyndman's suit for false imprisonment to draw attention to the continuing imbalance in government, an inheritance of the penal colony. They moved unsuccessfully to appoint their own visitors to Tarban Creek, and in debates and legislative amendments worked to diminish the power of the governor over the asylum and its population. The Select Committee inquiry, conducted after George Gipps had left the colony and before the arrival of his successor, rejected the authority of the visitors appointed by government, critiqued the staffing decisions of the governor and the secretary of state, and demonstrated that the Legislative Council was perfectly capable of overseeing even something so complex as the management of madness. And it went further. For all the rhetoric of Richard Bourke, he had made Tarban Creek a prison, or bastille, by entrusting it to those who could not possibly hope to cure madness. 'The time will come,' wrote 'Iatros', 'when the cure, not the imprisonment, of the maniac, even here in New South Wales, will be the policy of the statesman and the duty of the physician.' An immediate solution to the colonists' predicament was medicine, which confronted madness with the 'certainty of cure'. The more profound solution – which they had been pursuing for years – was to ensure that the lunatic asylum, and the colony itself, were governed by their elected representatives.[113]

EPILOGUE

In 1824, a young Dutch circus tumbler named Alexander Green stole 'a piece of brown stuff from a shop', and was transported to New South Wales for the term of his natural life. He managed to obtain a conditional pardon after a year, likely because he worked as a police informer, but he was promptly found guilty of bearing false witness in court and burned as a source. He found a form of refuge as a scourger, or flogger, at Sydney Gaol. The next year, at the age of twenty-six, Alexander Green became the hangman of New South Wales.[1] Over the next twenty-seven years, until his death, he would execute some 490 men and women at the 'place of atonement' – the sand hills near the Brickfields, in present-day Chippendale. The hills hosted ritual revenge combat among the Eora at the turn of the century, later becoming a burial ground before the dead made way in the middle of the century for Central Station.[2]

Execution was a wretched vocation. An axe-wielding prisoner left Green with a long scar down his cheek.[3] He tried to hang himself at thirty, when a woman he was courting rejected him, but he was cut down before death took him.[4] At thirty-nine, he moved into his first house, a small, whitewashed cottage outside

Darlinghurst Gaol, but the following year a mob enraged by the execution of some popular bushrangers surrounded the cottage and set fire to it. Green was almost burned alive. The number of executions in the colony began to fall rapidly, from 1838, and he began to drink heavily. He was drunk on the scaffold many times and once fell clean off it.[5] He had skirmishes with the law and was dismissed for intoxication and insolence, and then reinstated, dismissed and reinstated. Hangmen were hard to find.

In 1846, just forty-four years old, Green was described as 'a drooping figure' riding a coffin atop a cart to Goulburn.[6] Convicts no longer arrived each year, and executions were growing rare. Idle now for large swathes of time, he drank more heavily still. In 1853 he began to show signs of madness, and it may be that he hanged ten people in the company of his delusions.[7] After the first private execution in the colony in February 1855, within the walls of Darlinghurst Gaol, the sheriff reported that Green was 'now quite insane'. Two months later he suggested, more pointedly, that he be sent to Tarban Creek.[8] Eleven years later, Green was vigorously keeping the male dormitory of the asylum clean, and after another thirteen years a regional newspaper noted that 'Green, formerly the hangman, died at the Lunatic Asylum'.[9]

A local newspaper reported some years later a tale that was told at Tarban Creek about a former patient who had hanged his father and mother in a serial execution, only recognising them after they were dead. 'The result was madness.'[10] It seems a cruel story to tell of a man whose life had been so hard – but Tarban Creek was full of misery, and Sydney full of cruelty. 'It was a frightful city in which to contemplate madness,' writes Peter Carey, as his protagonist Lucinda feels herself slipping beyond reason, 'all hard with eucalyptus, snapping sticks, sandstone rocks with fractured faces and cutting edges. You could not, not in Sydney, dear God, allow yourself to fall into such a weakened state.'[11]

Alexander Green was a creature of Botany Bay. His story flows with the broader currents coursing through the colony: the isolation of transportation; the harshness of law enforcement in a penal society; the prosecution of a program of terror and class warfare; streets lit up by the fury of club law. The colony gave him a second chance, but it also took him in its grip and broke him, ending in drunkenness and madness. This book is partly an anthology of this sort of suffering, which by gathering together individual stories draws attention to the nature and scope of the colony's madness.

But it is more than an anthology. The history of madness in New South Wales is the history of madness in a penal colony, and it is cut through with striking revelations. Families were in general torn apart by transportation, and it took time for communities which were capable of supporting the ill to develop. Part of the grand experiment of shipping thousands of criminals across the seas was a new assertion of government responsibility for the physical health of the colonial population, and doctors and resources were deployed to preserve those who were transported. But madness, despite recurring discussions of its links with criminal behaviour, slipped through British courts, gaols, hulks and transport ships, and into the penal colony. There, in a society built around discipline, magistrates, officers, judges and governors charged with establishing order saw madness not as an illness, but as a perilous chaos. If they were sometimes moved to deal gently with the insane, at other times they were not, and the shifting structures of law and government left room for their discretion. There were many who suffered doubly, from the discipline and from the internal damage it wrought in them. Compounded suffering appeared to be the price of colonial order.

The government of New South Wales did take responsibility for madness when it posed a threat. The Heads marking the entrance to Sydney Harbour also marked an exit. They were a gateway to freedom, and shipping in and out of Sydney was carefully controlled. Governors were at times more concerned that the water was free of madness than the land, and found the means to apply their delegated powers over the bodies and minds of captains and supercargoes. They had been entrusted with the enormous discretionary power thought necessary to control a society of felons and soldiers. They did not do so with impunity, however, because even rumours of colonial despotism played poorly in British politics, and the empire was knit together by an endless stream of letters between the ranks of powerful families, patrons and protégés. Governors wrote late into the evenings, struggling to preserve their visions of the colony, which did not even internally cohere. Colonial policy in New South Wales had a persistently experimental aspect, fully conscious of the nightmare of North America but without a lucid vision for avoiding it. These autocratic experiments, in turn, frustrated the ambitions of officers and colonists, to whom the contradictions of a penal colony became violently clear.

For those wealthy, entitled, letter-writing colonists, strong government threatened their rights to personal liberty and private property. These were the core interests in the legal tests of madness, in which lawyers, witnesses, judges and jurors decided whether people were able to govern their selves and manage their estates. The rebellion which John Macarthur orchestrated in 1808 asked the same questions. It was a flashpoint of the tensions inherent in the penal colony, and an expression of the reach of colonists' power, of their capacity to change the course of empire. The drama – not only during the rebellion, but in the colourful skirmishes before and after it – affected its protagonists deeply, and left a trail of bitterness, madness and suicide.

Madness represents a slippage between the interior and

exterior; inhibitions and social graces fall away, the inner self erupts in startling behaviour and language. It is therefore a dexterous vehicle for navigating those borderlands between the inner world and outer world, sanity and insanity, self and history. It helps us see what the colony was – not from the perspective of theorists or administrators only, but also in the eyes of all those who made it. These stories of breakdown and suffering hardly absolve the guilt of colonisation, as a project, or of the theft, displacement and direct violence which constituted it. But they add to the complexity of our ideas of colonisation. What was it like to piece together a European society in Australia, working often from first principles, without a coherent program and at the mercy of a metropolitan government moved by distant concerns, and other constituents? We see the limits of consciousness drawn around the day-to-day life of a colony like New South Wales, as immediate needs and desires crowded out the cares and perspectives of others. But we see also the freedom of working without precedent, and the intimacy possible in a place where government, judiciary, church, citizenry and felonry lived on each other's streets and crossed paths frequently – where, indeed, a man like Samuel Marsden might act from hour to hour as a farmer, special adviser to government, judge, lobbyist, pastor, doctor, detective and evangelist. The history of madness shows that New South Wales was a village as well as a prison. Its power to disrupt demanded a response from the gamut of colonial society, from the leads – John Macarthur, Lachlan Macquarie, William Bland, William Wentworth – to the many who played bit parts in public life. As they responded to madness, they are revealed as complex and changeable, like ourselves. Madness similarly wreaked havoc on the inchoate structures of government, and as it did, revealed inconsistencies and vulnerabilities in the vast imperial machine.

The equivocal response from London after the 1808–09 rebellion revealed a deeper equivocation about the penal colony and the fabric of empire. After Lachlan Macquarie arrived, and set about establishing order, his own ambitions and policies did little to illuminate the nature of the colony, but they did force the ambiguity of the colony to a tipping point. Secretary of state for the colonies, Earl Bathurst, commissioned a thorough review, and specified what it was to find: a global terror emanating from Botany Bay, but one which did not compromise the prospects of New South Wales, a settler society of growing economic and political value. The voluminous reports of commissioner Bigge built upon the hundreds of interviews he conducted with colonists of every kind, and drew personal experiences of colonisation into the constitution of the society. Together they forged a path to prosperity through violence and terror.

IN AUSTRALIA, COLONIAL HISTORY ERUPTED AT THE TURN of the millennium in the History Wars (as the Culture Wars raged in the United States). Diverse moral assumptions and historical methodologies were set against each other, motivated by professional and political commitments. Historians and politicians fought not only about the interpretation of violence – the allocation of culpability – but about how we can be certain of the past. How, they asked, can we know how violent colonisation was? The stakes seemed terribly high. In Australia, one of the academic historians drawn unwillingly into the fray was Lyndall Ryan, whose research had helped clarify the relations between Aboriginal people and Europeans in Tasmania. 'Who is the Fabricator?', she fired back in a 2003 essay, and moved to establish the violence of colonisation upon a surer footing.[12] In 2017, a team of researchers led by Ryan at the University of Newcastle launched their Colonial Frontier Massacres Map. Like a wave of death the markers spread across the country, each representing the killing of six or more Aboriginal men, women or children by European colonists. It was a new and coldly visible archive, and it was alive. After thirteen months, the markers reached further north and further west, threatening to engulf the continent.[13]

Mapping the killing of Aboriginal people points to the attendant destruction of Aboriginal culture. The fear of this violence and the grief which followed it is certain to have left its own casualties, and a swathe of mental symptoms, but it was rarely identified with European notions of madness. Even in the 20th century, there were few Aboriginal patients admitted to the asylums that now spread around the continent, and it was well into the century before Aboriginal mental health and illness began to be seriously discussed.[14] In the present day, Aboriginal people are vulnerable to a range of mental symptoms, and a wide range of other indices measure their struggle to prosper in European Australia. Aboriginal community leaders, historians and mental health practitioners link these symptoms with intergenerational, systemic trauma.[15] Invasion, as Australian historian Patrick Wolfe made clear, is a structure and not an event.[16] 'We cannot allow ourselves to talk of loss,' Bruce Pascoe declared with force in October 2018 at the Australian Museum. He speaks instead of those who invented society, in the first known village, and agriculture – of discoveries and gains.[17]

This history of violence caused great consternation to Australians when it became unavoidable at the turn of the century. 'Why weren't we told?' asked Henry Reynolds bleakly, as he confronted the foundations of the country.[18] The researchers' fatal map prompts us to talk further of the killing of Aboriginal people – visualising, as it does, Wolfe's 'logic of elimination' – but it also demands other work.[19] It is clear to us now that violence affects perpetrators as well as victims, that it always bursts its bounds. What did men think and feel as they killed, and afterwards? What did they tell their wives and children? Aboriginal oral traditions preserve and wrestle with memories of war, but little enough was written down to enter the settler colonial consciousness – little commentary, certainly, on the scars it might leave. Even in the delusions and ravings of the mad there was a certain reservation, as if after the reticence insisted upon by reason was stripped away, some subjects were still protected by deeper codes of shame and silence, were taboo. But the cultural and physical violence of colonisation surrounded the European society it created; it was etched even into the ground and on the maps of the dispossessors. Poisoned Waterhole Creek, Carbine, Slaughter Creek, Blackfellas Leap.[20] It seems impossible that it did not also wound its participants; impossible that the madness of the colony was not in some way a mirror of the violence of colonisation. It is time to talk more about the ways in which the experience of colonisation turned back upon the colonisers – not to dismiss the continuing brutality of colonisation, but to more powerfully render the colonial present.

The concept of trauma was developed in the 20th century to describe the physical and mental effect of the near-global shock of the world wars, not because there had been no trauma before, but because its effects became unavoidable. The literature of cultural trauma draws from psychopathology to describe the effect of endemic violence upon a society.[21] The fact that trauma has, as historian of medicine Mark S. Micale writes, 'broken its original disciplinary boundaries' so strikingly and become something of a global obsession might suggest not only that violence is widespread, and broadcast everywhere in every media, but that we are increasingly haunted by our pasts. Trauma is a deeply historical concept, a metaphor borrowed from medicine to argue that the past remains with us.[22] This means that the trauma we might read into the history of madness – into the raving and boasting and crying and railing – emerged from colonial life, with all of its violence and terror, its loneliness and injustice, and its commonplace griefs in love and business. If cultural trauma is embedded in the literature of every society, we might conclude that violence bleeds into our culture in less clarified ways, including the fragmentation of minds under the weight of colonial burdens – and that to write and read history may be therapeutic.

NOTES

INTRODUCTION

1 *Morning Herald*, 11 November 1786, quoted in Emma Christopher and Hamish Maxwell-Stewart, 'Convict Transportation in Global Context, c. 1700–88,' in *The Cambridge History of Australia*, vol. 1, ed. A. Bashford and S. Macintyre (Melbourne: Cambridge University Press, 2013), 81.

2 Christopher and Maxwell-Stewart, 'Convict Transportation in Global Context,' 68–70.

3 Alan Frost, *Dreams of a Pacific Empire: Sir George Young's Proposal for a Colonization of New South Wales (1784–5)* (Sydney: Resolution Press, 1980), *Botany Bay Mirages: Illusions of Australia's Convict Beginnings* (Melbourne: Melbourne University Press, 1994), and *Botany Bay: The Real Story* (Melbourne: Black Inc., 2011); C. M. H. Clark, *A History of Australia, vol. 1* (Melbourne: Melbourne University Press, 1962); Robert Hughes, *The Fatal Shore: A History of the Transportation of Convicts to Australia, 1787–1868* (London: Collins Harvill, 1987); John Hirst, 'Changing My Mind,' in *The Historian's Conscience: Australian Historians on the Ethics of History*, ed. S. Macintyre (Melbourne: Melbourne University Press, 2004), 87–89 and *Freedom on the Fatal Shore: Australia's First Colony* (Melbourne: Black Inc., 2008); Grace Karskens, *The Colony: A History of Early Sydney* (Sydney: Allen & Unwin, 2009); Alan Atkinson, *The Europeans in Australia: A History, vol. 1* (Melbourne: Oxford University Press, 1997).

4 Douglas Hay, Peter Linebaugh, John G. Rule, E. P. Thompson and Cal Winslow, eds, *Albion's Fatal Tree: Crime and Punishment in Eighteenth-Century England* (London: Verso, 2011); Emma Christopher, *A Merciless Place: The Fate of Britain's Convicts after the American Revolution* (New York: Oxford University Press, 2011).

5 David Collins, *An Account of the English Colony in New South Wales* (London, 1798), 80.

6 'Jacob Nagle his Book A.D. One Thousand Eight Hundred and Twenty Nine May 19th. Canton. Stark County Ohio' (1775–1802, compiled 1829), SLNSW MLMSS 5954 (Safe 1/156), 85, 95–96, 101, 105–106.

7 Grace Karskens, 'The Early Colonial Presence, 1788–1825,' in *The Cambridge History of Australia*, vol. 1, 95; Lois Davey, Margaret Macpherson and F. W. Clements, *The Hungry Years: 1788–1792* (Canberra: Australian Institute of Anatomy, 1947).

8 Collins, *An Account of the English Colony*, 102–103.

9 I use Ralph Clark's spelling, but elsewhere Ascott is called Ancott or Escott: *Historical Records of New South Wales*, vol. 2, 416.

10 Ron Ringer, 'From Shea's Creek to Alexandra Canal,' *Dictionary of Sydney* (2013), <dictionaryofsydney.org/entry/from_sheas_creek_to_alexandra_canal>, accessed 6 October 2015.

11 Davey, Macpherson and Clements, *The Hungry Years*, 15.

12 Journal, 9 April 1791, *The Journal and Letters of Lt. Ralph Clark 1787–1792*, ed. by P. G. Fidlon and R. J. Ryan (Sydney: Australian Documents Library, 1981), 192.

13 Journal, 7 September 1791, *Journal and Letters of Lt. Ralph Clark*, 192, 212.

14 Karskens, *The Colony*, 314.

15 Christopher Lloyd and Jack L. S. Coulter, *Medicine and the Navy 1200–1900*, vol. 3 (Edinburgh: E. and S. Livingstone, 1961), 354–55.

16 Journal, 10 September 1791, *Journal and Letters of Lt. Ralph Clark*, 212.

17 Sic. R. Clark to Lieut. Creswell, Letterbook, 30 September 1791, *Journal and Letters of Lt. Ralph Clark*, 307.

18 I owe this insight to Sally Swartz, whose historical analysis incorporates a compelling psychoanalytical reading of colonial madness.

19 See the groundbreaking essay by Mark Finnane, 'Asylums, Families and the State,' *History Workshop Journal* 20, no. 1 (1985): 134–48, and, for instance, the essays collected in *Outside the Walls of the Asylum: The History of Care in the Community 1750–2000*, eds P. Bartlett and D. Wright (London: Athlone Press, 1999), 115–31, as well as Claire Edington, 'Going In and Getting Out of the Colonial Asylum: Families and Psychiatric Care in French Indochina,' *Comparative Studies in Society and History* 55, no. 3 (2013): 725–55; and see P. Savy, 'Outcry and Silence: The Social Implications of Asylum Closure in Australia,' *Health Sociology Review* 14, no. 3 (2005): 205–14 and other essays in the themed issue.

20 R. Darling to W. H. Huskisson, 29 May 1828, *Historical Records of Australia (HRA)* I, vol. 14, 211.

21 Sally Swartz, *Homeless Wanderers: Movement and Mental Illness in the Cape Colony in the Nineteenth Century* (Claremont: UCT Press, 2016); Harriet Deacon, 'Madness, Race and Moral Treatment: Robben Island Lunatic Asylum, Cape Colony, 1846–1890,' *History of Psychiatry* 7 (1996): 287–97.

22 John M. Ward, *Colonial Self-Government: The British Experience, 1759–1856* (London: Macmillan, 1976), 124–25.

23 Karskens, 'The Early Colonial Presence,' 112. Many women, however, ran small businesses which left few records and made them 'hidden in plain view': Catherine Bishop, *Minding Her Own Business: Colonial Businesswomen in Sydney* (Sydney: NewSouth, 2015).

24 Sally Swartz does some of this crucial work in the final chapter of her study of madness in South Africa: *Homeless Wanderers*, 183–205.

25 Laure Murat, *The Man Who Thought He Was Napoleon: Toward a Political History of Madness*, trans. Deke Dusinberre (Chicago: University of Chicago Press, 2014), 19; Ben Kafka, *The Demon of Writing* (New York: Zone Books, 2012).

26 'The Banks,' *Sydney Monitor*, 16 November 1836, Evening: 2.

27 Stijn Vanheule, *Diagnosis and the DSM: A Critical Review* (Basingstoke, U.K:

Palgrave Macmillan, 2014); Monica Greco, 'What is the DSM? Diagnostic Manual, Cultural Icon, Political Battleground: An Overview with Suggestions for a Critical Research Agenda,' *Psychology & Sexuality* 7, no. 1 (2016): 6–22.

28 Barbara Brookes, 'Papering Over Madness: Accountability and Resistance in Colonial Asylum Files: A New Zealand Case Study,' *Rethinking History* 22, no. 3 (2018): 356–74, 370, and see Sally Swartz, 'The Third Voice: Writing Case-notes,' *Feminism & Psychology* 16, no. 4 (2006): 427–44.

29 J. Grant to P. King, 1 May 1805, in *This Beauteous, Wicked Place: Letters and Journals of John Grant, Gentleman Convict*, ed. Y. Cramer (Canberra: National Library of Australia, 2000), 104.

30 Raymond Evans, '19 June 1822: Creating "an Object of Real Terror": The Tabling of the First Bigge Report,' in *Turning Points in Australian History*, eds M. Crotty and D. A. Roberts (Sydney: UNSW Press, 2009), 59.

31 R. Darling to W. H. Huskisson, 5 April 1828, *HRA* I, vol. 14, 119.

CHAPTER 1

1 'Old Bailey, May 26,' *Morning Post*, 27 May 1803: 3.

2 'D—d v—n' in the original: *The New Annual Register: Or General Repository of History, Politics, and Literature, for the Year 1803* (London, 1804), 47.

3 'Trial of John Grant, 25 May 1803 (t18030525-19), Old Bailey Proceedings Online, <www.oldbaileyonline.org>, accessed 11 March 2019; 'Old Bailey,' *E. Johnson's British Gazette and Sunday Monitor* 1230, 29 May 1803.

4 Ward v St Paul, Rolls, 28 April 1789 (Reg. Lib. 1788. B. fol. 323) in William Brown, *Reports of Cases Argued and Determined in the High Court of Chancery*, vol. 2 (Boston, 1844), 453–54; *The New Annual Register: Or General Repository of History, Politics, and Literature, for the Year 1803*, 48.

5 Yvonne Cramer, *This Beauteous, Wicked Place: Letters and Journals of John Grant, Gentleman Convict* (Canberra: National Library of Australia, 2000), 6.

6 Indenture of apprenticeship, 7 March 1791, Papers of John Grant, SLNSW MAV/FM4/114, item 2, AJCP Reel M462; Cramer, *This Beauteous, Wicked Place*, 6.

7 See Anthony Bruce, *The Purchase System in the British Army, 1660–1871* (London: Royal Historical Society, 1980).

8 W. H. Clinton to J. Grant, 21 October 1803, Papers of John Grant, NLA MS 737, item 8.

9 Cramer, *This Beauteous, Wicked Place*, 7.

10 Journal, 1805–10, quoted in Cramer, 7.

11 J. Grant to E. and M. Grant, 1–10 January 1805, in Cramer, 72.

12 Cramer, *This Beauteous, Wicked Place*, 7–8.

13 Samuel Stanton, *The Principles of Duelling; With Rules to Be Observed in Every Particular Respecting It* (London, 1790); J. M. Beattie, *Crime and the Courts in England, 1660–1800* (Princeton: Princeton University Press, 1986), 97–98; Donna T. Andrew, 'The Code of Honour and Its Critics: The Opposition to Duelling in England, 1700–1850,' *Social History* 5, no. 3 (1980): 412–13; Ruth Harris, *Murders and Madness: Medicine, Law, and Society in the Fin De Siècle* (Oxford: Clarendon, 1989), 288.

14 See Joel Peter Eigen, *Witnessing Insanity: Madness and Mad-Doctors in the English Court* (New Haven: Yale University Press, 1995), 82–107.
15 Akihito Suzuki, *Madness at Home: The Psychiatrist, the Patient, and the Family in England, 1820–1860* (Berkeley: University of California Press, 2006), 13–14, 37.
16 Rudolph J. Gerber, *The Insanity Defense* (New York: Associated Faculty Press, 1984), 9–12.
17 Matthew Hale, *The History of the Pleas of the Crown* (London, 1736), 25, 30.
18 See Roger Smith, *Trial by Medicine: Insanity and Responsibility in Victorian Trials* (Edinburgh: Edinburgh University Press, 1981), 94; Joel Peter Eigen, 'Intentionality and Insanity: What the Eighteenth-Century Juror Heard,' in *The Anatomy of Madness: Essays in the History of Psychiatry*, vol. II, eds W. F. Bynum, R. Porter and M. Shepherd (London: Tavistock Publications, 1985), 41.
19 Eigen, *Witnessing Insanity*, 110–20.
20 Jan Goldstein, *Console and Classify: The French Psychiatric Profession in the Nineteenth Century* (Cambridge, 1987), 152–57; Smith, *Trial by Medicine*, 37.
21 Bill Bynum, 'Discarded Diagnoses: Monomania,' *Lancet* 362 (25 October 2003): 1425.
22 Russell D. Covey, 'Temporary Insanity: The Strange Life and Times of the Perfect Defense,' *Boston University Law Review 91*, no. 5 (2011): 1624–28.
23 'Old Bailey,' *E. Johnson's British Gazette and Sunday Monitor*, 29 May 1803.
24 Tony Ballantyne, 'The Theory and Practice of Empire-Building: Edward Gibbon Wakefield and "Systematic Colonisation",' in *The Routledge History of Western Empires*, eds R. Aldrich and K. McKenzie (London: Routledge, 2014), 89–101.
25 Edward Gibbon Wakefield, *Facts Relating to the Punishment of Death in the Metropolis* (London, 1831), 147–48.
26 V. A. C. Gattrell, *The Hanging Tree: Execution and the English People 1770–1868* (Oxford: Oxford University Press, 1994), 29–40, 40–45.
27 Rudolph Ackerman, *The Microcosm of London, or London in Miniature*, vol. II, 1808 (London, 1904), 209.
28 Petition to King of John Grant in Newgate Prison, 1803 and Petition to the Princesses Augusta Sophia, Elizabeth, Mary, Sophia and Amelia Submitted by Matilda Grant, 1803, Papers of John Grant, NLA MS737, items 9 and 10.
29 'News in Brief,' *Times*, 14 July 1803: 4.
30 House of Commons, Report of the Select Committee on Transportation, printed 16 August 1838, 4.
31 House of Commons, Inquiry into the State of the Convict Establishment at Woolwich, Command Papers, vol. XVIII (London, 1847), xxv.
32 9 Geo. 1 c. 22 [1723]; L. Radzinowicz, 'The Waltham Black Act: A Study of the Legislative Attitude Towards Crime in the Eighteenth Century,' *Cambridge Law Journal* 9, no. 1 (1945): 56–81; Pat Rogers, 'The Waltham Blacks and the Black Act,' *Historical Journal* 17, no. 3 (1974): 465–86.
33 David D. Cooper, *The Lesson of the Scaffold: The Public Execution Controversy in Victorian England* (Athens: Ohio University Press, 1974).
34 Gatrell, *The Hanging Tree*, 6–8; Bruce Kercher, *An Unruly Child: A History of Law in Australia* (Sydney, 1995), xv; Douglas Hay, 'Property, Authority and the Criminal Law,' in *Albion's Fatal Tree: Crime and Punishment in Eighteenth-Century England*, eds

D. Hay, P. Linebaugh, J. G. Rule, E. P. Thompson, and C. Winslow (London: Verso, 2011), 17–63.

35 Gatrell, *The Hanging Tree*; Beattie, *Crime and the Courts in England*, 423–25.

36 J. Grant to E. and M. Grant, 2 May 1804, in Cramer, 24.

37 J. Grant to E. and M. Grant, 28 April 1805, in Cramer, 103.

38 'The Man Who Shot a Lawyer in the Buttock,' performed at the Old Magistrate's Court in Melbourne in December 2003; 'The Convict Harpsichordist,' <www.elizabethanderson.org/omc.pdf>, accessed 10 October 2015. But see also 'Appendix K: The First Harpsichord Brought to Australia: An Apocryphal Tale,' *The First Fleet Piano*, <press-files.anu.edu.au/downloads/press/p330471/html/AppK.xhtml#footnote-763>, accessed 26 February 2018.

39 Cramer, *This Beauteous, Wicked Place*, 13.

40 David S. Karr, '"The Embers of Expiring Sedition": Maurice Margarot, the Scottish Martyrs Monument and the Production of Radical Memory Across the British South Pacific,' *Historical Research* 86, no. 234 (2013): 644.

41 Karr, 'The Embers of Expiring Sedition,' 638–60.

42 Charles H. Bertie, *The Story of Vaucluse House and Sir Henry Browne Hayes*, 7th edn (Sydney: Vaucluse Park Trust, 1938), 8–9; Bruce Kercher, 'A Convict Conservative: George Crossley and the English Legal Tradition,' *Law in Context* 16, no. 1 (1998): 17.

43 J. Grant to P. King, October 1804, in Cramer, 70.

44 'Ship News,' *Sydney Gazette*, 13 May 1804: 1; J. Grant to E. and M. Grant, 2 May 1804, in Cramer, 23.

45 Alan Atkinson, 'The Free-Born Englishman Transported: Convict Rights as a Measure of Eighteenth-Century Empire,' *Past & Present* 144 (1994): 88–115.

46 Emma Christopher and Hamish Maxwell-Stewart, 'Convict Transportation in Global Context, c. 1700–88,' in *The Cambridge History of Australia, vol. 1*, eds A. Bashford and S. Macintyre (Cambridge: Cambridge University Press, 2013), 68–90.

47 Clare Anderson and Hamish Maxwell-Stuart, 'Convict Labour and the Western Empires, 1415–1954,' in *The Routledge History of Western Empires*, 102–17.

48 Original emphasis. L. Macquarie to Duke of York, 25 July 1817, *Historical Records of Australia (HRA)* I, vol. 9, 442–43.

49 J. Grant to E. and M. Grant, 7 May 1804, in Cramer, 27.

50 David Andrew Roberts, 'The Valley of Swells: "Special" or "Educated" Convicts on the Wellington Valley Settlement, 1827–1830,' *History Australia* 3 (2006): 11.5, 11.7–8; Sandra Blair, 'The Felonry and the Free? Divisions in Colonial Society in the Penal Era,' *Labour History* 45 (1983): 9.

51 J. Grant to E. and M. Grant, 8 May 1804, in Cramer, 30; J. Grant to E. and M. Grant, 13 May 1804, in Cramer, 39.

52 David Collins, *An Account of the English Colony in New South Wales*, vol. 1 (London, 1798), 327.

53 J. Grant to E. and M. Grant, 7 May 1804, in Cramer, 27.

54 Matthew Allen, 'Alcohol and Authority in Early New South Wales: The Symbolic Significance of the Spirit Trade, 1788–1808,' *History Australia* 9, no. 3 (2012): 11.

55 J. Grant to E. and M. Grant, 13 July 1804, in Cramer, 55.
56 J. Grant to E. and M. Grant, 13 July 1804, in Cramer, 55.
57 Cramer, *This Beauteous, Wicked Place*, 29; J. Grant to E. and M. Grant, 13 July 1804, in Cramer, 50.
58 J. Grant to E. and M. Grant, 9 May 1804, in Cramer, 35.
59 Atkins v. Harris [1799] NSWKR 4; [1799] NSWSupC 4, <www.law.mq.edu.au/research/colonial_case_law/nsw/cases/case_index/1799/atkins_esq_v_harris_esq/> , accessed 17 March 2015; Bruce Kercher, *Debt, Seduction, and Other Disasters: The Birth of Civil Law in Convict New South Wales* (Sydney, Federation Press, 1996), 30–31.
60 J. Grant to E. and M. Grant, 13 July 1804, in Cramer, 52; Kercher, *Debt, Seduction and Other Disasters*, 28–31.
61 Edna Hickson, 'Cox, William (1764–1837),' Australian Dictionary of Biography, <adb.anu.edu.au/biography/cox-william-1934/text2309>, accessed 8 August 2018; Cramer, *This Beauteous, Wicked Place*, 29.
62 Kent's petition was successful: J. Grant to E. and M. Grant, 28 April 1805, in Cramer, 100.
63 T. Fyshe Palmer, *A Narrative of the Sufferings of T. F. Palmer, and W. Skirving During a Voyage to New South Wales, 1794* (Cambridge, 1797), 15–16.
64 Karr, 'The Embers of Expiring Sedition,' 645.
65 Michael Roe, 'Margarot, Maurice (1745–1815),' *Australian Dictionary of Biography*, <adb.anu.edu.au/biography/margarot-maurice-2431/text3233>, accessed 21 November 2015.
66 J. Hunter to Duke of Portland, 25 October 1795, *Historical Records of NSW (HRNSW)*, vol. 2, 883; Unsigned opinion, no date, *HRNSW*, vol. 2, 886; R. Dundas to Duke of Portland, 5 September 1796, *HRNSW*, vol. 3, 112–13. See also Lisa Ford and David Andrew Roberts, 'New South Wales Penal Settlements and the Transformation of Secondary Punishment in the Nineteenth-Century British Empire,' *Journal of Colonialism and Colonial History* 15, no. 3 (2014): n.p.
67 J. Grant to E. and M. Grant, 13 July 1804, in Cramer, 50–51.
68 J. Grant to E. and M. Grant, 13 July 1804, in Cramer, 51.
69 Journal, 15 January 1809, in Cramer, 173.
70 Michael Roe, 'Bishop, Charles (1765–1810),' *Australian Dictionary of Biography*, <adb.anu.edu.au/biography/bishop-charles-1787/text2015>, accessed 8 May 2014. See also Michael Roe, ed., *The Journal and Letters of Captain Charles Bishop on the North-West Coast of America, in the Pacific and in New South Wales 1794–1799* (Nendeln, Liechtenstein: Kraus Reprint, 1974).
71 Jan Kociumbas, *The Oxford History of Australia*, vol. 2 (Melbourne: Oxford University Press, 1992), 99–100; Miriam Estensen, *The Life of George Bass: Surgeon and Sailor of the Enlightenment* (Sydney: Allen & Unwin, 2005), 121–23, 149–58.
72 J. Grant to E. and M. Grant, 28 April 1805, in Cramer, 98; Estensen, *Life of George Bass*, 173–82.
73 G. Bass to E. Bass, 15 November 1802, quoted in Estensen, *Life of George Bass*, 161.
74 G. Bass to W. Waterhouse, 5 January 1803, *HRNSW*, vol. 5, 2.
75 G. Bishop to W. Waterhouse, 2 February 1803, *HRNSW*, vol. 5, 15.

76 C. Bishop to P. King, 6 March 1804, SLNSW MLMSS 710, Philip Gidley King Letters received and other papers, 1794–1807, 74–78.
77 Grace Karskens, *The Colony: A History of Early Sydney* (Sydney: Allen & Unwin, 2009), 100, 105.
78 J. Grant to E. and M. Grant, 13 July 1804, in Cramer, 61, and 1–10 January 1805, in Cramer, 80–81.
79 J. Grant to E. and M. Grant, 1–10 January 1805, in Cramer, 81, and 13 July 1804, in Cramer, 62.
80 J. Grant to E. and M. Grant, 2 December 1803, in Cramer, 17; 13 July 1804, in Cramer, 61–62; 1–10 January 1805, in Cramer, 80–81; and Cramer, *This Beauteous, Wicked Place*, 47.
81 J. Grant to E. and M. Grant, 22 May 1804, in Cramer, 50.
82 Matthew Flinders, quoted in Estensen, *Life of George Bass*, 162.
83 Estensen, *Life of George Bass*, 183–94.
84 Keith Macrae Bowden, 'Bass, George (1771–1803),' *Australian Dictionary of Biography*, <adb.anu.edu.au/biography/bass-george-1748/text1939>, accessed 26 November 2015.
85 J. Grant to E. and M. Grant, 1–10 January 1805, in Cramer, 80; and see Roe, 'Bishop, Charles (1765–1810),' *Australian Dictionary of Biography*, and 'Charles Bishop, Pioneer of Pacific Commerce,' 14–15.
86 Norman S. Lynravn, 'Hayes, Sir Henry Browne (1762–1832),' *Australian Dictionary of Biography*, <adb.anu.edu.au/biography/hayes-sir-henry-browne-2172/text2787>, accessed 17 March 2014.
87 J. Grant to E. and M. Grant, 28 April 1805, in Cramer, 100–102.
88 Cramer, *This Beauteous, Wicked Place*, 89.
89 J. Grant to E. and M. Grant, 13 July 1804, in Cramer, 52, 63; J. Grant to E. and M. Grant, 1–10 January 1805, in Cramer, 72–73.
90 J. Grant to E. and M. Grant, 28 April 1805, in Cramer, 100.
91 J. Grant to E. and M. Grant, 1–10 January 1805, in Cramer, 68.
92 Alan Atkinson, *The Europeans in Australia: A History, vol. 1* (Melbourne: Oxford University Press, 1997), 265.
93 'Bellasis, George Bridges (?–1825),' *Australian Dictionary of Biography*, <adb.anu.edu.au/biography/bellasis-george-bridges-1766/text1909>, accessed 30 November 2015.
94 J. Grant to P. King, October 1804, reproduced in J. Grant to E. Grant and M. Grant, 1–10 January 1805, in Cramer, 70; J. Grant to E. and M. Grant, 21 May 1804, in Cramer, 48.
95 J. Grant to E. and M. Grant, 1–10 January 1805, in Cramer, 71.
96 J. Grant to H. B. Hayes, 27 January 1805, in Cramer, 90.
97 J. Grant to E. and M. Grant, 1–10 January 1805, in Cramer, 72.
98 J. Grant to P. King, 1 May 1805, in Cramer, 104–105.
99 Cramer, *This Beauteous, Wicked Place*, 60.
100 J. Grant to E. and M. Grant, 28 April 1805, in Cramer, 100–101; Lynravn, 'Hayes, Sir Henry Browne (1762–1832)'; Roe, 'Margarot, Maurice (1745–1815)'.
101 J. Grant to P. King, 1 May 1805, in Cramer, 104.
102 J. Grant to H. B. Hayes, 27 January 1805, in Cramer, 90.

103 'Bench of Magistrates,' *Sydney Gazette*, 19 May 1805: 3.
104 Journal, 19 May 1805, in Cramer, 121.
105 J. Grant to W. Kent, 19 May 1805, in Cramer, 122.
106 N. S. Lynravn, 'Grant, John (1776–?),' *Australian Dictionary of Biography*, <adb.anu.edu.au/biography/grant-john-2118/text2677>, accessed 8 May 2014.
107 J. Grant, 'Ode on His Majesty's Birthday 1805,' 4 June 1805, in Cramer, 130.
108 David Andrew Roberts, 'Dissent and Ill-Discipline: The Newcastle Penal Settlement, 1804–1823,' in *Radical Newcastle*, eds James Bennet, Nancy Cushing and Erik Eklund (Sydney, NewSouth Publishing, 2015), 18.
109 P. King to J. Sullivan, 21 August 1804, *HRA* I, vol. 5, 142; Atkinson, *The Europeans in Australia, vol. 1*, 254, 265–66.
110 'At a Meeting of His Excellency, the Governor, and the Magistrates for the County of Cumberland,' 13 July 1805, *HRA* I, vol. 5, 537–38; J. Grant to P. King, 8 May 1805, *HRA* I, vol. 5, 537; P. King to E. Cooke, 20 July 1805, *HRA* I, vol. 5, 534–36.
111 Atkinson, *The Europeans in Australia, vol. 1*, 73–75, 228–34; Valda Rigg, 'Convict Life: A "Tolerable Degree of Comfort"?,' in *Norfolk Island and Its First Settlement, 1788–1814*, ed. R. Nobbs (Sydney: Library of Australian History, 1988), 97, 100–101.
112 Journal, June 1805, in Cramer, 132–34.
113 Kercher, *An Unruly Child*, 60.
114 Malcolm Britts, 'The Commandants,' in *Norfolk Island and Its First Settlement, 1788–1814*, ed. R. Nobbs (Sydney: Library of Australian History, 1988), 78, 80; Anne-Maree Whitaker, *Joseph Foveaux: Power and Patronage in Early New South Wales* (Sydney: UNSW Press, 2000), 103–30.
115 Journal (French, this and subsequent French entries translated by Yvonne Cramer), in Cramer, 143–47.
116 Journal (French), October 1805, in Cramer, 148.
117 'Bond of Union,' October 1805, in Cramer, 149–50.
118 Journal (French), in Cramer, 154.
119 Petition to Captain Piper for John Morris, 19 July 1806, in Cramer, 158–59.
120 Journal, 10 August 1806, in Cramer, 159.
121 Journal, 23 May 1807, in Cramer, 160.
122 Hill-Reid, John Grant's Journey, 179.
123 W. Bligh to J. Piper, 27 December 1807, in Proceedings of a General Court-martial Held at Chelsea Hospital (Sherwood, UK, 1811), 349.
124 George Mackaness, *The Life of Vice-Admiral William Bligh, R.N., F.R.S.*, vol. 1 (New York: Farrar & Rinehart, 1931), 43, and see 2 & 3 Vict. c. 43 [1839].
125 Cramer, *This Beauteous, Wicked Place*, 165.
126 Ellis, *John Macarthur*, 381.
127 Mackaness, *Vice-Admiral William Bligh*, 297.
128 Journal, January 1809, in Cramer, 174.
129 Journal, 31 January 1809, in Cramer, 176; J. Grant to S. Lord, 17 February 1809, in Cramer, 179.
130 Journal, 5 February 1809, in Cramer, 177.
131 Journal, February 1809, in Cramer, 183.

132 Elizabeth Paterson, quoted in Cramer, 166.
133 Journal, February 1809, in Cramer, 181.
134 Cramer, *This Beauteous, Wicked Place*, 98.
135 Journal, March 1809, in Cramer, 184–85.
136 Cramer, *This Beauteous, Wicked Place*, 200; Testimonial to Macquarie, 3 May 1810, in Cramer, 202.
137 J. Grant to E. and M. and S. Grant, May 1810, in Cramer, 206–207.
138 Atkinson, 'The Free-Born Englishman Transported,' 879.
139 Testimony written by W. Bligh, copied in J. Grant to M. Grant, May 1809, in Cramer, 203.
140 J. Grant to W. Bligh and response, copied in journal, May 1810, in Cramer, 203–204.
141 Cramer, *This Beauteous, Wicked Place*, 200.
142 S. Marsden, 26 November 1811, in *Some Private Correspondence of the Rev. Samuel Marsden and Family 1794–1824*, ed. G. Mackaness (Sydney: self-published, 1942), 45–46.

CHAPTER 2

1 J. Grant to E. and M. Grant, 1–10 January 1805, in Yvonne Cramer, *This Beauteous, Wicked Place: Letters and Journals of John Grant, Gentleman Convict* (Canberra: National Library of Australia, 2000), 81 (hereafter Cramer).
2 David Collins, *An Account of the English Colony in New South Wales*, vol. 1 (London, 1798), 351–53.
3 *Memorandoms by James Martin: An Astonishing Escape from Early New South Wales*, ed. Tim Causer (London: UCL Press, 2017).
4 Grace Karskens and Richard Waterhouse, '"Too Sacred to be Taken Away": Property, Liberty, Tyranny and the "Rum Rebellion",' *Journal of Australian Colonial History* 12 (2010): 21; Ross Fitzgerald and Mark Hearn, *Bligh, Macarthur and the Rum Rebellion* (Sydney: Kangaroo Press, 1988), 24.
5 Linda Clark, 'Sydney Cove and the Indian Connection,' *Launceston Historical Society Papers and Proceedings* 23 (2011): 18–19; Michael Nash, *Sydney Cove: The History and Archaeology of an Eighteenth-century Shipwreck* (Hobart: Navarine Publishing, 2009).
6 Steven, Margaret, 'Campbell, Robert (1769–1846),' *Australian Dictionary of Biography*, <adb.anu.edu.au/biography/campbell-robert-1876/text2197>, accessed 20 November 2015.
7 See Felicity Grace Berry, 'Keeping the Home Fires Burning?: British Female Settlers' Conceptions of Home and Belonging in Colonial India, Van Diemen's Land and Western Australia, 1826–1860,' PhD thesis, University of Sydney, 2016.
8 'Classified Advertising,' *Sydney Gazette*, 24 November 1805: 3.
9 Anthony Highmore, *A Treatise on the Law of Idiocy and Lunacy* (Exeter, 1822), 20–22, 43–44.
10 Akihito Suzuki, *Madness at Home: The Psychiatrist, the Patient, and the Family in England, 1820–1860* (Berkeley: University of California Press, 2006), 68–69.
11 See Highmore, *A Treatise on the Law of Idiocy and Lunacy*, 42–72; Suzuki, Madness at Home, 18–19.

12 R. A. Houston, 'Legal Protection of the Mentally Incapable in Early Modern Scotland,' *Journal of Legal History* 24, no. 2 (2003): 165–86.
13 Michael Roe, 'Charles Bishop, Pioneer of Pacific Commerce,' *Papers and Proceedings (Tasmanian Historical Research Association)* 10, no. 1 (1962): 15.
14 'Classified Advertising,' *Sydney Gazette*, 24 November 1805: 3.
15 Vivienne Parsons, 'Jamison, Thomas (1753–1811),' *Australian Dictionary of Biography*, <adb.anu.edu.au/biography/jamison-thomas-2269/text2909>, accessed 24 November 2016; Roe, 'Charles Bishop,' 15.
16 'Classified Advertising,' *Sydney Gazette*, 18 May 1806: 3; Parsons, 'Jamison, Thomas (1753–1811)'.
17 'Classified Advertising,' *Sydney Gazette*, 23 August 1807: 3.
18 J. Grant, Journal, March 1809, in Cramer, 184–85.
19 W. Paterson to the Principal Officers and Commissioners of the Navy, 26 March 1809, *Historical Records of Australia (HRA)* I, vol. 7, 75.
20 J. Grant to M. Grant and E. Grant, 28 April 1805, in Cramer, 99, 81.
21 David Roger Hainsworth, *The Sydney Traders: Simeon Lord and His Contemporaries, 1788–1821*, 2nd edn (Melbourne: Melbourne University Press, 1981) and N. G. Butlin, 'Yo, Ho, and How Many Bottles of Rum?' *Australian Economic History Review* 23, no. 1 (1983): 1–27; Matthew Allen, 'Alcohol and Authority in Early New South Wales: The Symbolic Significance of the Spirit Trade, 1788–1808,' *History Australia* 9, no. 3 (2012): 7–26.
22 Alan Atkinson, 'The Little Revolution in New South Wales, 1808,' *International History Review* 12, no. 1 (1990): 65–75; Karskens and Waterhouse, 'Too Sacred to be Taken Away'; Richard Waterhouse, 'A Bastard Offspring of Tyranny under the Guise of Liberty: Liberty and Representative Government in Australia, 1788–1901,' in *Exclusionary Empire: English Liberty Overseas, 1600–1900*, ed. J. Greene (Cambridge: Cambridge University Press, 2010), 224.
23 Castlereagh to L. Macquarie, 14 May 1809, *HRA* I, vol. 7, 82.
24 C. H. Currey, 'Bent, Ellis (1783–1815),' *Australian Dictionary of Biography*, <adb.anu.edu.au/biography/bent-ellis-1772/text1985>, accessed 24 March 2016.
25 C. J. Cummins, *A History of Medical Administration in NSW 1788–1973*, 2nd edn (Sydney: NSW Department of Health, 2003), 17.
26 Proclamation, 4 January 1810, *Historical Records of NSW (HRNSW)*, vol. 7, 257.
27 Alan Atkinson, 'Jeremy Bentham and the Rum Rebellion,' *Journal of the Royal Australian Historical Society* 64, no. 1 (1978): 3–4.
28 Lisa Ford and David Andrew Roberts, 'Mr Peel's Amendments' in 'New South Wales: Imperial Criminal Reform in a Distant Penal Colony,' *Journal of Legal History* 37, no. 2 (2016): n.p.
29 Enid Campbell, 'Prerogative Rule in New South Wales, 1788–1823,' *Journal and Proceedings of the Royal Australian Historical Society* 50, no. 3 (1964): 162.
30 'Ship News,' *Sydney Gazette*, 27 October 1810: 3; R. F. Holder, 'Jenkins, Robert (1777–1822),' *Australian Dictionary of Biography*, <adb.anu.edu.au/biography/jenkins-robert-2274/text2919>, 24 November 2016.
31 *Macquarie's Journals of His Tours in New South Wales and Van Diemen's Land* (Sydney: Public Library of New South Wales, 1956), 18.
32 Garrison and General Order, 18 November 1810, Colonial Secretary's Papers, SRNSW NRS 898, 1–2.

33 Proclamation, 25 November 1810, Colonial Secretary's Papers, SRNSW NRS 898, 1–2.

34 Commission, 2 April 1787, *HRNSW* I, part 2, 64.

35 J. C. H. Gill, 'Genesis of the Australian Whaling Industry: Its Development up to 1850,' *Journal of the Royal Historical Society of Queensland* 8 (1965): 124.

36 J. T. Campbell to A. Bodie, April 1811, Colonial Secretary's Papers, SLNSW 4/3490D, 162.

37 J. T. Campbell to D. Wentworth and W. Redfern, 16 April 1811, Colonial Secretary's Papers, SLNSW 4/3490D, 160–61.

38 J. T. Campbell to S. Marsden and R. Jenkins, 18 April 1811, Colonial Secretary's Papers, SLNSW 4/3490D, 164–65.

39 Janet Holcomb, *Early Merchant Families of Sydney: Speculation and Risk Management on the Fringes of Empire* (London: Anthem Press, 2016), 29–41; C. E. T. Newman, *The Spirit of Wharf House: Campbell Enterprise from Calcutta to Canberra 1788–1930* (Sydney: Angus & Robertson, 1961), 108–10, 125–26.

40 J. T. Campbell to A. Bodie, 6 September 1811, Colonial Secretary's Papers, SLNSW 4/3491, 61–62.

41 Letters of marque, MLMSS 9367/BOX 1X.

42 Vincent O'Malley, *Haerenga: Early Māori Journeys Across the Globe* (Wellington: Bridget Williams Books, 2015), 25.

43 McHugo was also referred to as Jonathan Burke Hugo and this name survives in some documents. R. Jones to J. T. Campbell, 11 December 1817, *HRA* I, vol. 9, 547.

44 J. E. Calder, 'Paleological Sketch of Tasmania,' *Mercury*, 29 October 1874: 2.

45 L. Macquarie to Bathurst, 11 December 1817, *HRA* I, vol. 9, 545.

46 J. T. Campbell to D. Wentworth and W. Redfern, 30 January 1812, Colonial Secretary's Papers, SLNSW NRS 935 4/3491, Reel 6002, 172–73.

47 L. Macquarie to Bathurst, 11 December 1817, *HRA* I, vol. 9, 545–46.

48 Calder, 'Paleological Sketch,' 2.

49 'Gordon, George Alexander,' *Journeys in Time 1809–1822: The Journals of Lachlan & Elizabeth Macquarie*, <www.mq.edu.au/macquarie-archive/journeys/people/peopleg_k.html>, accessed 20 October 2016.

50 See Edgar Jones, 'Historical Approaches to Post-combat Disorders,' *Philosophical Transactions of the Royal Society* B 361, no. 1468 (2006): 533–42.

51 A. Gordon to H. Goulburn, 21 April 1817, *HRA* I, vol. 9, 413.

52 D. Wentworth and W. Redfern to J. T. Campbell, 1 February 1812, Colonial Secretary's Correspondence, SRNSW NRS897, 18–19.

53 E. Bent to L. Macquarie, 2 February 1812, Colonial Secretary's Papers, SRNSW NRS 897, 25.

54 E. Bent to L. Macquarie, no date, Colonial Secretary's Papers, SRNSW NRS 897, 21.

55 Information of Robert Mason, 3 February 1812, Colonial Secretary's Papers, SRNSW NRS 897, 13–14.

56 Affidavit of R. Mason and R. Ballard, 3 February 1812, Colonial Secretary's Papers, SRNSW NRS 897, 14–15.

57 Inquest on J. McHugo, 3 February 1812, Colonial Secretary's Papers, SRNSW NRS897, 27–28.
58 Inquisition into Johnathan Burke McHugo [sic], 4 February 1812, Colonial Secretary's Papers, SRNSW NRS897, 31–33.
59 Public Notice, 5 February 1812, Colonial Secretary's Papers, SRNSW NRS898, 281.
60 E. Bent to L. Macquarie, 3 February 1812, Colonial Secretary's Papers, SRNSW NRS897, 34–36.
61 Affidavit of J. Burke Hugo, 11 March 1817, *HRA* I, vol. 9, 389.
62 J. Burke McHugo to H. Goulburn, 11 January 1817, and J. Burke McHugo to J. Palmer, 1 January 1815, *HRA* I, vol. 9, 389–91.
63 Bathurst to L. Macquarie, 25 April 1817, *HRA* I, vol. 9, 388.
64 Houston, 'Legal Protection of the Mentally Incapable,' 171.
65 L. Macquarie to Bathurst, 11 December 1817, *HRA* I, vol. 9, 545–46, and enclosures 545–49.
66 Christine Shergold, 'Vice Admiralty Court of NSW, 1787–1911,' *NSW State Archives & Records*, <www.records.nsw.gov.au/archives/collections-and-research/guides-and-indexes/vice-admiralty-court-nsw-1787-1911>, accessed 25 October 2018.
67 Catharine Coleborne, *Insanity, Identity and Empire: Immigrants and Institutional Confinement in Australia and New Zealand, 1873–1910* (Manchester: Manchester University Press, 2015), 26–28.
68 Coleborne, *Insanity, Identity and Empire*, 9, and see Warwick Anderson, *The Cultivation of Whiteness* (Durham, NC: Duke University Press, 2006).
69 'Classified Advertising,' *Sydney Gazette*, 12 September 1812: 3.
70 Cindy McCreery and Kirsten McKenzie, 'The Australian Colonies in a Maritime World,' in *The Cambridge History of Australia*, vol. 1, eds A. Bashford and S. Macintyre (Melbourne: Cambridge University Press), 560–84.
71 Arthur Phillip's Commission, *HRNSW* I, part 2, 64.
72 See David Lambert and Alan Lester, eds, *Colonial Lives Across the British Empire: Imperial Careering in the Long Nineteenth Century* (Cambridge: Cambridge University Press, 2006); Zoe Laidlaw, *Colonial Connections, 1815–45: Patronage, the Information Revolution and Colonial Government* (Manchester: Manchester University Press, 2005).
73 Kirsten McKenzie, *Imperial Underworld: An Escaped Convict and the Transformation of the British Colonial Order* (Cambridge: Cambridge University Press, 2016), 23.
74 McKenzie, *Imperial Underworld*, 13.
75 Lauren Benton and Lisa Ford, *Rage for Order: The British Empire and the Origins of International Law 1800–1850* (Cambridge, MA: Harvard University Press, 2016), 32–33.

CHAPTER 3

1 Cassandra Pybus, *Black Founders: The Unknown Story of Australia's First Black Settlers* (Sydney: UNSW Press, 2006), 185; John Flood Nagle, *Collins, the Courts & the Colony: Law & Society in Colonial New South Wales 1788–1796* (Sydney: UNSW Press, 1996), 148.
2 John White, *Journal of a Voyage to New South Wales* (London, 1790), 128.

3 Nagle, *Collins, the Courts & the Colony*, 149; White, *Journal of a Voyage*, 128.
4 Pybus, *Black Founders*, 92–93.
5 White, *Journal of a Voyage*, 171.
6 Bruce Kercher, *An Unruly Child: A History of Law in Australia* (Sydney: Allen & Unwin, 1995), 24.
7 Watkin Tench, *A Narrative of the Expedition to Botany Bay* (London, 1789), 109.
8 Mollie Gillen, *The Founders of Australia: A Biographical Dictionary of the First Fleet* (Sydney: Library of Australian History, 1989), 145.
9 R. v. Gordon [1789] NSWKR 3; [1789] NSWSupC 3, <www.law.mq.edu.au/research/colonial_case_law/nsw/cases/case_index/1789/r_v_gordon/>, accessed 28 October 2018; Pybus, *Black Founders*, 103.
10 David Collins, *An Account of the English Colony in New South Wales* (London, 1789), 80.
11 J. Hunter to J. King, 20 August 1796, *Historical Records of NSW (HRNSW)*, vol. 3, 72; Nagle, *Collins, the Courts & the Colony*, 30, 38.
12 Alan Atkinson, *The Europeans in Australia: A History, vol. 1* (Melbourne: Oxford University Press, 1997), 89–91; 27 Geo. III c. 2 [1787]; and see David Neal, *The Rule of Law in a Penal Colony: Law and Power in Early New South Wales* (Cambridge: Cambridge University Press, 1992), 85–113.
13 Tench, *A Narrative of the Expedition to Botany Bay*, 70.
14 Pybus, *Black Founders*, 106, 121, 147, 185.
15 Norman J. Finkel, *Commonsense Justice: Jurors' Notions of the Law* (Cambridge, MA: Harvard University Press, 1995).
16 See Hamish Maxwell-Stewart, *Closing Hell's Gates: The Death of a Convict Station* (Sydney: Allen & Unwin, 2008).
17 Lisa Ford and David Andrew Roberts, 'New South Wales Penal Settlements and the Transformation of Secondary Punishment in the Nineteenth-Century British Empire,' *Journal of Colonialism and Colonial History* 15, no. 3 (2014): n.p.
18 See McGowan, Randall, 'A Powerful Sympathy: Terror, the Prison, and Humanitarian Reform in Early Nineteenth-Century Britain,' *Journal of British Studies* 25 (1986): 312–13.
19 *Memoirs of the Life of Sir James Mackintosh*, vol. 1, ed. R. J. Mackintosh (London, 1835), 343; Christian Giuseppe De Vito and Alex Lichtenstein, eds, *Global Convict Labour* (Leiden: Brill, 2015); Clare Anderson and Hamish Maxwell-Stewart, 'Convict Labour and the Western Empires,' in *The Routledge History of Western Empires*, eds R. Aldrich and K. McKenzie (London: Routledge, 2014), 102–17.
20 Atkinson, *Europeans in Australia, vol. 1*, 65–66.
21 Charles Bateson, *The Convict Ships, 1787–1868*, 2nd edn (Glasgow: Brown, Son & Ferguson, 1969); Gary L. Sturgess, Sara Rahmn and George Argyrous, 'Convict Transportation to New South Wales, 1787–1849: Mortality Rates Reconsidered,' *Australian Economic History Review* 58, no. 1 (2018): 62–86.
22 House of Commons, Instructions for Surgeons Superintendent on Board Convict Ships, Report from the Select Committee on Transportation, printed 14 July 1837, 344–45.
23 George Fairfowl, Surgeon's Journal, *Andromeda* 1830, quoted in Katharine Foxhall, 'From Convicts to Colonists: The Health of Prisoners and the Voyage to

Australia, 1823–1853,' *Journal of Imperial and Commonwealth History* 39, no. 1 (2011): 3. See also Beverley Earnshaw, 'The Lame, the Blind, the Mad, the Malingerers: Sick and Disabled Convicts within the Colonial Community,' *Journal of the Royal Australian Historical Society* 81, no. 1 (1995): 28.

24 Medical and Surgical Journal of the Convict Transport Ship Blackfriar, 1851, UKNA ADM101/12, 26–27.

25 Earnshaw, 'The Lame, the Blind, the Mad, the Malingerers,' 29, 33.

26 C. J. Cummins, *A History of Medical Administration in New South Wales 1788–1973*, 2nd edn (Sydney: NSW Department of Health, 2003); Angeline Brasier, 'Prisoners' Bodies: Methods and Advances in Convict Medicine in the Transportation Era,' *Health and History* 12, no. 2 (2010): 18–38.

27 E. Parry to A. McLeay, 13 April 1830, *In the Service of the Company: Letters of Sir Edward Parry, Commissioner to the Australian Agricultural Company, vol. 1* (Canberra: ANU ePress, 2005), 53–54.

28 Jaqui Newling, 'Dining with Strangeness: European Foodways on the Eora Frontier,' *Journal of Australian Colonial History* 13 (2011): 27–48; and 'Phillip's Table Food in the Early Sydney Settlement,' *Sydney Journal* 5, no. 1 (2016): 68–82.

29 John Hirst, *Convict Society and Its Enemies: A History of Early New South Wales* (Sydney: George Allen & Unwin, 1983), 47–50.

30 Earnshaw, 'The Lame, the Blind, the Mad, the Malingerers,' 33.

31 Hector Gavin, *On Feigned or Factitious Diseases, Chiefly of Soldiers and Seamen* (London, 1843), 11–12.

32 Henry Wentworth Acland, *Feigned Insanity, How Most Usually Simulated, and How Best Detected* (London, 1844), 4. On imitation see James Cowles Prichard, *A Treatise on Insanity and Other Disorders Affecting the Mind* (Philadelphia, 1837), 278–81. On feigning as a symptom: Henry Marshall, *Hints to Young Medical Officers of the Army on the Examination of Recruits* (London, 1828), 198; Gavin, *On Feigned or Factitious Diseases*, 12, 17.

33 'Lecture XXI: Corporeal Disablement, and Simulation,' *Lancet* 1 (25 February 1837): 769.

34 Thomas Blatchford, *An Inaugural Dissertation on Feigned Disease* (New York, 1817), 23.

35 Hirst, *Convict Society and Its Enemies*, 29.

36 H. Graham to A. Maconochie, 16 June 1842 and A. Maconochie to G. Gipps 16 September 1842, Despatch 42/54, UKNA CO 201/324, 147.

37 Henry Graham, 'A Criminal Lunatic,' *Medical Journal of Australia* (January 1857): 77.

38 Acland, *Feigned Insanity*, 9.

39 Watkin Tench, *A Complete Account of the Settlement at Port Jackson* (London, 1793), 17. Peter Burroughs, 'Crime and Punishment in the British Army, 1815–1870,' *English Historical Review* 100, no. 396 (1985): 545–46.

40 Blatchford, *An Inaugural Dissertation on Feigned Disease*, 23.

41 'Classified Advertising,' *Sydney Gazette*, 12 February 1804: 3.

42 'Sydney,' *Sydney Gazette*, 10 July 1808: 2.

43 'Classified Advertising,' *Sydney Gazette*, 6 January 1805: 3; 'Classified Advertising,' *Sydney Gazette*, 27 April 1806: 3.

44 'Court of Criminal Jurisdiction,' *Sydney Gazette*, 31 July 1808: 2.
45 See Nigel Walker, *Crime and Insanity in England*, vol. 1 (Edinburgh: Edinburgh University Press, 1967), 78–81 and Richard Moran, 'The Origin of Insanity as a Special Verdict: The Trial for Treason of James Hadfield (1800),' *Law & Society Review* 19, no. 3 (1985): 487–519.
46 'Court of Criminal Jurisdiction,' *Sydney Gazette*, 31 July 1808; B. H. Fletcher, 'Harris, John (1754–1838),' *Australian Dictionary of Biography*, <adb.anu.edu.au/biography/harris-john-2164/text2773>, accessed 18 February 2014.
47 Lord v Scott, 1 December 1808, quoted in Nagle, *Collins, the Courts & the Colony*, 30.
48 'Domestic Intelligence,' *Australian*, 7 November 1834: 2.
49 Grace Karskens, *The Colony: A History of Early Sydney* (Sydney: Allen & Unwin, 2009), 303.
50 L. Macquarie to Bathurst, 8 March 1819, *HRA* I, vol. 10, 43; 'Newcastle Penal Establishment,' NSW State Archives & Records, <www.records.nsw.gov.au/agency/2111>, accessed 27 July 2018.
51 J. Wallis to J. T. Campbell, 8 August 1817, Colonial Secretary's Papers, SRNSW 4/1806, Reel 6066, 82.
52 J. Wallis to J. T. Campbell, 8 November 1817, Colonial Secretary's Papers, SRNSW 4/1806, Reel 6066, 95.
53 J. T. Campbell to J. Jacques, 14 November 1817, Colonial Secretary's Papers, SRNSW 4/3497, Reel 6005, 137.
54 Original emphases. J. T. Morisset to J. T. Campbell, 21 July 1819, Colonial Secretary's Papers, SRNSW 4/1807, Reel 6067, 43–44.
55 J. T. Campbell to J. T. Morisset, 8 September 1819, Colonial Secretary's Papers, SRNSW 4/3500, Reel 6006, 251.
56 Paula J. Byrne, 'The Creation of Bushranging,' in *Criminal Law and Colonial Subject: New South Wales 1810–1830* (Melbourne: Cambridge University Press, 1993), 129–51.
57 'Sydney,' *Sydney Gazette*, 18 August 1821: 2.
58 Marcus Clarke, *For the Term of His Natural Life* (Floating Press, 2014), ProQuest Ebook Central, n.p.
59 On suicide lotteries, see Robert Hughes, *The Fatal Shore: A History of the Transportation of Convicts to Australia, 1787–1868* (London: Collins Harvill, 1987), 467–69, and Tim Causer, 'Norfolk Island's "Suicide Lotteries": Myth and Reality,' *Islands of History: Proceedings of the 25th Anniversary Conference, Professional Historians Association* (NSW) (Sydney: Anchor Books, 2011), 61–68.
60 Causer, 'Norfolk Island's "Suicide Lotteries",' 62, and see Barbara T. Gates, *Victorian Suicide: Mad Crimes and Sad Histories* (Princeton: Princeton University Press, 1988).
61 Henry Fielding, *An Enquiry into the Causes of the Late Increase of Robbers* (London, 1751), 96.
62 'Hints to Young Medical Officers of the Army on the Examination of Recruits, and respecting the feigned disabilities of soldiers [...] by Henry Marshall, Surgeon to the Forces [Review],' *London Medical and Physical Journal*, new series, 5 (1828): 152.

63 Mark Finnane, 'Law and Regulation,' in *The Cambridge History of Australia, vol. 1*, eds A. Bashford and S. Macintyre (Cambridge: Cambridge University Press, 2013), 411.

64 Byrne, *Criminal Law and Colonial Subject*, 148.

65 H. Macarthur to L. Macquarie, 15 February 1821, SRNSW NSW 4/1748, Reel 6051, 237–39; J. Redman to J. T. Campbell, 19 May 1821, SRNSW 4/1748, Reel 6051, 351–52; J. Redman to J. T. Campbell, 7 July 1821, SRNSW 4/1748, Reel 6051, 359; J. T. Campbell to F. Goulburn, SRNSW 4/1748, Reel 6051, 357; 'Sydney,' Sydney Gazette, 18 August 1821: 2; 'Supreme Court,' Sydney Gazette, 25 August 1821: 3; Death warrant, 24 August 1821, SRNSW 4/1265, Reel 6070, 38.

66 Joseph Mason Cox, *Practical Observation on Insanity* (London, 1806), 206.

67 Acland, *Feigned Insanity*, 6–7, 9–11.

68 Jeffrey L. Geller et al., 'Feigned Insanity in Nineteenth-Century America: Tactics, Trials, and Truth,' *Behavioral Sciences and the Law* 8, no. 1 (1990): 10–13.

69 Geller et al., 'Feigned Insanity in Nineteenth-Century America,' 13–15; 'Lecture XXII: Simulation of Diseases (Continued),' *Lancet* 1 (4 March 1837), 805.

70 Original emphasis. Acland, *Feigned Insanity*, 9.

71 See Geller et al., 'Feigned Insanity in Nineteenth-Century America,' 6.

72 Robert L. Martensen, 'The Detection of Feigned Insanity,' *Journal of the American Medical Association* 276, no. 16 (1996): 1357; Richard Rogers, 'Models of Feigned Mental Illness,' *Professional Psychology: Research and Practice* 21, no. 3 (1990): 182–88.

73 M. West, 26 September 1820, Appendix, Commission of Inquiry, SLNSW BT Box 6, Reel CY1551, 2590.

74 W. Bennett to J. T. Campbell, 1 January 1821, Colonial Secretary's Papers, SRNSW 4/1751, Reel 6052, 259.

75 W. Bennett to F. Goulburn, 2 July 1821, Colonial Secretary's Papers, SRNSW 4/1751, Reel 6052, 267.

76 W. Bland, 23 January 1821, in John Ritchie, *The Evidence to the Bigge Reports: New South Wales under Governor Macquarie*, vol. 1 (Melbourne: Heinemann, 1971), 144.

77 James Dunk, 'Authority and the Treatment of the Insane at Castle Hill Asylum, 1811–25,' *Health and History* 19, no. 2 (2017): 17–40.

78 'Hints to Young Medical Officers [Review]'.

79 L. L. Robson, *The Convict Settlers of Australia: An Enquiry into the Origin and Character of the Convicts Transported to New South Wales and Van Diemen's Land 1787–1852* (Melbourne: Melbourne University Press and Cambridge University Press, 1965).

80 House of Commons, 'Standing Instructions for the Regulation of the Penal Settlement on Tasman's Peninsula – (with a Plan),' 25 January 1833, in Secondary Punishment (Australia), printed 4 March 1834, *Parliamentary Accounts and Papers*, vol. 47, 62–63.

81 'Law,' *Australian*, 24 February 1837: 3.

82 'Quarter Sessions,' *Colonial Times*, 18 November 1845: 4.

83 'Responsibility of the Insane,' *Observer*, 28 November 1845: 2.

CHAPTER 4

1 L. Macquarie to Bathurst, 27 July 1822, *Historical Records of Australia (HRA)* I, vol. 10, 671.

2 Alan Atkinson, *The Europeans in Australia: A History, vol. 1* (Melbourne: Oxford University Press, 1997), 106.

3 *Memoirs of the Life of the Right Honourable Sir James Mackintosh*, vol. 1, ed. R. J. Mackintosh (London, 1835), 342–43.

4 Silvia Sebastiani, *The Scottish Enlightenment: Race, Gender, and the Limits of Progress* (New York: Palgrave Macmillan, 2013), 1–2.

5 Lenore Coltheart and Peter Bridges, 'The Elephant's Bed? Scottish Enlightenment Ideas and the Foundations of New South Wales,' *Journal of Australian Studies* 25, no. 68 (2001): 19–20.

6 Henry Lytton Bulwer, *Historical Characters: Talleyrand, Cobbett, Mackintosh, Canning*, vol. 2 (London, 1868), 93; G. Grey to Holland, 2 November 1835, quoted in Winifred Stokes and R. G. Thorne, 'Mackintosh, Sir James (1765–1832),' in *The History of Parliament: The House of Commons 1790–1820*, ed. R. G. Thorne (London, 1986), <www.historyofparliamentonline.org/volume/1790-1820/member/mackintosh-sir-james-1765-1832>, accessed 29 October 2015.

7 John Ritchie, *Lachlan Macquarie: A Biography* (Melbourne: Melbourne University Press, 1986), 131.

8 Malcolm Ellis, *Lachlan Macquarie: His Life, Adventures and Times, with Reference Notes and Bibliography* (Sydney: Angus & Robertson, 2010), 504.

9 L. Macquarie to Bathurst, 4 December 1817, *HRA* I, vol. 9, 506.

10 Colin Clair, *Lachlan Macquarie: Father of Australia* (Watford, UK: Bruce & Gawthorn, 1963); Marjorie Barnard, *Lachlan Macquarie* (Melbourne: Oxford University Press, 1964); John Ritchie, *The Governor: Lachlan Macquarie 1810 to 1821* (Sydney: State Library of New South Wales, 2010).

11 Diane Sylvester, 'Governor Lachlan Macquarie, Sir James Mackintosh and the Scottish Enlightenment,' *Journal of Australian Colonial History* 12 (2010): 32, 34–35; Atkinson, *The Europeans in Australia, vol. 1*, 324.

12 'Government and General Orders,' *Sydney Gazette*, 6 October 1810: 1.

13 Ritchie, *Lachlan Macquarie*, 155–56; Mary Casey, 'A Patina of Age: Elizabeth Macquarie (Née) Campbell and the Influence of the Buildings and Landscape of Argyll, Scotland, in Colonial New South Wales,' *International Journal of Historical Archaeology* 14, no. 3 (2010): 335–56.

14 Grace Karskens, *The Colony: A History of Early Sydney* (Sydney: Allen & Unwin, 2009), 89–90; Elizabeth Macarthur quoted in Tony Moore, *Death or Liberty: Rebels and Radicals Transported to Australia 1788–1868* (Sydney: Pier 9, 2010), 161.

15 J. T. Campbell to R. Durie, 15 April 1811, Colonial Secretary's Papers SRNSW 4/3490D, Reel 6002, 158–59.

16 'Sydney,' *Sydney Gazette*, 1 June 1811: 1.

17 W. D. Neil, *The Lunatic Asylum at Castle Hill: Australia's First Psychiatric Hospital, 1811–1826* (Sydney: Dryas, 1992); John Bostock, *The Dawn of Australian Psychiatry* (Sydney: Australian Medical Association, 1968).

18 W. Bland, 23 January 1821, *The Evidence to the Bigge Reports: New South Wales Under Governor Macquarie*, vol. I, ed. J. Ritchie (Melbourne: Heinemann, 1971), 143.

19 Neil, *The Lunatic Asylum*, 37–40, 52–54, 56, 59–60, 61–67.
20 W. Bennett to T. Allen, 1 April 1824, Colonial Secretary's Papers, SRNSW 4/1777, Reel 743, 153.
21 W. Bennett to F. Goulburn, 1 March 1822, Colonial Secretary's Papers, SRNSW 4/1756, Reel 743, 18.
22 John Thomas Bigge, *Report of the Commissioner of Inquiry into the State of the Colony of New South Wales* (London, 1822), 146.
23 Waltraud Ernst, 'Racial, Social and Cultural Factors in the Development of a Colonial Institution: The Bombay Lunatic Asylum (1670–1858),' *Internationales Asienforum* 22, no. 3–4 (1992): 63–64.
24 Waltraud Ernst, 'Idioms of Madness and Colonial Boundaries: The Case of the European and "Native" Mentally Ill in Early Nineteenth-Century British India,' *Comparative Studies in Society and History* 39, no. 1 (1997): 153–81.
25 Anouska Bhattacharyya, 'Indian Insanes: Lunacy in the "Native" Asylums of Colonial India, 1858–1912,' PhD thesis, Harvard University, 2013, 3.
26 See Bostock, *The Dawn of Australian Psychiatry*, 22; Neil, *The Lunatic Asylum*, 10.
27 'Classified Advertising,' *Sydney Gazette*, 31 October 1812: 1.
28 'Classified Advertising,' *Sydney Gazette*, 15 January 1814: 1.
29 A. T. Yarwood, 'Marsden, Samuel (1765–1838),' *Australian Dictionary of Biography*, <adb.anu.edu.au/biography/marsden-samuel-2433/text3237>, accessed 30 July 2014.
30 Meredith Lake, 'Samuel Marsden, Work and the Limits of Evangelical Humanitarianism,' *History Australia* 7, no. 3 (2010): 57.1–57.23; Andrew Sharp, *The World, the Flesh and the Devil: The Life and Opinions of Samuel Marsden in England and the Antipodes, 1765–1838* (Auckland: Auckland University Press, 2016).
31 *Memoirs of George Suttor, F.L.S.: Banksian Collector (1774–1859)*, ed. G. Mackaness (Sydney: self-published, 1948), 57.
32 Neil, *The Lunatic Asylum*, 11–12.
33 G. Suttor to L. Macquarie, 29 September 1814, Colonial Secretary's Papers, SRNSW 4/1730, Reel 6044, 303–306.
34 Neil, *The Lunatic Asylum*, 13.
35 Vivienne Parsons, 'Throsby, Charles (1777–1828),' *Australian Dictionary of Biography*, <adb.anu.edu.au/biography/throsby-charles-2735/text3861>, accessed 29 October 2018; Neil, *The Lunatic Asylum*, 14; *Memoirs of George Suttor*, 50.
36 Neil, *The Lunatic Asylum*, 14, 18–19.
37 See Penny Russell, *Savage or Civilised? Manners in Colonial Australia* (Sydney: UNSW Press, 2010), 165–89.
38 J. T. Campbell to G. Suttor, 12 September 1814, Colonial Secretary's Papers, SRNSW NRS937 4/3493, Reel 6004, 293–97.
39 J. T. Campbell to G. Suttor and to W. Bland, 12 September 1814, Colonial Secretary's Papers, SRNSW NRS937 4/3493, Reel 6004, 293, 295–97.
40 Monthly Reports of the Lunatic Asylum at Castle Hill, Colonial Secretary's Papers, SRNSW 4/1719.5, Reel 743, n.p.
41 J. T. Campbell to G. Suttor, 12 September 1814, Colonial Secretary's Papers, SRNSW NRS937 4/3493, Reel 6004, 294.
42 Neil, *The Lunatic Asylum*, 20.

43 G. Suttor to L. Macquarie, 27 February 1815, Colonial Secretary's Papers, SRNSW NRS 897 4/1732, Reel 6045, 83.
44 J. T. Campbell to G. Suttor, 2 March 1815 and to W. Bland, 2 March 1815, Colonial Secretary's Papers, SRNSW NRS 937 4/3493, Reel 6004, 474–75.
45 W. Bland, 23 January 1821, *The Evidence to the Bigge Reports*, ed. J. Ritchie, 143; J. T. Campbell to W. Bland, 28 August 1815, Colonial Secretary's Papers 4/3494, Reel 6004, 152; D. Richards, 'Transported to New South Wales: Medical Convicts 1788–1850,' *British Medical Journal (Clinical Research Edition)* 295, no. 6613 (1987), 1611.
46 Earl Spencer 1813, Convict Indents, SRNSW NRS 12188 4/4004, 478.
47 Neil, *The Lunatic Asylum*, 22–23; Rod Best, 'The Castle Hill Lunatic Asylum 1811–1826,' *Journal of the Royal Australian Historical Society 78*, no. 3–4 (1992): 9.
48 Doreen Lambert, *The Parmeter Story* (Sydney: Mini-Publishing, 2002), 5–11.
49 T. Parmeter to L. Macquarie, 24 May 1817, Wentworth Papers, SLNSW SAFE/A 753, Reel CY699, 105.
50 Andrew Scull, *The Most Solitary of Afflictions: Madness and Society in Britain, 1700–1900* (New Haven: Yale University Press, 1993), 263; Leonard Smith, *Cure, Comfort and Safe Custody: Public Lunatic Asylums in Early Nineteenth Century* (London: Leicester University Press, 1999), 137; Lee-Ann Monk, *Attending Madness: At Work in the Australian Colonial Asylum* (Amsterdam: Rodopi, 2008), 8–9; David Wright, 'The Dregs of Society? Occupational Patterns of Male Asylum Attendants in Victorian England,' *International History of Nursing Journal* 1, no. 4 (1996): 5–19.
51 Best, 'The Castle Hill Lunatic Asylum,' 17.
52 T. Parmeter to D. Wentworth, 2 October 1817, Appendix, Commission of Inquiry, SLNSW BT Box 16, Reel CY1553, 1983–85.
53 Thomas S. Kirkbride, *On the Construction, Organization and General Arrangements of Hospitals for the Insane* (Philadelphia, 1854), 42–43.
54 L. Macquarie to W. Wentworth, 30 December 1817, Wentworth Papers, SLNSW SAFE/A 753, 101.
55 T. Parmeter to D. Wentworth, 8 June 1818, Appendix, Commission of Inquiry, SLNSW BT Box 16, Reel CY1553, 2179–80.
56 Coroner's inquest on 'Francisco,' Appendix, Commission of Inquiry, SLNSW BT Box 16, Reel CY1553, 2192–93.
57 Thomas Parmeter, 'The Asylum,' SLNSW DLDOC 6.
58 Court of Inquiry, December 1818 – January 1819, Colonial Secretary's Papers, SLNSW NRS 897 (hereafter Court of Inquiry), 72–74.
59 G. Suttor, Court of Inquiry, 67.
60 T. McDougall, jnr, Court of Inquiry, 72.
61 Best, 'The Castle Hill Lunatic Asylum,' 12.
62 J. Cooper, Court of Inquiry, 79.
63 G. Suttor, Court of Inquiry, 67.
64 'Confessions of a Bookworm,' *Sydney Gazette*, 3 September 1831: 3.
65 Original emphasis. B. Newland, D. Tennant, and W. Maddox, Court of Inquiry, 69.
66 Michael Ignatieff, *A Just Measure of Pain: The Penitentiary in the Industrial Revolution, 1750–1850* (London: Penguin, 1978), 7.

67 Pieter Spierenburg, ed., *Violence and Punishment: Civilizing the Body Through Time* (Polity Press, 2013), ProQuest Ebook Central; Joy Damousi, *Depraved and Disorderly: Female Convicts, Sexuality and Gender in Colonial Australia* (Cambridge: Cambridge University Press, 1997), 85–86, 95–96; Wilbur R. Miller, ed., *The Social History of Crime and Punishment in America: An Encylopedia* (Sage, 2012), 1467.
68 W. Maddox, Court of Inquiry, 70.
69 J. Cooper, Court of Inquiry, 78–79.
70 David MacBride, *A Methodical Introduction to the Theory and Practice of Physick* (London, 1772), 592; Andrew Scull, 'The Domestication of Madness,' *Medical History* 27 (1983): 240.
71 Wilhelm Frydendahl, 26 July 1829, quoted in Bjørn Hamre, 'Disciplinary Power and the Role of the Subject at a Nineteenth-century Danish Asylum,' *PhaenEx* 5, no. 2 (2010): 11.
72 Scull, 'The Domestication of Madness,' 240.
73 Neil, *The Lunatic Asylum*, 21.
74 J. Cooper, Court of Inquiry, 79.
75 T. Parmeter to D. Wentworth, 2 October 1817, Appendix, Commission of Inquiry, SLNSW, BT Box 16, Reel CY1553, 1983–85.
76 Court of Inquiry, 65–66; Neil, *The Lunatic Asylum*, 28–29, 31.
77 Monk, *Attending Madness*, 10.
78 Nancy Tomes, 'A Generous Confidence: Thomas Story Kirkbride's Philosophy of Asylum Construction and Management,' in *Madhouses, Mad-Doctors, and Madmen: The Social History of Psychiatry in the Victorian Era*, ed. A. Scull (Philadelphia: University of Pennsylvania Press, 1981/2015), 137–38.
79 Tomes, 'A Generous Confidence,' 136.
80 Kirkbride, *On the Construction, Organization and General Arrangements of Hospitals for the Insane*, 42–43.
81 Tomes, 'A Generous Confidence,' 136.
82 Kirkbride, *On the Construction, Organization and General Arrangements of Hospitals for the Insane*, 42.
83 Best, 'The Castle Hill Lunatic Asylum,' 17.
84 John Thomas Bigge, *Report of the Commissioner of Inquiry on the State of Agriculture and Trade in the Colony of New South Wales* (London, 1823), 105.
85 Bigge, *Report of the Commissioner of Inquiry on the State of Agriculture and Trade*, 111.
86 Bigge, *Report of the Commissioner of Inquiry on the Judicial Establishments*, 89.
87 L. Macquarie to Bathurst, 27 July 1822, *HRA* I, vol. 10, 671.
88 L. Macquarie to Bathurst, 27 July 1822, *HRA* I, vol. 10, 671.
89 Bigge, *Report of the Commissioner of Inquiry on the Judicial Establishments*, 20.
90 E. S. Hall to G. Murray, 26 November 1828, *HRA* I, vol. 14, 597.
91 'Parramatta Quarter Sessions,' *Sydney Gazette*, 3 March 1825: 3. It was a grand jury, a rare formation of twelve to twenty-three men who gathered evidence and decided whether allegations should proceed to trial, employed in NSW 1824–28: G. D. Woods, *A History of Criminal Law in New South Wales: The Colonial Period, 1788–1900* (Sydney: Federation Press, 2002), 59–61; J. M. Bennett, 'The Establishment of Jury Trial in New South Wales,' *Sydney Law Review* 3, no. 3 (1961): 483.

92 'Parramatta Quarter Sessions,' *Sydney Gazette*, 25 August 1825: 3; W. Bennett to T. Allen, 1 April 1824, Colonial Secretary's Papers, SRNSW NRS 897 4/1777, Reel 743, 153.

CHAPTER 5

1 John Manning Ward, *Colonial Self-Government: The British Experience, 1759–1856* (London: Macmillan, 1976), 131; B. H. Fletcher, 'Phillip, Arthur (1738–1814),' *Australian Dictionary of Biography*, <adb.anu.edu.au/biography/phillip-arthur-2549/text3471>, accessed 11 February 2019.

2 The term 'crown colony' was introduced in 1828, but it is used here as a shorthand for the various iterations over the preceding fifty years, including 'royal colony': Ward, *Colonial Self-Government*, 82–83.

3 Thomas Keneally, *The Commonwealth of Thieves: The Sydney Experiment* (Sydney: Random House Australia, 2005); D. E. Fifer, 'The Australian Patriotic Association 1835–1841,' *Journal of the Royal Australian Historical Society*, 156.

4 Ward, *Colonial Self-Government*, 91, 131; Lauren Benton, *A Search for Sovereignty: Law and Geography in European Empires, 1400–1900* (Cambridge: Cambridge University Press, 2010), 208–21.

5 David Neal, *The Rule of Law in a Penal Colony: Law and Power in Early New South Wales* (Cambridge: Cambridge University Press, 1992).

6 F. Garling, A List of Prisoners Tried before the Court of Criminal Jurisdiction (16 January 1816), 20 March 1816, *Report from the Select Committee on the State of Gaols*, House of Commons, printed 12 July 1819, 521.

7 M. Hoare, 27 December 1820, in John Ritchie, ed., *The Evidence to the Bigge Reports: New South Wales Under Governor Macquarie*, vol. 2 (Melbourne: Heinemann, 1971), 102.

8 L. Macquarie to Bathurst, 4 December 1817, *Historical Records of Australia (HRA)* I, vol. 9, 503.

9 Zoë Laidlaw, *Colonial Connections, 1815–45: Patronage, the Information Revolution and Colonial Government* (Manchester: Manchester University Press, 2005), 49, 56 n50.

10 Alan Lester, *Imperial Networks: Creating Identities in Nineteenth-Century South Africa and Britain* (London: Routledge, 2001); Tony Ballantyne, *Orientalism and Race: Aryanism in the British Empire* (Houndmills, UK: Palgrave, 2002); Zoë Laidlaw, 'Breaking Britannia's Bounds? Law, Settlers, and Space in Britain's Imperial Historiography,' *Historical Journal* 55, no. 3 (2012): 807–30.

11 John Hirst, *Convict Society and Its Enemies: A History of Early New South Wales* (Sydney: George Allen & Unwin, 1983), 58–59; B. H. Fletcher, 'Bayly, Nicholas (1770–1823),' *Australian Dictionary of Biography*, <adb.anu.edu.au/biography/bayly-nicholas-1758/text1959>, accessed 28 May 2015.

12 Proclamation, 4 January 1810, *Historical Records of NSW (HRNSW)*, vol. 7, 255–57; Fletcher, 'Bayly, Nicholas (1770–1823)'.

13 Anonymous extracts, 13 March 1816, *HRA* I, vol. 9, 200.

14 Roy Porter, *Mind-Forg'd Manacles: A History of Madness in England from the Restoration to the Regency* (Cambridge, MA: Harvard University Press, 1987), 124–25 and 315 n72.

15 Samuel Tuke, *Description of The Retreat, an Institution Near York* (York, 1813).

16 Andrew Scull, *The Most Solitary of Afflictions: Madness and Society in Britain, 1700–1900* (New Haven: Yale University Press, 1993), 115–46; Seán McConville, *A History of English Prison Administration*, vol. 1 (Boston: Routledge & Kegan Paul, 1981), 78–104.

17 Lauren Benton, 'Just Despots: The Cultural Construction of Imperial Constitutionalism,' *Law, Culture and the Humanities* 9, no. 2 (2013): 214; Kirsten McKenzie, *Imperial Underworld: An Escaped Convict and the Transformation of the British Colonial Order* (Cambridge: Cambridge University Press, 2016); Mark Francis, *Governors and Settlers: Images of Authority in the British Colonies, 1820–60* (Houndmills, UK: Palgrave, 1992).

18 Bathurst to L. Macquarie, 24 January 1817, *HRA* I, vol. 9, 197; Ellis, *Lachlan Macquarie*, 401–402.

19 J. T. Bennett, 'The Day of Retribution – Commissioner Bigge's Enquiries in Colonial New South Wales,' *American Journal of Legal History* 15, no. 2 (1971): 87–88.

20 Elizabeth Macquarie to James Drummond, 12 December 1817, Lachlan Macquarie Papers, SLNSW A797, 135.

21 S. Marsden, 27 December 1820, in Ritchie, *The Evidence to the Bigge Reports*, vol. 2, 103, 105–106.

22 Deposition of G. Suttor, 22 October 1817, *HRA* I, vol. 9, 512.

23 G. Suttor, Evidence to the Commission of Inquiry, quoted in John Bostock, *The Dawn of Australian Psychiatry* (Sydney: Australian Medical Association, 1968), 24–25.

24 Deposition of G. Suttor, 22 October 1817, *HRA* I, vol. 9, 512.

25 S. Marsden to J. T. Campbell, 28 November 1817, *HRA* I, vol. 9, 538.

26 Anne Digby, 'Moral Treatment at The Retreat, 1796–1846,' in *The Anatomy of Madness: Essays in the History of Psychiatry, vol. II: Institutions and Society*, eds William F. Bynum, Roy Porter and Michael Shepherd (London: Tavistock Publications, 1985), 53.

27 S. Marsden to J. T. Campbell, 28 November 1817, *HRA* I, vol. 9, 538; Deposition of Michael Hoare, 22 October 1817, *HRA* I, vol. 9, 512–13.

28 U. R. Q. Henriques, 'The Rise and Decline of the Separate System of Prison Discipline,' *Past & Present* 54, no. 1 (1972): 64–65; Margaret Charleroy and Hilary Marland, 'Prisoners of Solitude: Bringing History to Bear on Prison Health Policy,' *Endeavour* 40, no. 3 (2016): 141–47.

29 William James Forsythe, *The Reform of Prisoners 1830–1900* (London: Croom Helm, 1987), 25–28; Henriques, 'The Rise and Decline of the Separate System,' 63–64.

30 F. Garling to L. Macquarie, 2 December 1817, *HRA* I, vol. 9, 514, and see John Ritchie, *Lachlan Macquarie: A Biography* (Melbourne: Melbourne University Press, 1986), 132–38.

31 See David Plater and Penny Crofts, 'Bushrangers, the Exercise of Mercy and the "Last Penalty of the Law" in New South Wales and Tasmania 1824–1856,' *University of Tasmania Law Review* 32, no. 2 (2013): 295–343; Paula J. Byrne, *Criminal Law and Colonial Subject: New South Wales 1810–1830* (Melbourne: Cambridge University Press, 1993), 129–51 and '"The Public Good":

Competing Visions of Freedom in Early Colonial New South Wales,' *Labour History* 58 (1990): 76–83; Neal, *The Rule of Law*, 150–64.

32 Jennifer Anne McKinnon, 'Convict Bushrangers in New South Wales, 1824–34,' MA thesis, La Trobe University, 1979.

33 Neal, *The Rule of Law*, 90.

34 John Thomas Bigge, *Report of the Commissioner of Inquiry on the Judicial Establishments of New South Wales, and Van Diemen's Land* (London, 1823), 19.

35 L. Macquarie to Bathurst, 4 December 1817, *HRA* I, vol. 9, 503, 513–14.

36 Ritchie, *Lachlan Macquarie*, 133.

37 L. Macquarie to Bathurst, 'Secret & confidential: List of names of discontented and seditious persons in N. S. Wales,' 1 December 1817, New South Wales Governors' despatches vol. 2, SLNSW ML A1191.

38 'Government and General Orders,' *Sydney Gazette*, 31 March 1810: 1.

39 L. Macquarie to S. Marsden, 8 January 1818, SLNSW A797, 141, transcription, <acms.sl.nsw.gov.au/_transcript/2015/D35658/a993.html>, accessed 7 November 2015.

40 John Ritchie, *Punishment and Profit: The Reports of Commissioner John Bigge on the Colonies of New South Wales and Van Diemen's Land, 1822–1823; Their Origins, Nature and Significance* (Melbourne: Heinemann, 1970), 1–30.

41 Bathurst to J. T. Bigge, 30 January 1819, *HRA* I, vol. 10, 7; Bennett, 'The Day of Retribution,' 88–89.

42 Bigge, *Report of the Commissioner of Inquiry on the Judicial Establishments*, 19; Rod Best, 'The Castle Hill Lunatic Asylum, 1811–1826,' *Journal of the Royal Australian Historical Society* 78, no. 3–4 (1992): 9.

43 Bigge, *Report of the Commissioner of Inquiry on the Judicial Establishments*, 20.

44 48 Geo III c 96 [1808].

45 Chantal Stebbings, 'Protecting the Property of the Mentally Ill: The Judicial Solution in Nineteenth Century Lunacy Law,' *Cambridge Law Journal* 71, no. 2 (2012): 388.

46 59 Geo III c 127 [1819]. See *The Parochial Lawyer; or Churchwarden and Overseer's Guide and Assistant* (London, 1829), 121–24. 9 Geo IV c 41 s 30 [1828] required two medical practitioners to separately certify insanity before committal could take place.

47 Ritchie, *Punishment and Profit*, 220; on Hannibal Macarthur's selling spirits, 191–92; on Marsden's character flaws, 201–204.

48 Lauren Benton and Lisa Ford, 'Magistrates in Empire: Convicts, Slaves, and the Remaking of the Plural Legal Order in the British Empire,' in *Legal Pluralism and Empires, 1500–1850*, eds R. J. Ross and L. Benton (New York: NYU Press, 2013), 186; Bruce Kercher, *An Unruly Child: A History of Law in Australia* (Sydney: Allen & Unwin, 1995), 25.

49 Benton and Ford, 'Magistrates in Empire,' 184.

50 See Byrne, *Criminal Law and Colonial Subject*, 169–70.

51 Benton and Ford, 'Magistrates in Empire,' 185; Neal, *The Rule of Law*, 137–38.

52 Circular to Magistrates, 20 April 1820, Commission of Inquiry, BT Box 24, 5270, quoted in Byrne, *Criminal Law and Colonial Subject*, 170.

53 4 Geo. IV c. 96 [1823]; Byrne, *Criminal Law and Colonial Subject*, 169–70; Kercher,

An Unruly Child, 69; Benton and Ford, 'Magistrates in Empire,' 185–86.

54 Neal, *The Rule of Law*, 109.

55 6 Geo. IV No. 5 NSW [1825], and see Kercher, *An Unruly Child*, 25.

56 H. Fulton to F. Goulburn, 5 July 1824, Colonial Secretary's Papers, SRNSW 4/1777, Reel 743, 144.

57 Catharine Coleborne, *Insanity, Identity and Empire: Immigrants and Institutional Confinement in Australia and New Zealand, 1873–1910* (Manchester: Manchester University Press, 2015); Sally Swartz, *Homeless Wanderers: Movement and Mental Illness in the Cape Colony in the Nineteenth Century* (Cape Town: UCT Press, 2016).

58 George F. J. Bergman, 'Solomon Levey in Sydney: From Convict Merchant to Prince,' *Royal Australian Historical Society: Journal and Proceedings* 49, no. 6 (1964): 401–403, and 'Levey, Solomon (1794–1833),' *Australian Dictionary of Biography*, <adb.anu.edu.au/biography/levey-solomon-2353/text3077>, accessed 5 May 2015.

59 George F. J. Bergman, 'Levey, Barnett (1798–1837),' *Australian Dictionary of Biography*, <adb.anu.edu.au/biography/levey-barnett-2352/text3075>, accessed 8 November 2015.

60 The surname appears in several spellings (Levy, Levi, Levey); Samuel was transported under the alias John Lee.

61 Conduct Register, TAS CON 31/1/27, 66, Founders & Survivors, <foundersandsurvivors.org/pubsearch/convict/chain/c31a31270341>, accessed 29 September 2014.

62 'The Governor's Court,' *Sydney Gazette*, 25 August 1821: 2.

63 Holder, 'Campbell, John Thomas (1770–1830),' *Australian Dictionary of Biography*, <adb.anu.edu.au/biography/campbell-john-thomas-1873/text2191>, accessed 30 April 2015.

64 J. T. Campbell to F. Goulburn, 26 March 1823, Colonial Secretary's Papers, SRNSW 4/1767, Reel 6057, 110.

65 John Maclehose, *The Picture of Sydney and Strangers' Guide in NSW for 1838* (Sydney, 1838), 136.

66 J. T. Campbell to T. Dunn and J. T. Campbell to S. Marsden, 20 January 1825, Colonial Secretary's Papers, SRNSW 4/3513, Reel 6014, 294–95.

67 Peter G. Bolt, *William Cowper (1778–1858): The Life and Influence of Australia's First Parish Clergyman* (Sydney: Bolt Publishing Services, 2009), 476–77.

68 James Bowman, not William, was the principal surgeon: S. Levey to F. Goulburn, 7 November 1823, Colonial Secretary's Papers, SRNSW 4/1773, 53.

69 Jeremy Bentham, *Principles of Penal Law* (Adelaide: University of Adelaide Library, 2016), <ebooks.adelaide.edu.au/b/bentham/jeremy/principles_of_penal_law/index.html>, accessed 8 November 2015.

70 F. Goulburn to W. Bennett, Colonial Secretary's Papers, SRNSW 4/3509, Reel 6011, 669.

71 W. Bennett to F. Goulburn, 24 January 1824, Colonial Secretary's Papers, SRNSW 4/1777, Reel 743, 145; W. Bennett to F. Goulburn, 24 February 1824, Colonial Secretary's Papers, SRNSW 4/1777, Reel 6060, 150.

72 F. Hely to R. Darling, 27 December 1812, quoted in Bostock, *The Dawn of Australian Psychiatry*, 35.

73 F. Goulburn to Parramatta Magistrate, 21 January 1824, Colonial Secretary's Papers, SRNSW 4/3510, Reel 6012, 222.
74 W. Bennett to F. Goulburn, 1 April 1824, Colonial Secretary's Papers, SRNSW 4/1777, Reel 6060, 152.
75 Monthly Return of Lunatics, 1 May 1826, Colonial Secretary's Papers, SRNSW 4/1917.5, Reel 743, n.p.
76 'Mr. Levey in England,' *Australian*, 20 June 1827: 3.
77 Mark Finnane, 'Asylums, Families and the State,' *History Workshop* 20 (1985): 142.
78 Catherine Coleborne, *Madness in the Family: Insanity and Institutions in the Australasian Colonial World, 1860–1914* (New York: Palgrave Macmillan, 2010), 52–54.
79 Finnane, 'Asylums, Families and the State,' 135.
80 David Wright, 'Family Strategies and the Institutional Confinement of "Idiot" Children in Victorian England,' *Journal of Family History* 23, no. 2 (1998): 204.
81 Finnane, 'Asylums, Families and the State,' 136.
82 Bergman, 'Solomon Levey in Sydney,' 403.
83 'John/Samuel Lee/Levi/Lee als. Saml. Levi,' Founders & Survivors, <foundersandsurvivors.org/pubsearch/convict/chain/c31a31270341>, accessed 29 September 2014.
84 Bergman, 'Levey, Solomon (1794–1833),' *Australian Dictionary of Biography*, <adb.anu.edu.au/biography/levey-solomon-2353/text3077>, accessed 5 May 2015.
85 'Family Notices,' *Sydney Monitor*, 18 February 1834: 3.
86 N. Horwood, 'James Birnie,' *Journal of the Royal Australian Historical Society* 59, no. 2 (1973): 95–113; David Roger Hainsworth, *The Sydney Traders: Simeon Lord and His Contemporaries, 1788–1821*, 2nd edn (Melbourne: Melbourne University Press, 1981).
87 'Supreme Court – In Equity,' *Australasian Chronicle*, 1 March 1842: 4; Hainsworth, *The Sydney Traders*, 60.
88 'Law,' *Australian*, 16 October 1838: 2.
89 'Domestic Intelligence,' *Sydney Herald*, 6 February 1839, 2.
90 'Commission of Lunacy,' *Australian*, 5 February 1839, 2.
91 'Domestic Intelligence,' *Sydney Herald*, 6 February 1839: 2.
92 'Commission of Lunacy,' *Australian*, 5 February 1839.
93 'Supreme Court – In Equity,' *Australasian Chronicle*, 1 March 1842; Editorial, *Sydney Morning Herald*, 24 December 1847: 2; 'Law Intelligence,' *Sydney Morning Herald*, 9 December 1848, 2.
94 John Davies, *The History of the Tahitian Mission, 1799–1830*, ed. C. W. Newbury (Cambridge: Hakluyt Society, 1961).
95 Niel Gunson, 'Oakes, Francis (1770–1844),' *Australian Dictionary of Biography*, <adb.anu.edu.au/biography/oakes-francis-2513/text3397>, accessed 16 November 2015.
96 'Commission of Lunacy,' *Australian*, 3 October 1840: 2.
97 Sally Swartz, 'The Regulation of British Colonial Lunatic Asylums and the Origins of Colonial Psychiatry, 1860–1864,' *History of Psychology* 13, no. 2 (2010): 160–77.
98 Benton, 'Just Despots,' 213–26.
99 Neal, *The Rule of Law*, 19.

100 Benton and Ford, 'Magistrates in Empire,' 187, 174.
101 Lauren Benton and Lisa Ford, *Rage for Order: The British Empire and the Origins of International Law 1800–1850* (Cambridge, MA: Harvard University Press, 2016).

CHAPTER 6

1 'Elizabeth Bay House,' Heritage Office 5045185, <www.environment.nsw.gov.au/heritageapp/ViewHeritageItemDetails.aspx?ID=5045185>, accessed 22 August 2018.
2 Clare Hickman, 'Cheerful Prospects and Tranquil Restoration: The Visual Experience of Landscape as Part of the Therapeutic Regime of the British Asylum, 1800–60,' *History of Psychiatry* 20, no. 4 (2009): 425–41.
3 John Ritchie, *Punishment and Profit: The Reports of Commissioner John Bigge on the Colonies of New South Wales and Van Diemen's Land, 1822–1823* (Melbourne: Heinemann, 1970), 249–50.
4 'Parramatta Quarter Sessions,' *Sydney Gazette*, 3 March 1825: 3.
5 Proceedings of a Medical Board held on Mr. Daniel Macdonnell, 15 January 1825, T. Brisbane to Bathurst, 5 July 1825, *Historical Records of Australia (HRA)* I, vol. 11, 687–88.
6 Proceedings of a Medical Board, T. Brisbane to Bathurst, 5 July 1825, *HRA* I, vol. 11, 688.
7 C. J. Cummins, *The Administration of Lunacy in New South Wales, 1788–1855* (Sydney: NSW Department of Public Health, 1967), 24.
8 T. Brisbane to Bathurst, 5 July 1825, *HRA* I, vol. 11, 687.
9 Original emphasis: Bathurst to R. Darling, 23 February 1826, *HRA* I, vol. 12, 185–86.
10 See the evocative play with the medieval trope of the 'Narrenschiff' in Michel Foucault's *History of Madness* (Basingstoke, UK: Routledge, 2006).
11 Ritchie, *Punishment and Profit*; Raymond Evans, '19 June 1822. Creating "an Object of Real Terror": The Tabling of the First Bigge Report,' in Martin Crotty and David Andrew Roberts, eds, *Turning Points in Australian History* (Sydney: UNSW Press, 2009), 48–49.
12 Bathurst to J. T. Bigge, 5 January 1819, *HRA* I, vol. 10, 3–4.
13 Bathurst to J. T. Bigge, 6 January 1819, *HRA* I, vol. 10, 9–11.
14 Ritchie, *Punishment and Profit*, 90–92, and see William Charles Wentworth, *A Statistical, Historical, and Political Description of the Colony of New South Wales* (London, 1819), 86.
15 Ritchie, *Punishment and Profit*, 64–65.
16 Lisa Ford and David Andrew Roberts, 'New South Wales Penal Settlements and the Transformation of Secondary Punishment in the Nineteenth-Century British Empire,' *Journal of Colonialism and Colonial History* 15, no. 3 (2014): n.p.
17 Evans, '19 June 1822,' 59–60, 48; Lisa Ford and David Andrew Roberts, 'Expansion, 1820–50,' in *The Cambridge History of Australia, vol. 1: Indigenous and Colonial Australia*, eds A. Bashford and S. Macintyre (Melbourne: Cambridge University Press, 2013), 126.
18 'Terms upon which Land is granted to Settlers,' April 1827, quoted in Angela

Woollacott, *Settler Society in the Australian Colonies: Self-Government and Imperial Culture* (Oxford: Oxford University Press, 2015), 25.

19 R. Darling to E. Dumaresq, Cheltenham, 7–8 December 1837, quoted in Woollacott, *Settler Society*, 27.

20 M. J. Warren, 'Unsettled Settlers: Fear and White Victimhood in New South Wales and Van Diemen's Land, 1788–1838,' PhD thesis, University of Sydney, 2016, 24–64.

21 Evans, '19 June 1822,' 49–54.

22 Douglas Hay, 'Property, Authority and Criminal Law,' in Douglas Hay, Peter Linebaugh, John G. Rule, E. P. Thompson and Cal Winslow, eds, *Albion's Fatal Tree: Crime and Punishment in Eighteenth-Century England* (London: Verso, 2011), 49.

23 Brian H. Fletcher, *Ralph Darling: A Governor Maligned* (Melbourne: Oxford University Press, 1984); A. G. L. Shaw, *Heroes and Villains in History: Governors Darling and Bourke in New South Wales* (Sydney: Sydney University Press, 1965).

24 Brian H. Fletcher, 'Administrative Reform in New South Wales under Governor Darling,' *Australian Journal of Public Administration* 38, no. 3 (1979): 246–62.

25 Mark Francis, *Governors and Settlers: Images of Authority in the British Colonies, 1820–60* (Basingstoke, UK: Palgrave, 1992), 84–93.

26 Colonial Secretary's Papers NRS 13836 7/449, Reel 2561, vol. 4, 78; 'To Major General Ralph Darling, Late Governor of New South Wales and Its Dependencies, &c. &c. &c.,' *Sydney Monitor*, 16 March 1833, Afternoon: 4.

27 House of Commons Debate, 30 July 1835, Hansard, vol. 29, c. 1254; 'Elizabeth Bay House,' Sydney Living Museums, <sydneylivingmuseums.com.au/elizabeth-bay-house>, accessed 22 August 2018.

28 'Parramatta Quarter Sessions,' *Sydney Gazette*, 12 April 1826: 3.

29 Editorial, *Australian*, 10 June 1826: 3.

30 L. Macquarie to Bathurst, 27 July 1822, *HRA* I, vol. 10, 692.

31 'Liverpool Grand Jury Presentment,' *Australian*, 6 July 1827: 2; Letter, *Australian*, 1 March 1827: 2.

32 Toby Raeburn et al., 'Liverpool "Lunatic Asylum": A Forgotten Chapter in the History of Australian Health Care,' *Collegian* 25 (2018): 347–53; R. Bourke to T. Spring Rice, 13 January 1835, *HRA* I, vol. 17, 631.

33 'Shipping Intelligence,' *Sydney Gazette*, 27 February 1827: 2; 'Home Intelligence,' *Asiatic Journal and Monthly Register for British and Foreign India, China and Australasia* 21 (1826): 815.

34 R. Darling to R. Hay, 31 January 1827, *HRA* I, vol. 13, 60.

35 'Police Report,' *Sydney Gazette*, 6 April 1827: 3.

36 'Mr Holland,' *Australian*, 20 June 1827: 2; 'Emigration,' *Sydney Gazette*, 1 August 1827: 3; 'Domestic Intelligence,' *Monitor*, 23 August 1827, Evening: 3.

37 Shepherd, Anne and David Wright, 'Madness, Suicide and the Victorian Asylum: Attempted Self-Murder in the Age of Non-Restraint,' *Medical History* 46, no. 2 (2002), 187–89, 191–92; Olive Anderson, *Suicide in Victorian and Edwardian England* (Oxford: Clarendon Press, 1987), 376–417.

38 'Parramatta,' *Sydney Gazette*, 21 August 1803: 2.

39 'Sydney,' *Sydney Gazette*, 19 April 1807: 2.

40 'Sydney,' *Sydney Gazette*, 30 March 1816: 2.

41 'Sydney,' *Sydney Gazette*, 28 October 1804: 2.

42 'Sydney,' *Sydney Gazette*, 29 October 1809: 2.

43 Georgina Laragy, '"A Peculiar Species of Felony": Suicide, Medicine, and the Law in Victorian Britain and Ireland,' *Journal of Social History* 46, no. 3 (2013): 733 n6.

44 R. A. Houston, 'Explanations for Death by Suicide in Northern Britain During the Long Eighteenth Century,' *History of Psychiatry* 23, no. 1 (2012): 54; Anderson, *Suicide in Victorian and Edwardian England*, 225–26.

45 Barbara T. Gates, *Victorian Suicide: Mad Crimes and Sad Histories* (Princeton: Princeton University Press, 1988), 3–7.

46 See 'Temporary Insanity,' *British Medical Journal* (26 August 1893): 484–85; Gates, *Victorian Suicide*, 7.

47 Maurice Floch, 'The Concept of Temporary Insanity Viewed by a Criminologist,' *Journal of Criminal Law and Criminology* 45, no. 6 (1955): 685–89.

48 Janet Holcomb, *Early Merchant Families of Sydney: Speculation and Risk Management on the Fringes of Empire* (London: Anthem Press, 2014), 83.

49 'Melancholy Occurrence,' *Australian*, 24 February 1825.

50 Ritchie, *Punishment and Profit*, 131.

51 'Melancholy Occurrence,' *Australian*, 24 February 1825: 3.

52 'Family Notices,' *Sydney Gazette*, 24 February 1825: 3.

53 'Riley, Edward (1784–1825),' *Australian Dictionary of Biography*, <adb.anu.edu.au/biography/riley-edward-2592/text3557>, accessed 13 November 2014.

54 'The Late Mr. Shennan,' *Sydney Gazette*, 5 July 1826: 4.

55 'Suicide,' *Australian*, 16 November 1827: 3.

56 Gates, *Victorian Suicide*; Rob M. Brown, *The Art of Suicide* (London: Reaktion Books, 2001).

57 Michael Persse, 'Wentworth, William Charles (1790–1872),' *Australian Dictionary of Biography*, <http://adb.anu.edu.au/biography/wentworth-william-charles-2782>, accessed 1 November 2018.

58 R. Darling to R. Hay, 10 January 1828, *HRA* I, vol. 13, 694.

59 M. J. B. Kenny, 'Hall, Edward Smith (1786–1860),' *Australian Dictionary of Biography*, <adb.anu.edu.au/biography/hall-edward-smith-2143/text2729>, accessed 25 August 2018.

60 Erin Ihde, *Edward Smith Hall and the Sydney Monitor 1826–1840* (Melbourne: Australian Scholarly Publishing, 2004), xviii–xix, xxiv, 36–68.

61 'To Major General Ralph Darling,' *Sydney Monitor*, 16 March 1833; Ihde, *Edward Smith Hall*, 143–75.

62 R. B. Walker, *The Newspaper Press in New South Wales 1803–1920* (Sydney: Sydney University Press, 1976), 6–19; Kenny, 'Hall, Edward Smith (1786–1860),' *Australian Dictionary of Biography*; John Hirst, *Convict Society and Its Enemies: A History of Early New South Wales* (Sydney: Allen & Unwin, 1983), 179.

63 John Macarthur, jnr, quoted in John Manning Ward, *Colonial Self-Government: The British Experience, 1759–1856* (London: Macmillan, 1976), 136; David Neal, *The Rule of Law in a Penal Colony: Law and Power in Early New South Wales* (Cambridge: Cambridge University Press, 1992), 177.

64 R. Darling to Goderich, 14 December 1827, *HRA* I, vol. 13, 638.

65 R. Darling to W. H. Huskisson, 26 February 1828, *HRA* I, vol. 13, 814.

66 Bruce Kercher, *An Unruly Child: A History of Law in Australia* (Sydney: Allen & Unwin, 1995), 85.
67 R. Darling to Bathurst, 15 December 1826, *HRA* I, vol. 12, 750–51.
68 Walker, *The Newspaper Press*, 9; Editorial, *Australian*, 27 September 1826: 2.
69 Francis, *Governors and Settlers*, 88.
70 Editorial, *Australian*, 27 September 1826: 2; 'New South Wales,' *Sydney Gazette*, 18 July 1827: 3; Hirst, *Convict Society*, 177.
71 Fletcher, *Ralph Darling*, 247–52.
72 R. Darling to Bathurst, 15 December 1826, *HRA* I, vol. 12, 750.
73 Kercher, *An Unruly Child*, 35–36; Fletcher, *Ralph Darling*, 315–33.
74 Editorial, *Monitor*, 13 January 1827: 4.
75 Bathurst to T. Brisbane, 5 January 1824, *HRA* I, vol. 11, 192; R. G. Thorne, 'Mills, George Galway (1765–1828), of Twickenham, Mdx. and Thoby Priory, Essex,' in R. G. Thorne, ed., *The History of Parliament: The House of Commons 1790–1820* (1986), <www.historyofparliamentonline.org/volume/1790-1820/member/mills-george-galway-1765-1828>, accessed 20 November 2014.
76 F. Forbes to W. H. Huskisson, 16 February 1828, *HRA* I, vol. 12, 820.
77 R. Darling, 1826, quoted in John Gascoigne, *The Enlightenment and the Origins of European Australia* (Cambridge: Cambridge University Press, 2002), 104.
78 R. Darling to R. Hay, 9 February 1827, *HRA* I, vol. 13, 98; R. Darling to R. Hay, 26 March 1827, *HRA* I, vol. 13, 191. See also Fletcher, *Ralph Darling*, 252.
79 R. Darling to J. Mackaness, 29 November 1827, printed in the *Monitor*, 28 May 1828, Evening: 4.
80 R. Darling to Goderich, 14 December 1827, *HRA* I, vol. 13, 638.
81 Darling wrote two letters to Viscount Goderich on the same day, both on the theme of his purge: R. Darling to Goderich, 14 December 1827, *HRA* I, vol. 13, 644.
82 Douglass was later one of the first teachers of clinical medicine, first parliamentarians, first supporters of the university, and one of the most prominent philanthropists in the colony: K. B. Noad, 'Douglass, Henry Grattan (1790–1865),' *Australian Dictionary of Biography*, <http://adb.anu.edu.au/biography/douglass-henry-grattan-1987>, accessed 1 November 2018.
83 L. Macquarie to Bathurst, 'Secret & confidential: List of names of discontented and seditious persons in N. S. Wales,' 1 December 1817, New South Wales Governors' Despatches, vol. 2, SLNSW ML A 1191.
84 R. Darling to Goderich, 14 December 1827, *HRA* I, vol. 13, 644.
85 'Coroner's Inquest,' *Australian*, 15 February 1828: 3; 'Coroner's Inquest on the Body of G. G. Mills, Esq.,' *Sydney Gazette*, 15 February 1828: 2.
86 F. Forbes, quoted in notes, Ex parte Raine (No. 1) (1828) NSW Sel Cas (Dowling) 732; [1828] NSWSupC 71., <www.law.mq.edu.au/research/colonial_case_law/nsw/cases/case_index/1828/ex_parte_raine_no_1_1828_nsw_sel_cas_dowling_732_1828_nswsupc_71/>, accessed 29 October 2014; Kercher, *An Unruly Child*, 83.
87 Editorial, *Australian*, 20 February 1828: 2.
88 'Domestic Intelligence,' *Monitor*, 21 February 1828, Evening: 4.
89 'Mr. Mackaness, the Ex-Sheriff, and the Editor of the *Sydney Gazette*,' *Sydney Gazette*, 25 February 1828: 2.

90 Paula J. Byrne, *Criminal Law and Colonial Subject: New South Wales 1810–1830, Studies in Australian History* (Melbourne: Cambridge University Press, 1993), 59; 'The Honorable Charles Throsby, Esq.,' *Sydney Gazette*, 4 April 1828: 2.
91 P. Helman, 'Droughts in the Murray Darling Basin Since European Settlement,' *Griffith Centre for Coastal Management Research Report* 100 (2009), 8.
92 'Agricultural and Horticultural Society of New South Wales,' *Sydney Gazette*, 7 April 1828: 2.
93 Editorial, *Australian*, 26 October 1827: 2; Elizabeth Macarthur to John Macarthur, jnr, March 1827, Macarthur Family Papers, SLNSW A2906, Reel CY940, n.p.
94 Vivienne Parsons, 'Throsby, Charles (1777–1828),' *Australian Dictionary of Biography*, <adb.anu.edu.au/biography/throsby-charles-2735/text3861>, accessed 29 October 2018.
95 R. Darling to W. H. Huskisson, 5 April 1828, *HRA* I, vol. 14, 119.
96 Editorial, *Sydney Monitor*, 15 August 1829, Afternoon: 3.
97 Parsons, 'Throsby, Charles (1777–1828),' *Australian Dictionary of Biography*.
98 'Coroner's Inquest,' *Sydney Gazette* 4 April 1828: 3.
99 'The Honorable Charles Throsby, Esq.,' *Sydney Gazette*, 4 April 1828.
100 'John Cullen,' *Sydney Monitor*, 24 July 1830, Afternoon: 3.
101 R. Bourke to Goderich, 24 September 1832, *HRA* I, vol. 16, 760–61.
102 Peter Doyle, 'The Brownes & O'Briens & Those Near Them,' *Illawarra Historical Society* (October 1990): 83.
103 R. Darling to W. H. Huskisson, 5 April 1828, *HRA* I, vol. 14, 119.
104 George Man Burrows, *Commentaries on the Causes, Forms, Symptoms, and Treatment, Moral and Medical, of Insanity. 1828* (New York: Arno Press, 1976), 235–38.
105 'Dreadful Suicide,' *Sydney Gazette*, 24 January 1829: 3.
106 'Captain Sturt's Expedition,' *Sydney Gazette*, 31 March 1829: 2.
107 'Shipping News,' *Australian*, 15 May 1829: 3.
108 Gates, *Victorian Suicide*, 38–42.
109 All articles in *Australian*, 12 May 1829: 3.
110 'Lamentable Catastrophe,' *Australian*, 12 August 1829: 2.
111 Original emphasis: 'Coroner's Inquest,' *Sydney Gazette*, 11 August 1829: 2.
112 Editorial, *Sydney Monitor*, 15 August 1829, Afternoon: 3.
113 'Coroner's Inquests,' *Sydney Gazette*, 14 April 1831: 2.
114 'Distressing Suicide,' *Sydney Gazette*, 18 August 1831: 3.
115 Burrows, *Commentaries*, 448.
116 'Attempts at Suicide,' *Sydney Gazette*, 25 August 1831: 3.
117 Editorial, *Australian*, 21 October 1831: 2.
118 'Neglect of the Early Symptoms of Insanity,' *Lancet* 203, no. 5250 (1924): 776.
119 Robert R. Desjarlais et al., *World Mental Health: Problems, and Priorities in Low-Income Countries* (New York: Oxford University Press, 1995), 74.
120 Emile Durkheim, *Suicide: A Study in Sociology*, trans. George Simpson and John A. Spaulding (London: Routledge, 2002), xliv; Benjamin Fincham, Susanne Langer, Jonathon Scourfield and Michael Shiner, *Understanding Suicide: A Sociological Autopsy* (Basingstoke, UK: Palgrave Macmillan, 2011), 8–9.

121 'Second Report of The Departmental Committee Appointed to Inquire into the Law Relating to Coroners and Coroners' Inquests, and into the Practice in Coroners' Courts,' *Lancet* 175, no. 4518 (1910): 944.

122 'Coroners' Law and Practice: The Departmental Committee's Report,' *British Medical Journal* 1, no. 3919 (1936): 322–24.

123 Houston, 'Explanations for Death by Suicide in Northern Britain,' 53, 55–56.

124 Russell D. Covey, 'Temporary Insanity: The Strange Life and Times of the Perfect Defense,' *Boston University Law Review* 91, no. 5 (2011): 1631.

125 Covey, 'Temporary Insanity,' 1602 and ff.

CHAPTER 7

1 A. G. L. Shaw, 'Bligh, William (1754–1817),' *Australian Dictionary of Biography*, <adb.anu.edu.au/biography/bligh-william-1797/text2037>, accessed 30 October 2018.

2 J. Banks to W. Bligh, 15 March 1805, quoted in George Mackaness, *The Life of Vice-Admiral William Bligh*, vol. 2 (Sydney: Angus & Robertson, 1931), 96–97.

3 Greg Dening, *Mr Bligh's Bad Language: Passion, Power and Theatre on the Bounty* (Cambridge: Cambridge University Press, 1994).

4 G. Caley to G. Johnston, 7 July 1808, *Historical Records of NSW (HRNSW)*, vol. 6, 687.

5 H. V. Evatt, *Rum Rebellion: A Study of the Overthrow of Governor Bligh by John Macarthur and the New South Wales Corps* (Sydney: Angus & Robertson, 1978); George Mackaness, *The Life of Vice-Admiral William Bligh, R.N., F.R.S.* (Sydney: Angus & Robertson, 1931).

6 M. H. Ellis, *John Macarthur* (Sydney: Discovery Press, 1972); Manning C. Clark, *A History of Australia*, vol. 1 (Melbourne: Melbourne University Press, 1968).

7 A. G. L. Shaw, *Heroes and Villains in History: Governors Darling and Bourke in New South Wales* (Sydney: Sydney University Press, 1965), 7; 'Violent Protest in Australian History,' *Historical Studies* 14, no. 60 (1968): 545–61; 'Some Aspects of the History of NSW 1788–1810,' *Journal of the Royal Australian Historical Society* 57, no. 2 (1971): 93–112.

8 Grace Karskens and Richard Waterhouse, ' "Too Sacred to Be Taken Away": Property, Liberty, Tyranny and the "Rum Rebellion",' *Journal of Australian Colonial History* 12 (2010): 1–3.

9 Alan Atkinson, 'The Little Revolution in New South Wales, 1808,' *The International History Review* 12, no. 1 (1990): 67–78.

10 Ross Fitzgerald and Mark Hearn, *Bligh, Macarthur and the Rum Rebellion* (Sydney: Kangaroo Press, 1988), 69.

11 J. Foveaux to Castlereagh, 6 September 1808, *Historical Records of Australia (HRA)* I, vol. 6, 642.

12 Karskens and Waterhouse, 'Too Sacred to Be Taken Away,' 4; Fitzgerald and Hearn, *Bligh, Macarthur and the Rum Rebellion*, 21, 101; Matthew Allen, 'Alcohol and Authority in Early New South Wales: The Symbolic Significance of the Spirit Trade, 1788–1808,' *History Australia* 9, no. 3 (2012): 7–26; Alan Atkinson, *The Europeans in Australia: A History, vol. 1* (Melbourne: Oxford University Press, 1997), 277.

13 Fitzgerald and Hearn, *Bligh, Macarthur and the Rum Rebellion*, 71; R. Townson to Castlereagh, 5 September 1808, *HRNSW*, vol. 6, 738–39.
14 Karskens and Waterhouse, 'Too Sacred to Be Taken Away,' 8–10.
15 D. R. Hainsworth, 'Kable, Henry (1763–1846),' *Australian Dictionary of Biography*, <adb.anu.edu.au/biography/kable-henry-2285/text2941>, accessed 18 March 2019; John Ritchie, *The Wentworths: Father and Son* (Melbourne: The Miegunyah Press, 1997), 105–8; Fitzgerald and Hearn, *Bligh, Macarthur and the Rum Rebellion*, 74–78; Evatt, *Rum Rebellion*, 89–92.
16 J. Blaxland, 16 October 1807, *HRNSW*, vol. 6, 312.
17 Ellis, *John Macarthur*, 273; Fitzgerald and Hearn, *Bligh, Macarthur and the Rum Rebellion*, 79–80.
18 C. J. Cummins, *A History of Medical Administration in NSW 1788–1973*, 2nd edn (Sydney: NSW Department of Health, 2003), 17.
19 Vivienne Parsons, 'Jamison, Thomas (1753–1811),' *Australian Dictionary of Biography*, <adb.anu.edu.au/biography/jamison-thomas-2269/text2909>, accessed 31 August 2018.
20 J. J. Auchmuty, 'Wentworth, D'Arcy (1762–1827),' *Australian Dictionary of Biography*, <adb.anu.edu.au/biography/wentworth-darcy-1545/text3917>, accessed 31 August 2018.
21 V. W. E. Goodin, 'Townson, Robert (1762–1827),' *Australian Dictionary of Biography*, <adb.anu.edu.au/biography/townson-robert-2743/text3879>, accessed 13 May 2015.
22 Grant spelled his name 'Draffen': Yvonne Cramer, *This Beauteous, Wicked Place: Letters and Journals of John Grant, Gentleman Convict* (Canberra: National Library of Australia, 2000), 23, 30, 45.
23 W. Bligh to Castlereagh, 10 June 1809, *HRNSW*, vol. 7, 174.
24 W. Bligh to Castlereagh, 30 June 1808, *HRA* I, vol. 6, 535–36; R. v. Gore [1808] NSWKR 2; [1808] NSWSupC 2, <www.law.mq.edu.au/research/colonial_case_law/nsw/cases/case_index/1808/r_v_gore>, accessed 3 June 2015; R. v. Blaxland, Blaxland and Lord [1808] NSWKR 5; [1808] NSWSupC 5, <www.law.mq.edu.au/research/colonial_case_law/nsw/cases/case_index/1808/r_v_blaxland/>, accessed 3 June 2015.
25 See P. King, 15 March 1805; P. King to G. Johnston, 15 March 1805, *HRNSW*, vol. 5, 570–71.
26 C. Throsby to P. King, 22 March 1805, *HRNSW*, vol. 5, 574–75.
27 Present State of His Majesty's New South Wales Corps, 22 April 1805, *HRNSW*, vol. 5, 592; John Ritchie, ed., *A Charge of Mutiny: The Court Martial of Colonel George Johnston for Deposing Governor William Bligh in the Rebellion of 26 January 1808* (Canberra: National Library of Australia, 1988), 268; and see Michael Duffy, *Man of Honour: John Macarthur – Duellist, Rebel, Founding Father* (Sydney: Macmillan, 2003), 294–95; Fitzgerald and Hearn, *Bligh, Macarthur and the Rum Rebellion*, 102.
28 J. Macarthur to J. Piper, 24 May 1808, *HRNSW*, vol. 6, 644.
29 Settlers' address to W. Paterson, 1 May 1808, *HRNSW*, vol. 6, 635.
30 Richard Neville, *Mr J. W. Lewin: Painter and Naturalist* (Sydney: UNSW Press, 2012), 134.
31 Settlers' address to W. Bligh, 22 September 1806, *HRNSW*, vol. 6, 189.

32 Settlers to G. Johnston, 18 April 1808, *HRNSW* vol. 6, 597.
33 Settlers to W. Paterson, 18 April 1808, *HRNSW* vol. 6, 597.
34 W. Bligh to Castlereagh, 10 June 1809, *HRA* I, vol. 7, p. 116.
35 R. v. Sutter [1808] NSWKR 4; [1808] NSWSupC 4, <www.law.mq.edu.au/research/colonial_case_law/nsw/cases/case_index/1808/r_v_sutter/>, accessed 27 May 2015.
36 *Memoirs of George Suttor, F.L.S.: Banksian Collector (1774–1859)*, ed. G. Mackaness (Sydney: self-published, 1948), 49–50.
37 See James Dunk, 'The Politics of Madness in a Penal Colony: New South Wales, 1788–1856,' PhD diss., University of Sydney, 2016, 269 n42, 272–73.
38 John West, *The History of Tasmania, vol. 1* (Hobart, 1852), 64; W. A. Townsley, 'Abbott, Edward (1766–1832),' *Australian Dictionary of Biography*, <adb.anu.edu.au/biography/abbott-edward-3/text1821>, accessed 6 November 2014.
39 'Demise of Major Abbott,' *Launceston Advertiser*, 7 August 1832: 254.
40 Parish Burial Registers, Textual Records, St John's Anglican Church Parramatta, 79. I owe this discovery to Michaela Cameron.
41 Editorial, *Sydney Gazette*, 22 May 1823: 2.
42 J. Palmer to W. Bligh, 31 August 1808, *HRA* I, vol. 6, 605; Fitzgerald and Hearn, *Bligh, Macarthur and the Rum Rebellion*, 115.
43 David Roger Hainsworth, *The Sydney Traders: Simeon Lord and His Contemporaries, 1788–1821*, 2nd edn (Melbourne: Melbourne University Press, 1981), 209; John Ritchie, *Punishment and Profit: The Reports of Commissioner John Bigge on the Colonies of New South Wales and Van Diemen's Land, 1822–1823; Their Origins, Nature and Significance* (Melbourne: Heinemann, 1970), 181.
44 E. W. Dunlop, 'Blaxcell, Garnham (1778–1817),' *Australian Dictionary of Biography*, <adb.anu.edu.au/biography/blaxcell-garnham-1794/text2029>, accessed 14 November 2014; E. Flinn, 'Jeffreys, Charles (1782–1826),' *Australian Dictionary of Biography*, <adb.anu.edu.au/biography/jeffreys-charles-2273/text2917>, accessed 27 March 2015.
45 G. Blaxland to E. Cooke, 24 October 1804, *HRNSW*, vol. 5, 479–80; W. Bligh to W. Windham, 31 October 1807, *HRA* I, vol. 6, 149.
46 Ron Buttrey, *A Short History of the Life of Gregory Blaxland* (Sydney: Brush Farm Historical Society, 2006), 37–50.
47 'Parramatta,' *Sydney Morning Herald*, 4 January 1853: 2; Jill Conway, 'Blaxland, Gregory (1778–1853),' *Australian Dictionary of Biography*, <adb.anu.edu.au/biography/blaxland-gregory-1795/text2031>, accessed 21 November 2014.
48 Evatt, *Rum Rebellion*, 47–51.
49 Fitzgerald and Hearn, *Bligh, Macarthur and the Rum Rebellion*, 104–105.
50 Fitzgerald and Hearn, *Bligh, Macarthur and the Rum Rebellion*, 17; G. Caley, 'An Open Letter to Johnston,' 7 July 1808, *HRNSW*, vol. 6, 688.
51 R. Townson to Castlereagh, 2 April 1808, *HRNSW*, vol. 6, 571; Goodin, 'Townson, Robert (1762–1827).'
52 E. Abbott to P. King, 13 February 1808, *HRNSW*, vol. 6, 834.
53 A. T. Yarwood, 'Johnston, George (1764–1823),' *Australian Dictionary of Biography*, <adb.anu.edu.au/biography/johnston-george-2277/text2925>, accessed 1 December 2015.

54 Evatt, *Rum Rebellion*, 336–38.
55 Stephen Dando-Collins, *Captain Bligh's Other Mutiny: The True Story of the Military Coup That Turned Australia into a Two-Year Rebel Republic* (Sydney: Random House, 2007), 228.
56 Fitzgerald and Hearn, *Bligh, Macarthur and the Rum Rebellion*, 119.
57 G. Johnston to J. MacMahon, June 1812, George Johnston Letterbook, Being Copies of Correspondence Between Johnston and the Duke of Northumberland, 1811–1812, Related Correspondence: SLNSW C474, <acms.sl.nsw.gov.au/_transcript/2011/D11961/a2252.htm>, accessed 14 November 2014, 106–107.
58 J. Adolphus to G. Johnston, 14 June 1811, Johnston Letters, SLNSW DLMSSQ22, quoted in Yarwood, 'Johnston, George (1764–1823)'.
59 Fitzgerald and Hearn, *Bligh, Macarthur and the Rum Rebellion*, 124; Ellis, *John Macarthur*, 418.
60 G. Johnston to the Duke of Northumberland, 3 January 1812, George Johnston Letterbook, 18–19; Anne-Maree Whitaker, *Joseph Foveaux: Power and Patronage in Early New South Wales* (Sydney: UNSW Press, 2000), 145–47.
61 Yarwood, 'Johnston, George (1764–1823)'; Alan Roberts, *Marine Officer, Convict Wife: The Johnstons of Annandale* (Sydney: Annandale Urban Research Association and Barbara Beckett Publishing, 2008), 130. In their *Bligh, Macarthur and the Rum Rebellion* (124), Fitzgerald and Hearn draw on a reference in Ellis's *John Macarthur* (402), which in turn draws upon an opaque reference in Lachlan Macquarie's journal from 1821.
62 *Memoirs of George Suttor*, 50. As Andrew Sharp's comprehensive biography of Marsden makes no reference to Johnston's confession there are likely no corroborating sources.
63 See Roberts, *Marine Officer, Convict Wife*, 135–42.
64 In re Johnstone [1829] NSWSupC 15, <www.law.mq.edu.au/research/colonial_case_law/nsw/cases/case_index/1829/in_re_johnstone/>, accessed 13 May 2014.
65 Moss v Johnstone (1830) NSW Sel Cas (Dowling) 373; [1830] NSWSupC 24, <www.law.mq.edu.au/research/colonial_case_law/nsw/cases/case_index/1830/moss_v_johnstone/>, accessed 14 May 2014.
66 J. Macarthur to E. Macarthur, April 1808, *HRNSW*, vol. 6, 594.
67 Memorandum, 8 February 1808, *HRNSW*, vol. 6, 512–13.
68 J. Macarthur to E. Macarthur, April 1808, *HRNSW*, vol. 6, 594.
69 Alan Atkinson, 'John Macarthur Before Australia Knew Him,' *Journal of Australian Studies* 3, no. 4 (1979): 27, 29; Margaret Steven, 'Macarthur, John (1767–1834),' *Australian Dictionary of Biography*, <adb.anu.edu.au/biography/macarthur-john-2390/text3153>, accessed 14 September 2018.
70 Atkinson, 'John Macarthur Before Australia Knew Him,' 33–34.
71 E. Macarthur, Journal, April 1790, in Sibella Macarthur Onslow, ed., *Some Early Records of the Macarthurs of Camden* (Sydney: Angus & Robertson, 1914), 14.
72 Onslow, *Some Early Records*, 4.
73 Atkinson, 'John Macarthur Before Australia Knew Him,' 29–30.
74 Fitzgerald and Hearn, *Bligh, Macarthur and the Rum Rebellion*, 76–78, 99; Evatt, *Rum Rebellion*.

75 P. King to J. King, 8 November 1801, *HRA* I, vol. 3, 322, 325; J. Hunter to the Duke of Portland, 14 September 1796, *HRNSW*, vol. 3, 130.
76 Lauren Benton, 'Just Despots: The Cultural Construction of Imperial Constitutionalism,' *Law, Culture and the Humanities* 9, no. 2 (2013): 223.
77 Jeremy Bentham, *A Plea for the Constitution* (London, 1803).
78 Alan Atkinson, 'Jeremy Bentham and the Rum Rebellion,' *Journal of the Royal Australian Historical Society* 64, no. 1 (1978): 6–7; David Godfrey Matthew Llewellyn, 'Australia Felix: Jeremy Bentham and Australian Colonial Democracy,' PhD diss., University of Melbourne, 2016.
79 Lauren Benton and Lisa Ford, *Rage for Order: The British Empire and the Origins of International Law 1800–1850* (Cambridge, MA: Harvard University Press, 2016), 41.
80 Atkinson, 'Jeremy Bentham and the Rum Rebellion,' 3–5.
81 J. Macarthur to E. Macarthur, 30 July 1809, in Onslow, *Some Early Records*, 181.
82 Atkinson, 'Jeremy Bentham and the Rum Rebellion,' 8–9.
83 Atkinson, 'Jeremy Bentham and the Rum Rebellion,' 9; Fitzgerald and Hearn, *Bligh, Macarthur and the Rum Rebellion*, 107–108.
84 Ritchie, *A Charge of Mutiny*, 90.
85 Atkinson, 'John Macarthur Before Australia Knew Him,' 34.
86 J. Macarthur to E. Macarthur, 4 March 1812, Macarthur Papers, vol. 3, SLNSW A2898, Reel CY832, 117–18, 120.
87 Ellis, *John Macarthur*, 402.
88 J. Macarthur to E. Macarthur, 16 October 1812, in Onslow, *Some Early Records*, 225; see James Broadbent, *Elizabeth Farm Parramatta: A History and a Guide* (Sydney: Historic Houses Trust, 1984), 12; Ellis, *John Macarthur*, xv.
89 Fitzgerald and Hearn, *Bligh, Macarthur and the Rum Rebellion*, 121–22.
90 J. Macarthur to Edward Macarthur, 8 December 1814, in Onslow, *Some Early Records*, 245.
91 Ellis, *Lachlan Macquarie*, 177.
92 J. Macarthur to E. Macarthur, 21 April 1811, in Onslow, *Some Early Records*, 215.
93 J. Macarthur to W. Davidson, 3 September 1818, in Onslow, *Some Early Records*, 315–20.
94 Zoë Laidlaw, *Colonial Connections, 1815–45: Patronage, the Information Revolution and Colonial Government* (Manchester: Manchester University Press, 2005), 131–38.
95 Ellis, *John Macarthur*, 277, 450, 477.
96 See C. A. Liston, 'New South Wales Under Governor Brisbane, 1821–1825,' PhD diss., University of Sydney, 1980, 355–403.
97 Ellis, *John Macarthur*, 489, 496.
98 Hazel King, *Richard Bourke* (Melbourne: Oxford University Press, 1971), 143.
99 F. Macleay to W. Macleay, 28 May 1826, in *Fanny to William: The Letters of Frances Leonora Macleay 1812–1836*, eds B. Earnshaw and J. Hughes (Sydney: Historic Houses Trust of New South Wales and Macleay Museum, University of Sydney, 1993), 56.
100 John Manning Ward, *Colonial Self-Government: The British Experience, 1759–1856* (London: Macmillan, 1976), 136–41.
101 R. Darling to R. Hay, 1 May 1826, *HRA* I, vol. 12, 254–55.

102 R. Darling to R. Hay, 2 September 1826, *HRA* I, vol. 12, 523.
103 Ellis, *John Macarthur*, 496.
104 F. Macleay to W. Macleay, 10 May 1826, in *Fanny to William*, 54–55.
105 R. Scott to his mother, 14 May 1822, Scott Papers, SLNSW A2263, quoted in Rebecca Catherine Ruth Geraghty, 'A Change in Circumstance: Individual Responses to Colonial Life,' BA (Hons) thesis, University of Sydney, 2006, 24.
106 Original emphases. R. Darling to R. Hay, 2 September 1826, *HRA* I, vol. 12, 523.
107 F. Macleay to W. Macleay, 28 May 1826, in *Fanny to William*, 56.
108 E. Macarthur to Edward Macarthur, 27 December 1830, Macarthur Papers, vol. 10, SLNSW A2906, Reel CY940, n.p., and see Lennard Bickel, *Australia's First Lady: The Story of Elizabeth Macarthur* (Sydney: Allen & Unwin, 1991), 158–59, 163–66.
109 Hazel King, *Elizabeth Macarthur and Her World* (Sydney: Sydney University Press, 1980), 149.
110 W. Taylor to J. Macarthur, April 1831, quoted in Bickel, *Australia's First Lady*, 170. See also King, *Elizabeth Macarthur*, 147–48 and n5.
111 J. Macarthur to Edward Macarthur, 26 March 1832, Macarthur Papers, vol. 3, SLNSW A2899, Reel CY832, 209a.
112 E. Macarthur to Edward Macarthur, 23 March 1832, Macarthur Papers, vol. 10, SLNSW A2906, Reel CY940, n.p.
113 E. Macarthur to Edward Macarthur, May 1832. Macarthur Papers, vol. 10, SLNSW A2906, Reel CY940, 2–3.
114 E. Macarthur to Edward Macarthur, 30 June 1832, Macarthur Papers, vol. 10, SLNSW A2906, Reel CY940, n.p.
115 Ellis, *John Macarthur*, 504–507.
116 I owe this insight to Ross Fitzgerald and Mark Hearn, in *Bligh, Macarthur and the Rum Rebellion*, 124.
117 J. Macarthur to Edward Macarthur, 26 March 1832, Macarthur Papers, vol. 3, SLNSW A2899, Reel CY832, 209.
118 Damaris Bairstow, *A Million Pounds, a Million Acres: The Pioneer Settlement of the Australian Agricultural Company* (Sydney: self-published, 2003).
119 Ellis, *John Macarthur*, 511–15; Broadbent, *Elizabeth Farm Parramatta*, 13, 15.
120 Jesse Gregson, quoted in Ellis, *John Macarthur*, 513.
121 E. Macarthur to Edward Macarthur, 26 May 1832, Macarthur Papers, vol. 10, SLNSW A2906, Reel CY940, n.p.
122 Ellis, *John Macarthur*, 527.
123 E. Macarthur to Edward Macarthur, 30 June 1832, Macarthur Papers, vol. 10, SLNSW A2906, Reel CY940, n.p.
124 E. Macarthur to Edward Macarthur, 30 June 1832, Macarthur Papers, vol. 10, SLNSW A2906, Reel CY940, n.p.; Michelle Scott Tucker, *Elizabeth Macarthur: A Life at the Edge of the World* (Melbourne: Text, 2018), 282.
125 *Australian*, 10 August 1832: 3.
126 Documents Relating to the Committal of John Macarthur for Lunacy, SRNSW NRS13524, 17–19.
127 Ellis, *John Macarthur*, 524–25.

128 Documents Relating to the Committal of John Macarthur for Lunacy, SRNSW NRS13524, 5–6.
129 *The Australian*, 10 August 1832: 3; 'New South Wales Intelligence,' *Tasmanian*, 7 September 1832: 7.
130 R. Bourke to Goderich, 24 September 1832, *HRA* I, vol. 16, 760.
131 For example: J. Macarthur to E. Macarthur, 6 April 1811, in Onslow, *Some Early Records*, 212; J. Macarthur to E. Macarthur, 26 July 1814, in Onslow, *Some Early Records*, 240.
132 Scott Hill, 'Remembering John Macarthur,' Sydney Living Museums, <sydneylivingmuseums.com.au/stories/remembering-john-macarthur>, accessed 30 October 2018.
133 Original emphases. E. Macarthur to Edward Macarthur, May 1832, Macarthur Papers, vol. 10, SLNSW A2906, Reel CY940, 2–3.
134 E. Macarthur to Edward Macarthur, 3 July 1832, Macarthur Papers, vol. 10, SLNSW A2906, Reel CY940, n.p.

CHAPTER 8

1 The term 'Australian party' is used in a short biography of George Robert Nichols, and although it is otherwise uncommon, I use it as a helpful shorthand for those who gathered around Wentworth and *The Australian*, united by their politics and ambition: G. P. Walsh, 'Nichols, George Robert (Bob) (1809–1857),' *Australian Dictionary of Biography*, <adb.anu.edu.au/biography/nichols-george-robert-bob-4296/text6957>, accessed 17 October 2015.
2 J. H. McClemens and J. M. Bennett, 'Historical Notes on the Law of Mental Illness in New South Wales,' *Sydney Law Review* 4, no. 1 (1964): 49–74.
3 R. W. Hay to H. Prinsep, 30 July 1828, UKNA CO 324/86, quoted in Hazel King, *Richard Bourke* (Melbourne: Melbourne University Press, 1971), 13.
4 King, *Richard Bourke*, 134, 196–98; L. L. Robson, *The Convict Settlers of Australia: An Enquiry into the Origin and Character of the Convicts Transported to New South Wales and Van Diemen's Land 1787–1852* (Melbourne: Melbourne University Press and Cambridge University Press, 1965), 168.
5 R. Bourke to T. Spring Rice, 11 October 1836, Bourke Papers, vol. 9, SLNSW, quoted in King, *Richard Bourke*, 178.
6 Lisa Ford and David Andrew Roberts, 'Expansion, 1820–50,' in *The Cambridge History of Australia*, vol. 1, eds A. Bashford and S. Macintyre (Melbourne: Cambridge University Press, 2013).
7 R. Bourke to T. Spring Rice, 13 January 1835, *Historical Records of Australia (HRA)* I, vol. 17, 631; R. Bourke to Glenelg, 24 April 1837, *HRA* I, vol. 18, 737.
8 Sic. 'Notice to Correspondents,' *Sydney Gazette*, 29 November 1836: 2.
9 Editorial, *Sydney Gazette*, 21 October 1837: 2; Editorial, *Sydney Gazette*, 24 September 1836: 2.
10 Editorial, *Australian*, 3 November 1837: 2.
11 'To Builders, Masons, Carpenters, and Others,' *Sydney Gazette*, 10 October 1835: 4; 'Minutes of Evidence Taken Before the Committee on Immigration,' *Sydney Herald*, 26 October 1835: 2; 'Domestic Intelligence,' *Sydney Herald*, 30 March 1837: 3.

12 'New Lunatic Asylum,' *Sydney Herald*, 5 November 1835: 2.

13 N. G. Butlin, *Forming a Colonial Economy, Australia 1810–1850* (Cambridge: Cambridge University Press, 1994), 223; Frank Decker, 'Monetary Recovery Measures in the New South Wales 1840s Depression – a New Assessment,' Paper Delivered at Bremen University, December 2009, 1.

14 D. I. McDonald, 'Gladesville Hospital: The Formative Years, 1838–1850,' *Journal of the Royal Australian Historical Society* 51, no. 3 (1965): 275.

15 R. Bourke to Glenelg, 24 April 1837, *HRA* I, vol. 18, 736.

16 'Legislative Council,' *Sydney Morning Herald*, 13 May 1847: 3.

17 Glenelg to G. Gipps, 31 October 1837, *HRA* I, vol. 19, 142; John Bostock, *The Dawn of Australian Psychiatry* (Sydney: Australian Medical Association, 1968), 41.

18 Bostock, *The Dawn of Australian Psychiatry*, 42.

19 Letters between J. Digby and E. D. Thompson, with annotations by G. Gipps, November 1838, Colonial Secretary's Correspondence, SRNSW 4/2401 Reel 743; Bostock, *The Dawn of Australian Psychiatry*, 43.

20 J. Digby to Colonial Secretary, with Gipps's annotation, 14 April 1842, Colonial Secretary's Papers, quoted in McDonald, 'Gladesville Hospital,' 276.

21 J. Digby, Minutes of Evidence, Report from the Select Committee on the Lunatic Asylum Tarban Creek, printed 21 October 1846, New South Wales Legislative Council Votes and Proceedings (hereafter Minutes), 13.

22 Board Proceedings, 23 April 1839, *HRA* I, vol. 20, 389–90.

23 G. Gipps to Normanby, 8 November 1839, *HRA* I, vol. 20, 387–90.

24 'Mr. Blaxland's Protests,' *Sydney Monitor*, 10 October 1838, Morning: 1; T. H. Irving, 'Blaxland, John (1769–1845),' *Australian Dictionary of Biography*, <adb.anu.edu.au/biography/blaxland-john-1796/text2033>, accessed 7 October 2018; Medical and Surgical Journal of the Convict Transport Ship Blackfriar, 1851, UKNA ADM101/12, 26-27.

25 William Charles Wentworth, *A Statistical, Historical, and Political Description of the Colony of New South Wales* (London, 1819), 172–73.

26 On William Bland's duelling, see Penny Russell, *Savage or Civilised? Manners in Colonial Australia* (Sydney: UNSW Press, 2010), 165–89.

27 D. E. Fifer, 'The Australian Patriotic Association 1835–1841,' *Journal of the Royal Australian Historical Society* 73, no. 3 (1987): 155.

28 'Legislative Council,' *Sydney Morning Herald*, 2 July 1849: 2; William Charles Wentworth,' *Sydney Morning Herald*, 6 May 1872: 5; John Dunmore Lang, *An Historical and Statistical Account of New South Wales*, vol. 2 (London, 1875), 321.

29 See John Ritchie, 'Towards Ending an Unclean Thing: The Molesworth Committee and the Abolition of Transportation to N.S.W., 1837–40,' *Historical Studies* (Melbourne) 17, no. 67 (1976): 144–64; Isobelle Barrett Meyering, 'Abolitionism, Settler Violence and the Case against Flogging: A Reassessment of Sir William Molesworth's Contribution to the Transportation Debate,' *History Australia* 7, no. 1 (2010): 6.1–6.18.

30 William Bland, *Letters to Charles Buller, Junior, Esq., M.P., From the Australian Patriotic Association* (Sydney, 1849).

31 *Empire*, 21 January 1862: 8.

32 Fifer, 'The Australian Patriotic Association,' 168.

33 5 & 6 Vic. C. 76 [1842].
34 M. M. H. Thompson, *The Seeds of Democracy: Early Elections in Colonial New South Wales* (Sydney: Federation Press, 2006), 4.
35 'Sydney Quarter Sessions,' *Sydney Gazette*, 29 February 1840: 2.
36 Hyndman in fact never made captain, and retired as lieutenant on 31 August 1832: Henry Stooks Smith, *An Alphabetical List of the Officers of the Eleventh, or Prince Albert's Own, Regiment of Hussars, from 1800 to 1850* (London, 1850), 14–15; Graham A. Edwards, 'The Mental Illness of Captain Hyndman,' *Australian and New Zealand Journal of Psychiatry* 13, no. 2 (1979): 147.
37 'Title Deeds,' *Sydney Gazette*, 3 June 1837: 4; 'Law Intelligence,' *Sydney Morning Herald*, 18 November 1843: 2; Advertising, *Sydney Monitor*, 9 February 1838, Evening: 2; 'Country News,' *Australian*, 13 February 1841: 2.
38 'Port Macquarie,' *New South Wales Examiner*, 4 June 1842: 3.
39 Editorial, *Australian*, 9 April 1840: 2.
40 'Port Macquarie,' *Australian*, 10 February 1843: 2.
41 'Sydney News,' *Maitland Mercury*, 8 July 1843: 4; 'County of Cumberland Election,' *Australasian Chronicle*, 4 July 1843: 2. See also 'The Cumberland Election,' *Australian*, 10 July 1843: 2.
42 'Hyndman v Innes and Another,' *Sydney Morning Herald*, 18 November 1843: 2. All quotes and references to Hyndman's trial are from this source.
43 Godfrey Mundy, *Our Antipodes; Or, Residence and Rambles in the Australian Colonies*, vol. 1 (London, 1852), 53–54.
44 Melissa Bellanta, *Larrikins: A History* (Brisbane: University of Queensland Press, 2012), 63.
45 Both Weston and Johnstone were grandsons of George and Esther Johnston; the family had acquired an 'e'. 'Legislative Council,' *Weekly Register of Politics, Facts and General Literature*, 9 December 1843: 308.
46 Paul D. Halliday, *Habeas Corpus: From England to Empire* (Cambridge, MA: Belknap Press of Harvard University Press, 2011), 127, 130.
47 R. B. Walker, *The Newspaper Press in New South Wales 1803–1920* (Sydney: Sydney University Press, 1976), 23; G. P. Walsh, 'Nichols, George Robert (Bob) (1809–1857),' *Australian Dictionary of Biography*, <http://adb.anu.edu.au/biography/nichols-george-robert-bob-4296>, accessed 1 November 2019.
48 John Dunmore Lang, *An Historical and Statistical Account of New South Wales*, vol. 2 (London, 1875), 321.
49 'Public Meeting,' *Sydney Gazette*, 1 March 1842: 2; 'Second Public Meeting,' *Courier*, 1 April 1842: 4.
50 J. B. Windeyer, 'Windeyer, Richard (1806–1847),' *Australian Dictionary of Biography*, <adb.anu.edu.au/biography/windeyer-richard-1060/text4017>, accessed 17 October 2015; J. M. Bennett, 'The Establishment of Jury Trial in New South Wales,' *Sydney Law Review* 3, no. 3 (1961): 480.
51 7 Vic. No. 14 [22 December 1843].
52 Peter Shea, *Defining Madness* (Sydney: Hawkins Press, 1999), 26–27.
53 'Legislative Council,' *Weekly Register of Politics, Facts and General Literature*, 9 December 1843: 308.
54 'Legislative Council – Progress of the Session,' *Australian*, 2 December 1843: 2.

55 'Thursday, December 7, 1843,' *Australian*, 9 December 1843: 3.
56 Original emphasis. 'Legislative Council,' *Sydney Morning Herald*, 8 December 1843: 2.
57 48 George 3, c. 96 [1808].
58 'Thursday, December 7, 1843,' *Australian*, 9 December 1843: 3.
59 'Departures,' *Morning Chronicle*, 31 January 1844: 3.
60 Casenotes of Francis Campbell, quoted in Edwards, 'The Mental Illness of Captain Hyndman,' 151.
61 R. Jones, solicitor, quoted in Edwards, 'The Mental Illness of Captain Hyndman,' 151.
62 Edwards, 'The Mental Illness of Captain Hyndman,' 150.
63 J. L. Innes to E. D. Thomson, 13 March 1846, Colonial Secretary's Papers, quoted in McDonald, 'Gladesville Hospital,' 283–84.
64 Anon., 'Robinson, Joseph Phelps (1815–1848),' *Australian Dictionary of Biography*, <adb.anu.edu.au/biography/robinson-joseph-phelps-2597/text3567>, accessed 10 September 2015.
65 McDonald, 'Gladesville Hospital,' 283–84; Bostock, *The Dawn of Psychiatry in Australia*, 92–94.
66 9 Vic. 34 [13 June 1846].
67 Appendix, Report from the Select Committee on the Lunatic Asylum Tarban Creek, 6.
68 'The Lunacy Bill. No. I,' *Sydney Morning Herald*, 29 May 1846: 3; 'The Lunatic Bill. No II,' *Sydney Morning Herald*, 2 June 1846: 3.
69 'The Lunacy Bill,' 8 June 1846, suppl.: 1; 'Lunatic Asylums. No IV,' 12 June 1846: 3; 'Lunatic Asylums. No V,' 15 June 1846: 3; 'Lunatic Asylums. No VI,' 17 June 1846: 2; 'Lunatic Asylums. No VII,' 10 September 1846: 3; 'Lunatic Asylums. No VIII,' 11 September 1846: 3; 'Lunatic Asylums. No IX,' 22 September 1846: 4 – all in *Sydney Morning Herald*.
70 'Lunatic Asylums,' *Sydney Morning Herald*, 9 June 1846: 2; Editorial, *Sydney Morning Herald*, 4 September 1846: 2.
71 J. Eckford, Minutes, 34–35.
72 Justin A. Frank, jnr, 'Non-Restraint and Robert Gardiner Hill,' *Bulletin of the History of Medicine* 41, no. 2 (1967): 140–60.
73 G. Turner, Minutes, 21.
74 T. Lee, Minutes, 19.
75 'Review: State of the Lunatic Asylum, Tarban Creek,' *Sydney Morning Herald*, 20 May 1847: 3.
76 See Roger G. Parker, *Cockatoo Island: A History* (Melbourne: Thomas Nelson Australia, 1977), 1–4.
77 'Review: State of the Lunatic Asylum, Tarban Creek,' *Sydney Morning Herald*, 20 May 1847.
78 Roy Porter, *Mind Forg'd Manacles: A History of Madness in England from the Restoration to the Regency* (Cambridge, MA: Harvard University Press, 1987), 176.
79 'Sydney Races,' *Australian*, 9 May 1837: 2.
80 Appendix to Minutes, Report from the Select Committee on the Lunatic Asylum Tarban Creek, 15.

81 Toby Raeburn et al., 'Liverpool "Lunatic Asylum": A Forgotten Chapter in the History of Australian Health Care,' *Collegian* 25 (2018): 347–53.
82 Samuel Tuke, *Description of the Retreat, an Institution Near York* (York, 1813); Porter, *Mind Forg'd Manacles*, 143; Anne Digby, *Madness, Morality and Medicine: A Study of the York Retreat 1796–1914* (Cambridge: Cambridge University Press, 1985).
83 Andrew Scull, *The Most Solitary of Afflictions: Madness and Society in Britain, 1700–1900* (New Haven: Yale University Press, 1993), 188–89, 224–30.
84 James Dunk, 'Work, Paperwork and the Imaginary Tarban Creek Lunatic Asylum, 1846,' *Rethinking History: The Journal of Theory and Practice* 22, no. 3 (2018): 326–55.
85 'The Lunatic Asylum,' *Sydney Morning Herald*, 8 June 1847: 2.
86 'Original Correspondence,' *Sydney Morning Herald*, 11 June 1847: 3.
87 'To the Editors of the Sydney Morning Herald,' *Sydney Morning Herald*, 29 June 1847: 3.
88 T. Lee to E. D. Thompson, 12 January 1848, with Gipps's annotation, SLNSW 48/832, quoted in Bostock, *The Dawn of Australian Psychiatry*, 112.
89 John Dunmore Lang, *Phillipsland; Country Hitherto Designated Port Phillip* (London, 1847), 320.
90 'Legislative Council,' *Sydney Morning Herald*, 13 May 1847: 2; 'Council Papers,' *Sydney Morning Herald*, 30 September 1847: 2; 'Lunatic Asylum, Tarban Creek,' *Australian*, 21 December 1847: 3.
91 W. Dawson to F. Campbell, 1 January 1848, quoted in Bostock, *The Dawn of Australian Psychiatry*, 112.
92 Donald I. McDonald, 'Gladesville Hospital: The Formative Years, 1838–1850,' *Journal of the Royal Australian Historical Society* 51, no. 3 (1965): 289–92; Bostock, *The Dawn of Australian Psychiatry*, 107–12.
93 Report from the Select Committee on the Lunatic Asylum Tarban Creek, 4; 'Lunatic Asylum – Tarban Creek,' *Sydney Morning Herald*, 7 July 1847: 3.
94 'Original Correspondence,' *Freeman's Journal*, 4 September 1851: 10.
95 'The Herald on Charles Cowper,' *Bell's Life in Sydney and Sporting Reviewer*, 16 August 1851: 2; 'Original Correspondence,' *Australian*, 10 September 1846: 3.
96 John Hirst, 'Cowper, Charles,' in *The Oxford Companion to Australian History*, eds G. Davison, J. Hirst and S. Macintyre (Oxford University Press, 2003), DOI:10.1093/acref/9780195515039.001.0001.
97 'Original Correspondence,' *Freeman's Journal*, 4 September 1851.
98 See Leonard D. Smith, 'Ellis, Sir William Charles (1780–1839),' *Oxford Dictionary of National Biography*, <www.oxforddnb.com/view/article/53734>, accessed 20 October 2015.
99 'State of the Lunatic Asylum, Tarban Creek,' *Sydney Morning Herald*, 17 June 1847: 2; William Charles Ellis, *A Treatise on the Nature, Symptoms, Causes, and Treatment of Insanity* (London, 1838), 314.
100 'State of the Lunatic Asylum, Tarban Creek,' *Sydney Morning Herald*, 17 June 1847: 2.
101 Ellis, *A Treatise*, 315.
102 Scull, *The Most Solitary of Afflictions*, 164.
103 Editorial, *Morning Chronicle*, 27 December 1843: 4.

104 'Public meeting,' *Sydney Gazette*, 1 March 1842; Victor Windeyer, *Sir Charles Nicholson: A Place in History* (Brisbane: University of Queensland Press, 1978), 16–20 and David S. Macmillan, 'Nicholson, Sir Charles (1808–1903),' *Australian Dictionary of Biography*, <adb.anu.edu.au/biography/nicholson-sir-charles-2508/text3387>, accessed 20 October 2015.

105 Stanley to G. Gipps, 28 October 1844, *HRA* I, vol. 24, 58.

106 9 Vic. IV [11 September 1845].

107 'Legislative Council,' *Sydney Morning Herald*, 4 September 1845: 2; 9 Vic. 4 [1845].

108 Editorial, *Sydney Morning Herald*, 6 December 1845: 2.

109 H. H. Browne, Minutes, 28.

110 J. Innes, Minutes, 1; Bostock, *The Dawn of Australian Psychiatry*, 80–81.

111 Original emphasis: 'Review: State of the Lunatic Asylum, Tarban Creek,' *Sydney Morning Herald*, 20 May 1847: 3.

112 Samuel Sidney, *The Three Colonies of Australia: New South Wales, Victoria, South Australia*, 2nd edn (London, 1853); Stanley Tick, 'Sidney, Samuel (1813–1883),' *Australian Dictionary of Biography*, <adb.anu.edu.au/biography/sidney-samuel-2662/text3599>, accessed 6 December 2015.

113 'Lunatic Asylums. No V,' *Sydney Morning Herald*, 15 June 1846; and see A. W. Ireland, 'The Select Committee on the Lunatic Asylum, Tarban Creek, 1846,' *Medical Journal of Australia* 51 (1964): 91.

EPILOGUE

1 Ray Beckett and Richard Beckett, *Hangman: The Life and Times of Alexander Green, Public Executioner to the Colony of New South Wales* (Melbourne: Nelson, 1980), 13–14, 27.

2 Keith Vincent Smith, 'Redfern in Time,' *Eora People*, <www.eorapeople.com.au/tag/the-sandhills-cemetery/>, accessed 12 February 2019.

3 K. K. Mcnab, 'Green, Alexander (1802–?),' *Australian Dictionary of Biography*, <adb.anu.edu.au/biography/green-alexander-12949>, accessed 19 March 2019.

4 'Wednesday,' *Sydney Herald*, 8 October 1832, suppl.: 2.

5 Beckett and Beckett, *Hangman*, 68, 149, 155–57.

6 Beckett and Beckett, *Hangman*, 171.

7 Beckett and Beckett, *Hangman*, 175–76.

8 Beckett and Beckett, *Hangman*, 179–80.

9 'Ministerial Visit to Parramatta,' *Sydney Mail*, 11 August 1866: 5; 'Parramatta,' *Maitland Mercury* and *Hunter River General Advertiser*, 4 September 1879: 3.

10 'A Mad Executioner,' *Mount Alexander Mail*, 20 January 1894: 2.

11 Peter Carey, *Oscar and Lucinda* (Brisbane: Queensland University Press, 1988), 295.

12 Lyndall Ryan, 'Who Is the Fabricator?' in *Whitewash: On Keith Windschuttle's Fabrication of Aboriginal History*, ed. R. Manne (Melbourne: Black Inc., 2003), 230–57.

13 'Colonial Frontier Massacres in Eastern Australia 1788–1872,' Centre for 21st Century Humanities, University of Newcastle, <c21ch.newcastle.edu.au/colonialmassacres/>, accessed 15 October 2018.

14 Philippa Martyr and Sophie Davison, 'Aboriginal People in Western Australian Mental Hospitals, 1903–1966,' *Social History of Medicine* 31, no. 3 (2018): 462–84; Philippa Martyr, '"Behaving Wildly": Diagnoses of Lunacy among Indigenous Persons in Western Australia, 1870 –1914,' *Social History of Medicine* 24, no. 2 (2011): 316–33.

15 Pat Dudgeon, Helen Milroy and Roz Walker, eds, *Working Together: Aboriginal and Torres Strait Islander Mental Health and Wellbeing Principles and Practice*, 2nd edn (Canberra: Commonwealth of Australia, 2014); John Boulton, 'History Branded on the Mind: Trans-Generational Trauma in Aboriginal Australia,' *Health and History* 20, no. 2 (2018): 100–105, DOI: 10.5401/healthhist.20.2.0100.

16 Patrick Wolfe, 'Settler Colonialism and the Elimination of the Native,' *Journal of Genocide Research* 8, no. 4 (2006): 388.

17 Bruce Pascoe, 'Dark Emu,' HumanNature lecture series, Australian Museum, 18 October 2018; *Dark Emu: Aboriginal Australia and the Birth of Agriculture* (Broome: Magabala Books, 2018).

18 Henry Reynolds, *Why Weren't We Told? A Personal Search for the Truth About Our History* (Melbourne: Viking, 1999).

19 Wolfe, 'Settler Colonialism and the Elimination of the Native,' 387.

20 See Robert Foster and Amanda Nettleback's study of the culture of the South Australian frontier in *Out of the Silence: The History and Memory of South Australia's Frontier Wars* (Adelaide: Wakefield Press, 2012), especially 78–86; Lorenzo Veracini's 'Settler Collective, Founding Violence and Disavowal: The Settler Colonial Situation,' *Journal of Intercultural Studies* 29, no. 4 (2008): 363–79, DOI:10.1080/07256860802372246; Michael Sturma's psychological profile in 'Myall Creek and the Psychology of Mass Murder,' *Journal of Australian Studies* 9, no. 16 (1985): 62–70, DOI:10.1080/14443058509386904; and the essays collected in Estela Schindel and Pamela Colombo, eds, *Space and the Memories of Violence: Landscapes of Erasure, Disappearance and Exception* (Basingstoke, UK: Palgrave Macmillan, 2014).

21 Jeffrey C. Alexander, *Trauma: A Social Theory* (Cambridge: Polity, 2012).

22 Mark S. Micale, 'Toward a Global History of Trauma,' in *Psychological Trauma and the Legacies of the First World War*, eds J. Crouthamel and P. Leese (Springer International Publishing): 289–310.

SELECT BIBLIOGRAPHY

The *Australian Dictionary of Biography*, published by the National Centre for Biography at the Australian National University, has been invaluable; I thank its editors and owe debts to numerous contributors including J. J. Auchmuty, George F. J. Bergman, Keith Macrae Bowden, Jill Conway, C. H. Currey, Norman J. Dunlop, Brian H. Fletcher, V. W. E. Goodin, Niel Gunson, R. F. Holder, T. H. Irving, M. J. B. Kenny, Norman S. Lynravn, David S. Macmillan, K. B. Noad, Vivienne Parsons, Michael Persse, Michael Roe, A. G. L. Shaw, Margaret Steven, W. A. Townsley, G. P. Walsh, John Manning Ward, J. B. Windeyer, and A. T. Yarwood.

This book was only possible though the enormous amount of work that went into the preparation of the *Historical Records of New South Wales* edited by F. M. Bladen and published by the New South Wales Government in 1892–1901 and the *Historical Records of Australia*, published by the Commonwealth Government in 1914–25. Equally valuable is the superb online database of digitised newspapers Trove, published and maintained by the National Library of Australia and corrected daily by countless generous readers.

This book draws on extensive archival material including, at Mitchell Library, State Library of New South Wales, the papers of John Grant (MAV/FM4/1411), the Bonwick Transcripts of the Commission of Inquiry 1819–21, Lachlan Macquarie papers (A797), Macarthur Papers (A2899 and A2906), the letterbook of George Johnston (C474 George Johnston), and Philip Gidley King's correspondence (MSS 710). Collections consulted at State Records, New South Wales include Colonial Secretary's Papers (NRS 897, NRS 898) and the documents of John Macarthur's Commission of Inquiry (NRS 13524). National Archives UK collections include Colonial Office dispatches (CGO 201/324) and Surgeon's Reports, Convict Transport Ships (ADM101).

PUBLISHED JOURNALS, MEMOIRS AND DOCUMENTS

A Charge of Mutiny: The Court Martial of Colonel George Johnston for Deposing Governor William Bligh in the Rebellion of 26 January 1808, edited by John Ritchie (Canberra: National Library of Australia, 1988).

Bishop, Charles, *The Journal and Letters of Captain Charles Bishop on the North-West Coast of America, in the Pacific and in New South Wales 1794–1799*, edited by Michael Roe (Nendeln, Liechtenstein: Kraus Reprint, 1974).
Clark, Ralph, *The Journal and Letters of Lt Ralph Clark 1787–1792,* edited by Paul G. Fidlon and R. J. Ryan (Sydney: Australian Documents Library, 1981).
Collins, David, *An Account of the English Colony in New South Wales* (London, 1798).
The Evidence to the Bigge Reports: New South Wales Under Governor Macquarie, 2 vols, edited by John Ritchie (Melbourne: Heinemann, 1971).
Grant, John, *This Beauteous, Wicked Place: Letters and Journals of John Grant, Gentleman Convict*, edited by Yvonne Cramer (Canberra: National Library of Australia, 2000).
Mackintosh, James, *Memoirs of the Life of the Right Honourable Sir James Mackintosh, Vol. 1*, edited by Robert James Mackintosh (London, 1835).
Macleay, Frances, *Fanny to William: The Letters of Frances Leonora Macleay 1812–1836*, edited by Beverley Earnshaw and Joy Hughes (Sydney: Historic Houses Trust of New South Wales and Macleay Museum, 1993).
Macquarie, Lachlan, *Macquarie's Journals of His Tours in New South Wales and Van Diemen's Land* (Sydney: Public Library of New South Wales, 1956).
Nagle, Jacob, *The Nagle Journal: A Diary of the Life of Jacob Nagle, Sailor, from the Year 1775 to 1841*, edited by John C. Dann (New York: Weidenfeld & Nicolson, 1988).
Some Private Correspondence of the Rev. Samuel Marsden and Family 1794–1824, edited by George Mackaness (Sydney: self-published, 1942).
Some Early Records of the Macarthurs of Camden, edited by Sibella Onslow Macarthur (Sydney: Angus & Robertson, 1914).
Suttor, George, *Memoirs of George Suttor, F.L.S.: Banksian Collector (1774–1859)*, edited by George Mackaness (Sydney: self-published, 1948).
Tench, Watkin, *A Narrative of the Expedition to Botany Bay* (London, 1789).
———, *A Complete Account of the Settlement at Port Jackson* (London, 1793).
Wentworth, William Charles, *A Statistical, Historical, and Political Description of the Colony of New South Wales and Its Dependent Settlements in Van Diemen's Land* (London, 1819).
White, John, *Journal of a Voyage to New South Wales.* 1790 (Sydney: University of Sydney Library, 2001).

OTHER PUBLISHED PRIMARY SOURCES

Acland, Henry Wentworth, *Feigned Insanity, How Most Usually Simulated, and How Best Detected* (London, 1844).
Bentham, Jeremy, *A Plea for the Constitution* (London, 1803).
———, *Principles of Penal Law* (Adelaide: University of Adelaide Library, 2016).
Bland, William, *Letters to Charles Buller, Junior, Esq., M.P., from the Australian Patriotic Association* (Sydney, 1849).
Blatchford, Thomas W., *An Inaugural Dissertation on Feigned Disease* (New York, 1817).
Burrows, George Man, *Commentaries on the Causes, Forms, Symptoms, and Treatment, Moral and Medical, of Insanity* (New York: Arno Press, 1976, first published 1828).
Cox, Joseph Mason, *Practical Observation on Insanity* (London, 1806).
Ellis, William Charles, *A Treatise on the Nature, Symptoms, Causes, and Treatment of Insanity* (London, 1838).
Gavin, Hector, *On Feigned or Factitious Diseases, Chiefly of Soldiers and Seamen; On the Means*

Used to Simulate or Produce Them; And on the Best Modes of Discovering Impostors (London, 1843).

Graham, Henry, 'A Criminal Lunatic,' *Medical Journal of Australia* (January 1857): 76–78.

Highmore, Anthony, *A Treatise on the Law of Idiocy and Lunacy* (Exeter, 1822).

Lang, John Dunmore, *An Historical and Statistical Account of New South Wales, From the Founding of the Colony in 1788, to the Present Day, Vol. 2* (London, 1875).

Marshall, Henry, *Hints to Young Medical Officers of the Army on the Examination of Recruits, and Respecting the Feigned Disabilities of Soldiers* (London, 1828).

James Cowles Prichard, *A Treatise on Insanity and Other Disorders Affecting the Mind* (Philadelphia, 1837).

Sidney, Samuel, *The Three Colonies of Australia: New South Wales, Victoria, South Australia; Their Pastures, Copper Mines, & Gold Fields*. 2nd edn (London, 1853).

Tuke, Samuel, *Description of The Retreat, an Institution Near York, for Insane Persons of the Society of Friends* (York, 1813).

SECONDARY ARTICLES AND BOOKS

Allen, Matthew, 'Alcohol and Authority in Early New South Wales: The Symbolic Significance of the Spirit Trade, 1788–1808,' *History Australia* 9, no. 3 (2012): 7–26.

Anderson, Warwick, *The Cultivation of Whiteness: Science, Health, and Racial Destiny in Australia* (Durham, NC: Duke University Press, 2006).

Andrew, Donna T., 'The Code of Honour and Its Critics: The Opposition to Duelling in England, 1700–1850,' *Social History* 5, no. 3 (1980): 409–34.

Atkinson, Alan, 'Jeremy Bentham and the Rum Rebellion,' *Journal of the Royal Australian Historical Society* 64, no. 1 (1978): 1–13.

———, 'John Macarthur Before Australia Knew Him,' *Journal of Australian Studies* 3, no. 4 (1979): 22–37.

———, 'The Little Revolution in New South Wales, 1808,' *International History Review* 12, no. 1 (1990): 65–75.

———, 'The Free-Born Englishman Transported: Convict Rights as a Measure of Eighteenth-Century Empire,' *Past & Present*, no. 144 (1994): 88–115.

———, *The Europeans in Australia: A History, Vol. 1: The Beginning* (Melbourne: Oxford University Press, 1997).

Ballantyne, Tony, 'The Theory and Practice of Empire-Building: Edward Gibbon Wakefield and "Systematic Colonisation",' in *The Routledge History of Western Empires*, edited by R. Aldrich and K. McKenzie (London: Routledge, 2014), 89–101.

Bennett, J. M., 'The Establishment of Jury Trial in New South Wales,' *Sydney Law Review* 3, no. 3 (1961): 463–85.

———, 'The Day of Retribution – Commissioner Bigge's Enquiries in Colonial New South Wales,' *American Journal of Legal History* 15, no. 2 (1971): 85–196.

Benton, Lauren, 'Just Despots: The Cultural Construction of Imperial Constitutionalism,' *Law, Culture and the Humanities* 9, no. 2 (2013): 213–26.

———, *A Search for Sovereignty: Law and Geography in European Empires, 1400–1900* (Cambridge: Cambridge University Press, 2010).

Benton, Lauren and Lisa Ford, 'Magistrates in Empire: Convicts, Slaves, and the

Remaking of the Plural Legal Order in the British Empire,' in *Legal Pluralism and Empires, 1500–1850*, edited by Lauren A. Benton and Richard Jeffrey Ross (New York: New York University Press, 2013): 173–97.
———, *Rage for Order: The British Empire and the Origins of International Law 1800–1850* (Cambridge, MA: Harvard University Press, 2016).
Bergman, George F. J., 'Solomon Levey in Sydney: From Convict Merchant to Prince,' *Royal Australian Historical Society: Journal and Proceedings* 49, no. 6 (1964): 401–22.
Berry, Felicity Grace, 'Keeping the Home Fires Burning?: British Female Settlers' Conceptions of Home and Belonging in Colonial India, Van Diemen's Land and Western Australia, 1826–1860,' PhD thesis, University of Sydney, 2016.
Best, Rod, 'The Castle Hill Lunatic Asylum, 1811–1826,' *Journal of the Royal Australian Historical Society* 78, no. 3–4 (1992): 1–18.
Blair, Sandra, 'The Felonry and the Free? Divisions in Colonial Society in the Penal Era,' *Labour History*, no. 45 (1983): 1–16.
Bolt, Peter G., *William Cowper (1778–1858): The Life and Influence of Australia's First Parish Clergyman* (Sydney: Bolt Publishing Services, 2009).
Bostock, John, *The Dawn of Australian Psychiatry: An Account of the Measures Taken for Mental Invalids from the Time of the First Fleet, 1788, to the Year 1850* (Sydney: Australian Medical Association, 1968).
Boulton, John, 'History Branded on the Mind: Trans-Generational Trauma in Aboriginal Australia,' *Health and History* 20, no. 2 (2018): 100–105.
Brasier, Angeline, 'Prisoners' Bodies: Methods and Advances in Convict Medicine in the Transportation Era,' *Health and History* 12, no. 2 (2010): 18–38.
Brookes, Barbara, 'Papering Over Madness: Accountability and Resistance in Colonial Asylum Files: A New Zealand Case Study,' *Rethinking History* 22, no. 3 (2018): 356–74.
Butlin, N. G., *Forming a Colonial Economy: Australia 1810–1850* (Cambridge: Cambridge University Press, 1994).
———, 'Yo, Ho, and How Many Bottles of Rum?,' *Australian Economic History Review* 23, no. 1 (1983): 1–27.
Byrne, Paula J., *Criminal Law and Colonial Subject: New South Wales 1810–1830, Studies in Australian History* (Melbourne: Cambridge University Press, 1993).
Castle, Tim, 'Constructing Death: Newspaper Reports of Executions in Colonial New South Wales, 1826–1837,' *Journal of Australian Colonial History* 9 (2007): 51–68.
Causer, Tim, 'Norfolk Island's "Suicide Lotteries": Myth and Reality,' *Islands of History: Proceedings of the 25th Anniversary Conference, Professional Historians Association (NSW)* (Sydney: Anchor Books Australia, 1997), 61–68.
Christopher, Emma, *A Merciless Place: The Fate of Britain's Convicts after the American Revolution* (New York: Oxford University Press, 2011).
Christopher, Emma and Hamish Maxwell-Stewart, 'Convict Transportation in Global Context, c. 1700–88,' in *The Cambridge History of Australia, Vol. 1: Indigenous and Colonial Australia*, edited by Alison Bashford and Stuart Macintyre (Melbourne: Cambridge University Press, 2013), 68–90.
Clark, Manning C., *A History of Australia, Vol. 1: From the Earliest Times to the Age of Macquarie* (Melbourne: Melbourne University Press, 1968).
Coleborne, Catharine, *Madness in the Family: Insanity and Institutions in the Australasian*

Colonial World, 1860–1914 (New York: Palgrave Macmillan, 2010).

———, *Insanity, Identity and Empire: Immigrants and Institutional Confinement in Australia and New Zealand, 1873–1910* (Manchester: Manchester University Press, 2015).

Coleborne, Catharine and Dolly MacKinnon, eds, *'Madness' in Australia: Histories, Heritage and the Asylum* (Brisbane: University of Queensland Press, 2003).

Coltheart, Lenore and Peter Bridges, 'The Elephant's Bed? Scottish Enlightenment Ideas and the Foundations of New South Wales,' *Journal of Australian Studies* 25, no. 68 (2001): 19–33.

Covey, Russell D., 'Temporary Insanity: The Strange Life and Times of the Perfect Defense,' *Boston University Law Review* 91, no. 5 (2011): 1597–668.

Cummins, C. J., *The Administration of Lunacy and Idiocy in New South Wales 1788–1855* (Sydney: NSW Department of Public Health, 1967).

———, *A History of Medical Administration in NSW 1788–1973*, 2nd edn (Sydney: NSW Department of Health, 2003).

Damousi, Joy, *Depraved and Disorderly: Female Convicts, Sexuality and Gender in Colonial Australia* (Cambridge: Cambridge University Press, 1997).

Davey, Lois, Margaret Macpherson, and F. W. Clements, *The Hungry Years: 1788–1792* (Canberra: Australian Institute of Anatomy, 1947).

Deacon, Harriet Jane, 'Madness, Race and Moral Treatment: Robben Island Lunatic Asylum, Cape Colony, 1846–1890,' *History of Psychiatry* 7, no. 26 (1996): 287–97.

Digby, Anne, *Madness, Morality and Medicine: A Study of the York Retreat 1796–1914* (Cambridge: Cambridge University Press, 1985).

Dunk, James, 'Work, Paperwork and the Imaginary Tarban Creek Lunatic Asylum, 1846,' *Rethinking History: The Journal of Theory and Practice* 22, no. 3 (2018): 326–55.

———, 'Authority and the Treatment of the Insane at Castle Hill Asylum, 1811–25,' *Health and History* 19, no. 2 (2017): 17–40.

———, 'The Politics of Madness in a Penal Colony: New South Wales, 1788–1856,' PhD thesis, University of Sydney, 2016.

Earnshaw, Beverley, 'The Lame, the Blind, the Mad, the Malingerers: Sick and Disabled Convicts within the Colonial Community,' *Journal of the Royal Australian Historical Society* 81, no. 1 (1995): 25–38.

Edwards, Graham A., 'The Mental Illness of Captain Hyndman,' *Australian and New Zealand Journal of Psychiatry* 13, no. 2 (1979): 147–52.

Eigen, Joel Peter, *Witnessing Insanity: Madness and Mad-Doctors in the English Court* (New Haven: Yale University Press, 1995).

Ellis, Malcolm Henry, *John Macarthur* (Penrith: Discovery Press, 1972).

———, *Lachlan Macquarie: His Life, Adventures and Times, with Reference Notes and Bibliography* (Sydney: Angus & Robertson, 2010).

Ernst, Waltraud, 'Idioms of Madness and Colonial Boundaries: The Case of the European and "Native" Mentally Ill in Early Nineteenth-Century British India,' *Comparative Studies in Society and History* 39, no. 1 (1997): 153–81.

Estensen, Miriam, *The Life of George Bass: Surgeon and Sailor of the Enlightenment* (Sydney: Allen & Unwin, 2005).

Evans, Raymond, '19 June 1822 Creating "an Object of Real Terror": The Tabling of the First Bigge Report,' in *Turning Points in Australian History*, edited by Martin Crotty and David Andrew Roberts (Sydney: UNSW Press, 2009), 48–61.

Select bibliography

Evatt, H. V., *Rum Rebellion: A Study of the Overthrow of Governor Bligh by John Macarthur and the New South Wales Corps* (London: Angus & Robertson, 1978).

Fifer, D. E., 'The Australian Patriotic Association 1835–1841,' *Journal of the Royal Australian Historical Society* 73, no. 3 (1987): 155–72.

Finnane, Mark, 'Asylums, Families and the State,' *History Workshop* 17, no. 1 (1985): 134–48.

———, 'Law and Regulation,' in *The Cambridge History of Australia, Vol. 1: Indigenous and Colonial Australia*, edited by Alison Bashford and Stuart Macintyre (Cambridge: Cambridge University Press, 2013), 391–413.

Fitzgerald, Ross and Mark Hearn, *Bligh, Macarthur and the Rum Rebellion* (Sydney: Kangaroo Press, 1988).

Fletcher, Brian H., 'Administrative Reform in New South Wales under Governor Darling,' *Australian Journal of Public Administration* 38, no. 3 (1979): 246–62.

Ford, Lisa and David Andrew Roberts, 'Expansion, 1820–50,' in *The Cambridge History of Australia, Vol. 1: Indigenous and Colonial Australia*, edited by Alison Bashford and Stuart Macintyre (Melbourne: Cambridge University Press, 2013).

———, 'New South Wales Penal Settlements and the Transformation of Secondary Punishment in the Nineteenth-Century British Empire,' *Journal of Colonialism and Colonial History* 15, no. 3 (2014): n.p.

Forsythe, William James, *The Reform of Prisoners 1830–1900* (London: Croom Helm, 1987).

Foxhall, Katherine, *Health, Medicine, and the Sea: Australian Voyages, c.1815–1860* (Manchester: Manchester University Press, 2012).

———, 'From Convicts to Colonists: The Health of Prisoners and the Voyage to Australia, 1823–1853,' *Journal of Imperial and Commonwealth History* 39, no. 1 (2011): 3.

Francis, Mark, *Governors and Settlers: Images of Authority in the British Colonies, 1820–60* (Basingstoke, UK: Palgrave, 1992).

Garton, Stephen, *Medicine and Madness: A Social History of Insanity in New South Wales, 1880–1940* (Sydney: UNSW Press, 1988).

———, 'Asylum Histories: Reconsidering Australia's Lunatic Past,' in *Madness in Australia: Histories, Heritage and the Asylum*, edited by C. Coleborne and D. MacKinnon (Brisbane: University of Queensland Press, 2003), 11–22.

Gatrell, V. A. C., *The Hanging Tree: Execution and the English People 1770–1868* (Oxford: Oxford University Press, 1994).

Geller, Jeffrey L., Jonathon Erlen, Neil S. Kaye, and William H. Fisher, 'Feigned Insanity in Nineteenth-Century America: Tactics, Trials, and Truth,' *Behavioral Sciences and the Law* 8, no. 1 (1990): 3–26.

Hainsworth, David Roger, *The Sydney Traders: Simeon Lord and His Contemporaries, 1788–1821*, 2nd edn (Melbourne: Melbourne University Press, 1981).

Halliday, Paul D., *Habeas Corpus: From England to Empire* (Cambridge, MA: The Belknap Press of Harvard University Press, 2011).

Hay, Douglas, 'Property, Authority and the Criminal Law,' in *Albion's Fatal Tree: Crime and Punishment in Eighteenth-Century England*, edited by Douglas Hay, Peter Linebaugh, John G. Rule, E. P. Thompson and Cal Winslow (London: Verso, 2011), 17–63.

Henriques, U. R. Q., 'The Rise and Decline of the Separate System of Prison Discipline,' *Past & Present* 54, no. 1 (1972): 61–93.

Hill-Reid, William, *John Grant's Journey: A Convict Story 1803–1811* (London: Heinemann, 1957).

Hirst, John, *Convict Society and Its Enemies: A History of Early New South Wales* (Sydney: Allen & Unwin, 1983).

Holcomb, Janet, *Early Merchant Families of Sydney: Speculation and Risk Management on the Fringes of Empire* (London: Anthem Press, 2014).

Houston, R. A., 'Explanations for Death by Suicide in Northern Britain During the Long Eighteenth Century,' *History of Psychiatry* 23, no. 1 (2012): 52–64.

———, 'Legal Protection of the Mentally Incapable in Early Modern Scotland,' *Journal of Legal History*, 24, no. 2 (2003): 165–86.

Hughes, Robert, *The Fatal Shore: A History of the Transportation of Convicts to Australia, 1787–1868* (London: Vintage Books, 2003).

Ihde, Erin, *Edward Smith Hall and the Sydney Monitor 1826–1840* (Melbourne: Australian Scholarly Publishing, 2004).

Ireland, A. W., 'The Select Committee on the Lunatic Asylum, Tarban Creek, 1846,' *Medical Journal of Australia* 51 (1964): 90–97.

Kafka, Ben, *The Demon of Writing* (New York: Zone Books, 2012).

Karr, David S., '"The Embers of Expiring Sedition": Maurice Margarot, the Scottish Martyrs Monument and the Production of Radical Memory across the British South Pacific,' *Historical Research* 86, no. 234 (2013): 638–60.

Karskens, Grace, *The Colony: A History of Early Sydney* (Sydney: Allen & Unwin, 2009).

———, 'The Early Colonial Presence, 1788–1822,' in *The Cambridge History of Australia, Vol. 1: Indigenous and Colonial Australia*, edited by Alison Bashford and Stuart Macintyre (Melbourne: Cambridge University Press, 2013), 91–120.

Karskens, Grace and Richard Waterhouse, '"Too Sacred to Be Taken Away": Property, Liberty, Tyranny and the "Rum Rebellion",' *Journal of Australian Colonial History* 12 (2010): 1–22.

Kercher, Bruce, *An Unruly Child: A History of Law in Australia* (Sydney: Allen & Unwin, 1995).

———, *Debt, Seduction, and Other Disasters: The Birth of Civil Law in Convict New South Wales* (Sydney: Federation Press, 1996).

Lewis, Milton, *Managing Madness: Psychiatry and Society in Australia 1788–1980* (Canberra: AGPS Press, 1988).

Laidlaw, Zoë, 'Breaking Britannia's Bounds? Law, Settlers, and Space in Britain's Imperial Historiography,' *Historical Journal* 55, no. 3 (2012): 807–30.

———, *Colonial Connections, 1815–45: Patronage, the Information Revolution and Colonial Government* (Manchester: Manchester University Press, 2005).

Lambert, Doreen and Thomas William Parmeter, *The Parmeter Story* (Sydney: Mini-Publishing, 2002).

Laragy, Georgina, '"A Peculiar Species of Felony": Suicide, Medicine, and the Law in Victorian Britain and Ireland,' *Journal of Social History* 46, no. 3 (2013): 732–43.

Lester, Alan, *Imperial Networks: Creating Identities in Nineteenth-Century South Africa and Britain* (London: Routledge, 2001).

McClemens, J. H. and J. M. Bennett, 'Historical Notes on the Law of Mental Illness in

New South Wales,' *Sydney Law Review* 4, no. 1 (1964): 49–74.
McConville, Seán, *A History of English Prison Administration, Vol. I: 1751–1877* (Boston: Routledge & Kegan Paul, 1981).
McCreery, Cindy, and Kirsten McKenzie, 'The Australian Colonies in a Maritime World,' in *The Cambridge History of Australia, Vol. 1,* edited by Alison Bashford and Stuart Macintyre (Melbourne: Cambridge University Press), 560–84.
McDonald, Donald I., 'Gladesville Hospital: The Formative Years, 1838–1850,' *Journal of the Royal Australian Historical Society* 51, no. 3 (1965): 273–95.
McGowan, Randall, 'A Powerful Sympathy: Terror, the Prison, and Humanitarian Reform in Early Nineteenth-Century Britain,' *Journal of British Studies* 25 (1986): 312–13.
McKenzie, Kirsten, *Imperial Underworld: An Escaped Convict and the Transformation of the British Colonial Order* (Cambridge: Cambridge University Press, 2016).
McKinnon, Jennifer Anne, 'Convict Bushrangers in New South Wales, 1824–34,' MA thesis, La Trobe University, 1979.
Martensen, Robert L., 'The Detection of Feigned Insanity,' *Journal of the American Medical Association* 276, no. 16 (1996): 1357.
Martyr, Philippa and Sophie Davison, 'Aboriginal People in Western Australian Mental Hospitals, 1903–1966,' *Social History of Medicine* 31, no. 3 (2018): 462–84.
Meyering, Isobelle Barrett, 'Abolitionism, Settler Violence and the Case against Flogging: A Reassessment of Sir William Molesworth's Contribution to the Transportation Debate,' *History Australia* 7, no. 1 (2010): 6.1–6.18.
Micale, Mark S., 'Toward A Global History of Trauma,' in *Psychological Trauma and the Legacies of the First World War*, edited by J. Crouthamel and P. Leese (Springer International Publishing): 289–310.
Monk, Lee-Ann, *Attending Madness: At Work in the Australian Colonial Asylum* (Amsterdam: Rodopi, 2008).
Moore, Tony, *Death or Liberty: Rebels and Radicals Transported to Australia 1788–1868* (Sydney: Pier 9, 2010).
Murat, Laure, *The Man Who Thought He Was Napoleon: Toward a Political History of Madness*, translated by Deke Dusinberre (Chicago: University of Chicago Press, 2014).
Nagle, John Flood, *Collins, the Courts and the Colony: Law and Society in Colonial New South Wales, 1788–1796* (Sydney: UNSW Press, 1996).
Neal, David, *The Rule of Law in a Penal Colony: Law and Power in Early New South Wales* (Cambridge: Cambridge University Press, 1992).
Neil, W. D., *The Lunatic Asylum at Castle Hill: Australia's First Psychiatric Hospital 1811–1826* (Sydney: Dryas, 1992).
Newling, Jaqui, 'Dining with Strangeness: European Foodways on the Eora Frontier,' *Journal of Australian Colonial History* 13 (2011): 27–48.
Newman, C. E. T., *The Spirit of Wharf House: Campbell Enterprise from Calcutta to Canberra 1788–1930* (Sydney: Angus & Robertson, 1961).
Parry-Jones, William L., *The Trade in Lunacy* (London: Routledge & Kegan Paul, 1972).
Pascoe, Bruce, *Dark Emu: Aboriginal Australia and the Birth of Agriculture* (Broome: Magabala Books, 2018).
Porter, Roy, *Mind Forg'd Manacles: A History of Madness in England from the Restoration to the Regency* (Cambridge, MA: Harvard University Press, 1987).

Pybus, Cassandra, *Black Founders: The Unknown Story of Australia's First Black Settlers* (Sydney: UNSW Press, 2006).
Raeburn, T., C. Liston, J. Hickmott and M. Cleary, 'Liverpool "Lunatic Asylum": A Forgotten Chapter in the History of Australian Health Care,' *Collegian* 25 (2018): 347–53.
Reynolds, Henry, *Why Weren't We Told? A Personal Search for the Truth About Our History* (Melbourne: Viking, 1999).
Richards, D., 'Transported to New South Wales: Medical Convicts 1788–1850,' *British Medical Journal (Clinical Research Edition)* 295, no. 6613 (1987): 1609–12.
Ritchie, John, *Punishment and Profit: The Reports of Commissioner John Bigge on the Colonies of New South Wales and Van Diemen's Land, 1822–1823; Their Origins, Nature and Significance* (Melbourne: Heinemann, 1970).
Roberts, David Andrew, 'The Valley of Swells: "Special" or "Educated" Convicts on the Wellington Valley Settlement, 1827–1830,' *History Australia* 3 (2006): 11.1–11.21.
Robson, L. L., *The Convict Settlers of Australia: An Enquiry into the Origin and Character of the Convicts Transported to New South Wales and Van Diemen's Land 1787–1852* (Melbourne: Melbourne University Press and Cambridge University Press, 1965).
Roe, Michael, 'Charles Bishop, Pioneer of Pacific Commerce,' *Papers and Proceedings (Tasmanian Historical Research Association)* 10, no. 1 (1962): 6–15.
Russell, Penny, *Savage or Civilised?: Manners in Colonial Australia* (Sydney: UNSW Press, 2010).
Scull, Andrew, *The Most Solitary of Afflictions: Madness and Society in Britain, 1700–1900* (New Haven: Yale University Press, 1993).
———, 'The Domestication of Madness,' *Medical History* 27 (1983): 233–48.
Sharp, Andrew, *The World, the Flesh and the Devil: The Life and Opinions of Samuel Marsden in England and the Antipodes, 1765–1838* (Auckland: Auckland University Press, 2016).
Shaw, A. G. L., *Heroes and Villains in History: Governors Darling and Bourke in New South Wales* (Sydney: Sydney University Press, 1965).
Shea, Peter, *Defining Madness* (Sydney: Hawkins Press, 1999).
Shepherd, Anne and David Wright, 'Madness, Suicide and the Victorian Asylum: Attempted Self-Murder in the Age of Non-Restraint,' *Medical History* 46, no. 2 (2002): 175–96.
Smith, Roger, *Trial by Medicine: Insanity and Responsibility in Victorian Trials* (Edinburgh: Edinburgh University Press, 1981).
Stebbings, Chantal, 'Protecting the Property of the Mentally Ill: The Judicial Solution in Nineteenth Century Lunacy Law,' *Cambridge Law Journal* 71, no. 2 (2012): 384–411.
Sturma, Michael, 'Myall Creek and the Psychology of Mass Murder,' *Journal of Australian Studies* 9, no. 16 (1985): 62–70.
Suzuki, Akihito, *Madness at Home: The Psychiatrist, the Patient, and the Family in England, 1820–1860* (Berkeley: University of California Press, 2006).
Swartz, Sally, *Homeless Wanderers: Movement and Mental Illness in the Cape Colony in the Nineteenth Century* (Claremont: UCT Press, 2016).
———, 'The Regulation of British Colonial Lunatic Asylums and the Origins of

Colonial Psychiatry, 1860–1864,' *History of Psychology* 13, no. 2 (2010): 160–77.
———, 'The Third Voice: Writing Case-notes,' *Feminism & Psychology* 16, no. 4 (2006): 427–44.
Sylvester, Diane, 'Governor Lachlan Macquarie, Sir James Mackintosh and the Scottish Enlightenment,' *Journal of Australian Colonial History* 12 (2010): 23–38.
Thompson, M. M. H., *The Seeds of Democracy: Early Elections in Colonial New South Wales* (Sydney: Federation Press, 2006).
Tomes, Nancy, *The Art of Asylum-Keeping: Thomas Story Kirkbride and the Origins of American Psychiatry* (Philadelphia: University of Pennsylvania Press, 1994).
Tucker, Michelle Scott, *Elizabeth Macarthur: A Life at the Edge of the World* (Melbourne: Text, 2018).
Vanheule, Stijn, *Diagnosis and the DSM: A Critical Review* (Basingstoke, UK: Palgrave Macmillan, 2014).
Veracini, Lorenzo, 'Settler Collective, Founding Violence and Disavowal: The Settler Colonial Situation,' *Journal of Intercultural Studies* 29, no. 4 (2008): 363–79.
Walker, R. B., *The Newspaper Press in New South Wales 1803–1920* (Sydney: Sydney University Press, 1976).
Ward, John Manning, *Colonial Self-Government: The British Experience, 1759–1856* (London: Macmillan, 1976).
Warren, M. J., 'Unsettled Settlers: Fear and White Victimhood in New South Wales and Van Diemen's Land, 1788–1838,' PhD thesis, University of Sydney, 2016.
Waterhouse, Richard, 'A Bastard Offspring of Tyranny under the Guise of Liberty: Liberty and Representative Government in Australia, 1788–1901,' in *Exclusionary Empire: English Liberty Overseas, 1600–1900* edited by Jack P. Greene (Cambridge: Cambridge University Press, 2010), 220–47.
Wolfe, Patrick, 'Settler Colonialism and the Elimination of the Native,' *Journal of Genocide Research* 8, no. 4 (2006): 387–409
Woods, G. D., *A History of Criminal Law in New South Wales: The Colonial Period, 1788–1900* (Sydney: Federation Press, 2002).
Woollacott, Angela, *Settler Society in the Australian Colonies: Self-Government and Imperial Culture* (Oxford: Oxford University Press, 2015).
Wright, David and Peter Bartlett, eds, *Outside the Walls of the Asylum: The History of Care in the Community 1750–2000* (London: Athlone Press, 1999) Acknowledgments

INDEX

Index

Index

Index

Index

FSC
www.fsc.org
MIX
Papier | Fördert
gute Waldnutzung
FSC® C083411

Zeitfracht Medien GmbH
Ferdinand-Jühlke-Straße 7
99095 Erfurt, Deutschland
produktsicherheit@kolibri360.de